NSNA Review Series

D0082466

Medical-Surgical Nursing

Consulting Editors

Ardelina A. Baldonado, Ph.D., R.N.
Associate Professor
Loyola University
Marcella Niehoff School of Nursing
Chicago, Illinois

Karen R. Williams, R.N., D.N.Sc.
Associate Professor
San Francisco State University
Department of Nursing
San Francisco, California

Reviewer

Deborah A. Davis, R.N.C., M.S.N., F.N.C.P.S.
Former Assistant Professor of Nursing
East Tennessee State University
Johnson City, Tennessee

Delmar Publishers Inc.™
I(T)P™

Developed for Delmar Publishers Inc. by Visual Education Corporation,
    Princeton, New Jersey.
Publisher: David Gordon
Sponsoring Editor: Patricia Casey
Project Director: Susan J. Garver
Developmental Editor: Amy B. Lewis
Production Supervisor: Amy Davis
Proofreading Management: Christine Osborne
Word Processing: Cynthia C. Feldner
Composition: Maxson Crandall, Lisa Evans-Skopas
Cover Designer: Paul C. Uhl, DESIGNASSOCIATES
Text Designer: Circa 86

For information, address
Delmar Publishers Inc.
3 Columbia Circle
Box 15015
Albany, New York 12212

Printed in the United States of America
Published simultaneously in Canada by Nelson Canada, a division of
The Thomson Corporation

10 9 8 7 6 5 4 3 2

Library of Congress Cataloging-in-Publication Data

Medical-surgical nursing / consulting editor, Ardelina A. Baldonado; reviewers,
    Deborah A. Davis, Karen R. Williams.
        p.   cm. — (NSNA review series)
    Developed for Delmar Publishers Inc. by Visual Education Corporation.
    ISBN 0-8273-5673-0
    1. Nursing—Outlines, syllabi, etc.   I. Baldonado, Ardelina A.   II. Davis,
Deborah A.   III. Williams, Karen R., 1943– .   IV. Visual Education Corporation.
V. Series.
    [DNLM: 1. Nursing Service, Hospital—outlines. 2. Nursing Service, Hospital—
nurses' instruction. 3. Surgical Nursing—outlines. 4. Surgical Nursing—nurses'
instruction. WY 18 M4896 1994]
RT52.M43 1994
610.73—dc20
DNLM/DLC
for Library of Congress   93-33600
                                                                            CIP

Titles in Series

Maternal-Newborn Nursing

Pediatric Nursing

Nursing Pharmacology

Medical-Surgical Nursing

Psychiatric Nursing

Gerontologic Nursing
(available in 1995)

Health Assessment/Physical Assessment
(available in 1995)

Series Advisory Board

Series Review Board

Contents

Notice to the Reader...vi

Preface...vii

Chapter 1   General Medical-Surgical Nursing Management 1

Chapter 2   Electrolytes, Fluids, Acid Balance 23

Chapter 3   Immune System Function 42

Chapter 4   Care of Patient with Infectious Disease 55

Chapter 5   Care of Cancer Patient 69

Chapter 6   Respiratory Function...82

Chapter 7   Cardiovascular Function 111

Chapter 8   Hematologic and Lymphatic Function 148

Chapter 9   Nervous System Function 170

Chapter 10 Musculoskeletal Function 196

Chapter 11 Senses (Eyes, Ears)...212

Chapter 12 Gastrointestinal Tract Function 230

Chapter 13 Hepatic, Biliary, and Pancreatic Function 258

Chapter 14 Endocrine System Function 278

Chapter 15 Reproductive and Sexual Function..295

Chapter 16 Urinary and Renal Function 314

Chapter 17 Integumentary Function 332

Medical-Surgical Nursing Comprehensive Review Questions 349

Notice to the Reader

The publisher, editors, advisors, and reviewers do not warrant or guarantee any of the products described herein nor have they performed any independent analysis in connection with any of the product information contained herein. The publisher, editors, advisors, and reviewers do not assume, and each expressly disclaims, any obligation to obtain and include information other than that provided to them by the manufacturer.

The reader is expressly warned to consider and **adopt** all safety precautions that might be indicated by the activities described herein and to avoid all potential hazards. By following the instructions contained herein, the reader willingly assumes all risks in connection with such instructions.

The publisher, editors, advisors, and reviewers make no representations or warranties of any kind, including but not limited to the warranties of fitness for particular purpose or merchantability, nor are any such representations implied with respect to the material set forth herein, and the publisher, editors, advisors, and reviewers take no responsibility with respect to such material. The publisher, editors, advisors, and reviewers shall not be liable for any special, consequential, or exemplary damages resulting, in whole or in part, from readers' use of, or reliance upon, this material.

A conscientious effort has been made to ensure that the drug information and recommended dosages in this book are accurate and in accord with accepted standards at the time of publication. However, pharmacology is a rapidly changing science, so readers are advised, before administering any drug, to check the package insert provided by the manufacturer for the recommended dose, for contraindications for administration, and for added warnings and precautions. This recommendation is especially important for new, infrequently used, or highly toxic drugs.

CPR standards are subject to frequent change due to ongoing research. The American Heart Association can verify changing CPR standards when applicable. Recommended Schedules for Immunization are also subject to frequent change. The American Academy of Pediatrics, Committee on Infectious Diseases can verify changing recommendations.

Preface

The NSNA Review Series is a multiple-volume series designed to help nursing students review course content and prepare for course tests.

Chapter elements include:

Overview—lists the main topic headings for the chapter

Nursing Highlights—gives significant nursing care concepts relevant to the chapter

Glossary—features key terms used in the chapter that are not defined within the chapter

Enhanced Outline—consists of short, concise phrases, clauses, and sentences that summarize the main topics of course content; focuses on nursing care and the nursing process; includes the following elements:
* *Client Teaching Checklists:* shaded boxes that feature important issues to discuss with clients; designed to help students prepare client education sections of nursing care plans
* *Nurse Alerts:* shaded boxes that provide information that is of critical importance to the nurse, such as danger signs or emergency measures connected with a particular condition or situation
* *Locators:* finding aids placed across the top of the page that indicate the main outline section that is being covered on a particular 2-page spread within the context of other main section heads
* *Textbook reference aids:* boxes labeled "See text pages ___," which appear in the margin next to each main head, to be used by students to list the page numbers in their textbook that cover the material presented in that section of the outline
* *Cross references:* references to other parts of the outline, which identify the relevant section of the outline by using the numbered and lettered outline levels (e.g., "same as section I,A,1,b" or "see section II,B,3")

Chapter Tests—review and reinforce chapter material through questions in a format similar to that of the National Council Licensure Examination for Registered Nurses (NCLEX-RN); answers follow the questions and contain rationales for both correct and incorrect answers

Comprehensive Test—appears at the end of the book and includes items that review material from each chapter

1

General Medical-Surgical Nursing Management

OVERVIEW

I. Management of pain
A. Types
B. Mechanisms of pain
C. Pain relief measures
D. Essential nursing care for patients in pain

II. Management of shock
A. General issues
B. Stages of shock
C. Types of shock
D. Symptoms of shock
E. Prevention of shock
F. Medical treatment of shock
G. Essential nursing care for patients in shock

III. Preoperative nursing management
A. Nursing assessment
B. Nursing diagnoses
C. Nursing intervention
D. Nursing evaluation

IV. Intraoperative nursing management
A. General operating room procedures
B. Essential intraoperative nursing care

V. Postoperative nursing management
A. Nursing assessment
B. Nursing diagnoses
C. Nursing intervention
D. Nursing evaluation

VI. Special gerontologic considerations
A. Drugs and the elderly
B. Hospital and physical care
C. Patient education

NURSING HIGHLIGHTS

1. Nurse should develop a philosophy about pain management that is caring and respectful of the patient in pain.
2. Nurse should recognize cultural differences in the expression of pain and not evaluate a patient from his/her own cultural expectations.
3. Onset of shock is often insidious and requires careful evaluation of clinical data and patient risk factors.

4. Preoperative care consists primarily of patient and family education directed at reducing anxiety and postoperative complications and assuring adequate physical preparation.

5. Nurse should be aware that the surgical experience subjects the patient and family to both psychologic and physiologic stress.

6. Nurse should encourage self-care in activities of daily living for elderly patients when they are capable of performing these activities themselves in an effort to maintain independence.

GLOSSARY

cordotomy—surgical procedure to relieve intractable pain by sectioning pain pathway in spinal cord

dehiscence—partial or total separation of the layers of a wound

epidural analgesic—method in which a narcotic or local anesthetic is infused into the epidural space of the spinal cord

evisceration—displacement of internal organs or viscera through an open wound

extravasation—the escape of fluids into surrounding tissues

gram-negative bacteria—bacteria that lose the stain and take the color of the red counterstain in Gram's method of staining

intrathecal analgesic—method in which a narcotic or local anesthetic is introduced into the space between the arachnoid mater and the pia mater of the spinal cord via spinal catheter

malignant hyperthermia—a rare and life-threatening complication of general anesthesia marked by tachycardia, continual increase in body temperature, hypotension, cyanosis, muscular rigidity, and arrhythmias

necrosis—death of areas of tissue or bone surrounded by healthy tissue

rhizotomy—surgical procedure to relieve intractable pain by sectioning posterior nerve root just before it enters the spinal cord

vasopressor—an agent that stimulates contraction of muscles or capillaries and arteries, causing a rise in blood pressure

ENHANCED OUTLINE

See text pages
_____

I. Management of pain

A. Types
   1. Acute pain: serves as the body's "warning signal"; decreases as healing progresses
   2. Chronic pain: persists or recurs for more than 6 months; often does not respond to treatment

3. Chronic pain syndrome: persistent pain whose source or cause is unknown
4. Cancer-related pain: often severe, may be caused by nerve compression, infection, inflammation, necrosis, arterial ischemia, venous engorgement, or ulceration
5. Postoperative pain: after surgery; highly influenced by psychosocial variables

B. Mechanisms of pain
1. Theories of pain and pain transmission
   a) Specificity theory: Pain occurs because specific pain receptors transmit the sensation of pain to higher centers of the brain.
   b) Pattern theory: Pain receptors share nerve endings with other sensory modalities, and the same nerve can transmit both painful and nonpainful stimuli.
   c) Gate control theory: Simultaneous firing of large nerve fibers that transmit nonpainful sensations and small nerve fibers that transmit pain can block the transmission of pain impulses going to the brain.
   d) Endorphins and enkephalins: These morphinelike substances are manufactured by the body and bind to receptor sites in the brain, providing analgesic by raising the body's threshold for pain.
2. Psychosocial influences on pain
   a) Age, sex, sociocultural background, personality, and mood affect a patient's ability to process and react to pain.
   b) Past experiences influence present perception of pain; the more experience a person has with pain, the more frightened he/she may be about subsequent painful events.

C. Pain relief measures
1. Cognitive and behavioral methods
   a) Application of cold
      (1) Cold relieves pain faster than heat, and relief lasts longer.
      (2) Cold is used to reduce bleeding and swelling.
   b) Application of pressure or massage
      (1) Direct stimulation may be applied near pain site.
      (2) If massage near site is painful, ineffective, or contraindicated, side of the body opposite painful area may be stimulated (contralateral stimulation).
      (3) Stimulation should be of moderate intensity.
   c) Transcutaneous electrical nerve stimulation (TENS): a device either worn or applied that delivers small electrical currents to the skin and underlying tissues, interfering with transmission of pain stimuli
   d) Imagery or distraction: pain relief increased in direct relation to patient's active participation (see Client Teaching Checklist, "Distraction Techniques for Handling Pain")
   e) Acupuncture: needles inserted into skin and subcutaneous tissues at specific acupuncture sites and manually vibrated or electrically stimulated

2. Analgesic methods
   a) Types of analgesics
     (1) Nonnarcotics
       (a) Aspirin (Ecotrin), acetaminophen (Tylenol), and nonsteroidal anti-inflammatory agents (NSAIAs) such as ibuprofen (Motrin) may work as well as some narcotics for mild to moderate pain.
       (b) Side effects include gastrointestinal bleeding, hemorrhagic disorders, and decreased renal function.
     (2) Narcotics
       (a) Codeine, meperidine (Demerol), oxycodone (Percodan), morphine, and hydromorphone (Dilaudid) are a few commonly prescribed narcotics.
       (b) Side effects may include constipation, nausea, lowering of blood pressure, tachycardia, and decreased respirations.
       (c) Improper use of narcotics may lead to physical dependency, drug tolerance, and addiction.
   b) Methods of administration
     (1) Oral: preferred because it is easy, noninvasive, and nonpainful
     (2) Parenteral: used when a drug cannot be given orally
       (a) Intramuscular (IM) injection: absorption uncertain; painful if given frequently
       (b) Subcutaneous (SC) administration: used when patient requires frequent pain relief but cannot tolerate oral administration or repeated IM injections

---

✔ CLIENT TEACHING CHECKLIST ✔

Distraction Techniques for Handling Pain

Explain these two distraction techniques to the client:

Active Listening

✔ Listen to music on tape recorder with earphone or headset.
✔ Keep time by tapping finger or nodding head.
✔ Focus on object or close eyes and imagine something about the music.

Concentration Method

✔ Stare at a spot on the wall or ceiling.
✔ Rub or massage part of the body with firm, circular motion on bare skin.
✔ Breathe in and out slowly, repeating: "Breathe in slowly, breathe out slowly."
✔ Never rub the legs because of risk of forming emboli and/or causing embolism.

    (c) Intravenous (IV) administration: medication metabolized more quickly than with other methods of administration

      i) Injection ("push"): immediate delivery of medication

      ii) Continuous drip: uses infusion pump to deliver a steady flow of medication

      iii) Patient-controlled analgesic (PCA): allows patient to administer analgesic using an IV pump system

    (d) Intraspinal analgesic infusion: includes epidural analgesic and intrathecal analgesic; minimal systemic side effects

   (3) Transdermal: medication absorbed directly through skin by means of an adhesive patch

   (4) Rectal: may be indicated if patient is not allowed oral intake or has bleeding problems

 3. Surgical methods

  a) Types include rhizotomy, cordotomy, and nerve block.

  b) Such invasive measures are performed only when pain is intractable or cannot be controlled by any other means.

D. Essential nursing care for patients in pain

 1. Nursing assessment

  a) Determine onset and location of pain.

  b) Obtain description of pain (e.g., sharp, stabbing, dull, throbbing, shooting, stinging, hot, sickening, squeezing, radiating, intermittent, steady, severe, mild, bearable, superficial).

  c) Assess relation to circumstances: what brings on and relieves pain.

  d) Assess patient's response to pain.

  e) Assess patient's pain with self-rating tools such as verbal descriptor scales ("none, moderate, or severe"), visual analogue scales (using a continuum of pain intensity), or numeric scales (rating pain from 0–10).

 2. Nursing diagnoses

  a) Pain or discomfort related to illness or injury

  b) Anxiety related to anticipation of pain or inability to obtain relief

  c) Self-care deficits related to pain and central nervous system (CNS) depressant effects of a narcotic analgesic

  d) Potential for injury related to the CNS depressant effects of a narcotic analgesic

  e) Ineffective individual coping related to chronic pain

 3. Nursing intervention

  a) Explain to patient and family the mechanism of any drugs prescribed.

  b) Administer analgesics promptly as ordered by physician.

  c) When giving narcotics, watch for sudden drop in blood pressure or respiration; be prepared to administer naloxone (Narcan) to offset narcotic overdose.

  d) Identify and encourage strategies of pain relief that patient has used successfully before.

  e) Teach patient new strategies to relieve pain and discomfort (see Client Teaching Checklist, "Distraction Techniques for Handling Pain").

f) Protect patient from injury: assist patient with activities of daily living as needed; raise side rails of bed; use restraints only when absolutely necessary.

4. Nursing evaluation
   a) Patient states that pain and discomfort are reduced or eliminated.
   b) Patient performs activities of daily living alone or with assistance.
   c) Injuries are avoided.
   d) Patient exhibits an ability to cope with pain and understands concern of health care team in relieving pain.
   e) Patient demonstrates or states an understanding of postdischarge care of the surgical site and of analgesic use and other pain-relief measures.

II. Management of shock

See text pages
_____

A. General issues
   1. Inadequate blood flow throughout the body tissues decreases oxygen flow to tissues and organs and impedes the removal of waste products of metabolism.
   2. Untreated shock may lead to collapse, coma, and death.
   3. Complications include failure of the kidneys to resume work after the blood pressure improves; other complications, such as peripheral and pulmonary edema due to fluid overload, may not appear until the patient recovers from shock.
   4. Secondary prevention (early detection) is a major nursing responsibility; development of shock should always be considered a possibility.

B. Stages of shock
   1. Early (nonprogressive) stage
      a) Signs and symptoms of this stage are hard to detect.
      b) Increase in heart rate may be the only symptom.
      c) Orthostatic changes may occur.
   2. Compensatory stage
      a) Stage occurs when blood pressure drops 10–15 mm Hg; if this stage does not progress to the intermediate stage, patient can remain in this stage for hours without sustaining permanent damage.
      b) Conditions that initiated shock must be reversed, or progression of shock must be prevented through supportive interventions.
   3. Intermediate stage
      a) This is a life-threatening emergency characterized by sustained drop in blood pressure of more than 20 mm Hg.
      b) Cell damage and cell death occur as a result of inadequate oxygenation and toxic metabolite buildup.

c) Immediate interventions are required to reverse effects of this stage of shock; the patient's life can be saved if this stage of shock can be corrected within an hour.
    4. Irreversible stage
        a) Widespread tissue anoxia and cell death occur, causing overwhelming functional changes in vital organs.
        b) Patient will die even if the underlying cause of shock is corrected and blood pressure returns to normal.
C. Types of shock
    1. Hypovolemic shock: caused by reduced fluid volume due to loss of blood, plasma, or body fluids
    2. Vasogenic shock: caused by diffuse vasodilatation and an increase in the size of the vascular bed, trapping blood in small vessels and viscera, where it is temporarily lost to the mainstream of circulating fluid
    3. Septic (bacteremic) shock: caused by an overwhelming bacterial infection, usually caused by gram-negative organisms (e.g., *Escherichia coli*)
    4. Cardiogenic shock: caused by direct (e.g., myocardial infarction, cardiac arrest, or arrhythmias) or indirect (e.g., cardiac tamponade, head trauma, or drug overdose) impairment of pumping ability of the heart, reducing blood flow and decreasing oxygen to body tissues and organs
D. Symptoms of shock
    1. Drop in blood pressure due to decreased cardiac output
    2. Inability to maintain blood pressure when upright (orthostatic hypotension) due to decreased cardiac output
    3. Pale, clammy skin due to constriction of peripheral blood vessels
    4. Reduced urinary output due to reduced renal blood flow
    5. Tachycardia and cardiac dysrhythmias due to decreased cardiac output
    6. Rapid, thready pulse due to fall in systolic blood pressure and rise in diastolic blood pressure
    7. Tachypnea due to decreased oxygen in the tissues
    8. Subnormal temperature due to depression of heat-regulating mechanisms
    9. Increased temperature in septic shock due to bacterial infection
E. Prevention of shock
    1. Recognize early signs of shock.
    2. Recognize conditions that may lead to shock.
    3. Monitor vital signs of *all* postoperative patients until danger of shock is no longer probable.
F. Medical treatment of shock
    1. Keeping patient warm but not overheated
    2. Placing patient in supine position with legs elevated at a 20° angle
    3. Continuously monitoring patient's respiratory and circulatory status
    4. Measuring patient's blood gas levels to assess pulmonary function
    5. Starting oxygen therapy

6. Replacing fluids with electrolyte solutions and/or blood, plasma, or blood products
7. Administering drugs (e.g., vasodilators, cardiotonics, diuretics, steroids) to reverse shock

G. Essential nursing care for patients in shock
    1. Nursing assessment
        a) Assess patient's level of consciousness and orientation to time, place, and person.
        b) Assess central and peripheral pulses for rate and quality.
        c) Monitor patient's blood pressure for changes from baseline and changes from the previous measurement; measure blood pressure with patient in lying, sitting, and standing positions (depending on stage of shock).
        d) Assess temperature and color of skin and mucous membranes.
        e) Assess rate, depth, and ease of respiration; auscultate the lungs for presence of abnormal breath sounds.
        f) Measure urinary output every hour.
        g) Assess urine for color, specific gravity, and the presence of blood or protein; if septic shock is suspected, send a sample of urine for microscopic examination and culture.
        h) Assess patient's muscle strength.
            (1) Have patient squeeze nurse's hand.
            (2) Tell patient to try to keep arms flexed while nurse pulls downward on lower arms.
            (3) Have patient push both feet against palms of nurse's hands while nurse applies resistance.
    2. Nursing diagnoses
        a) Anxiety related to a change in physical status
        b) Hypothermia related to hypovolemic, vasogenic, and cardiogenic shock
        c) Hyperthermia related to bacteremic shock
        d) Pain related to initial disorder, decreased tissue oxygenation, or treatment procedures for shock
        e) Fluid volume deficit related to blood loss
    3. Nursing intervention
        a) Provide emotional support and information to patient and family and calmly provide care.
        b) Administer vasopressors as ordered (see Nurse Alert, "Administering Vasopressors").
        c) Provide hypothermia blanket if patient does not respond to medication.
        d) Administer narcotic analgesic after consultation with physician; avoid multiple doses of narcotics.

Administering Vasopressors

- Patient must be under constant nursing supervision.
- Monitor blood pressure every 2–5 minutes if levarterenol (Levophed) is being administered; every 3–8 minutes for all other vasopressors.
- Adjust rate of IV administration according to blood pressure.
- Frequently inspect site of IV infusion and surrounding areas for signs of extravasation or infiltration.
- If extravasation or infiltration occurs, discontinue IV as ordered by physician (especially if levarterenol is being administered). Start another infusion in another extremity before the original infusion is discontinued (even though extravasation is occurring), or circulatory collapse may result.
- Obtain phentolamine (usually 10 mg in 15 ml saline) to use as antidote for extravasation of levarterenol.

    e) Administer fluid and electrolytes as well as blood and blood products as ordered.

  4. Nursing evaluation

    a) Patient states that anxiety is reduced.

    b) Patient's body temperature is at or near normal.

    c) Patient states that pain and discomfort are reduced or eliminated.

    d) Fluid volume deficit is corrected.

III. Preoperative nursing management

See text pages
_____

A. Nursing assessment

  1. Obtain a health and surgical history on the patient.

  2. Obtain complete set of vital signs as baseline to assess postoperative complications.

  3. Perform physical assessment focusing on problem areas and all body systems that could be affected by surgical procedure.

  4. Assess cardiovascular system.

    a) Palpate peripheral pulses.

    b) Auscultate heart sounds.

    c) Assess for hypertension or preexisting heart conditions.

  5. Assess respiratory system.

    a) Assess for special risks: age, smoking history, and chronic illness.

    b) Observe posture; respiratory rate, depth, and rhythm; and lung expansion.

    c) Establish baseline for incentive spirometer.

    d) Auscultate to determine quality and presence of adventitious sounds and congestion.

  6. Assess renal system.

    a) Observe for frequent urination, dysuria, anuria; check appearance and odor of urine.

          b) Abnormal renal function can slow the excretion of preoperative medications and alter their effectiveness.

    7. Assess neurologic system.

        a) Assess level of consciousness, orientation, and ability to follow commands.

        b) Note gait steadiness and ability to ambulate for use in analysis of postoperative and discharge goal attainment.

    8. Obtain a psychosocial assessment of the patient in order to determine patient's coping ability, provide information, and offer support.

    9. Examine results of laboratory and diagnostic tests to detect abnormal findings.

B. Nursing diagnoses

    1. Knowledge deficit related to impending surgical procedure and preoperative protocol

    2. Anxiety related to surgical procedure and outcome

    3. Ineffective individual coping related to the potential results of surgery

    4. Altered family processes related to the possible outcome of the surgical procedure

C. Nursing intervention

    1. Present information about surgical procedures and preparations required beforehand.

    2. Present information on pain control; explanation and description of recovery room; how to perform deep breathing, relaxation, and coughing exercises; and how and why to change positions after surgery.

    3. Present information on discharge planning, home care, referrals, and community agencies.

    4. Ensure that patient or a legal guardian is fully informed about surgical procedures and voluntarily signs the consent form.

    5. Perform preoperative skin preparation by cleaning a wide area above and below the surgical site and, if required, by shaving the area.

    6. Administer preanesthetic medication according to physician's instructions.

    7. Provide emotional support to patient and family.

    8. Complete preoperative checklist.

D. Nursing evaluation

    1. Patient states an understanding of type and purpose of surgical procedure, preoperative preparations, and postoperative tasks performed by self and nursing personnel.

    2. Patient's preoperative anxiety is reduced or eliminated.

    3. Patient demonstrates ability to cope with the potential results of surgery.

    4. Patient's family demonstrates evidence of coping with the potential results of surgery.

IV. Intraoperative nursing management

See text pages

A. General operating room procedures
1. Asepsis procedures
    a) Scrubbing
        (1) Hold hands above level of elbows and away from body so contaminated water flows away from hands.
        (2) Use a scrub brush or sponge impregnated with antimicrobial solution, applying friction from the fingertips and hands to the arms and elbows for 5 to 10 minutes.
        (3) Dry hands and arms from fingertips to elbow with sterile towel to prevent contamination of sterile gown.
    b) Dress code
        (1) Surgical attire (cap or hood, mask, pantsuit or dress, and shoe coverings) must be worn by all members of surgical team to decrease contamination from microorganisms.
        (2) Cap or hood should be put on first; hair (including facial hair) must be covered.
        (3) Circulating nurse should wear jacket to prevent shedding from bare arms.
        (4) Scrub tops should be tucked into pants or conform to the waist.
        (5) Surgical mask should be tied securely in place, and sterile gloves should extend over the cuffs of the gown when sterile attire is worn over a scrub suit.
        (6) Scrub attire should be changed daily, when it is wet or soiled, or after leaving surgical suite without a cover gown.
        (7) Shoe covers, masks, and clean attire should be changed between surgical procedures.
        (8) Jewelry should be removed before entering surgical suite.
2. Anesthesia
    a) General
        (1) Methods of administration and types
            (a) Inhalation: includes nitrous oxide, halothane (Fluothane), enflurane (Ethrane), methoxyflurane (Penthrane), isoflurane (Forane), and diethyl ether
            (b) Intravenous: includes thiopental sodium (Pentothal), fentanyl citrate (Sublimaze), fentanyl citrate with droperidal (Innovar), and ketamine (Ketalar, Ketaject)
        (2) Anesthetic agent(s) inhibit neuronal impulses in the brain and cause a subsequent loss of consciousness.
        (3) Retching, vomiting, and restlessness may occur as the patient emerges from anesthesia.
        (4) Complications (rare) include broken or injured teeth or caps or trauma to vocal cords due to intubation technique; overdose; malignant hyperthermia.
    b) Regional
        (1) Spinal anesthesia (epidural anesthesia)
            (a) This type is administered for surgery of lower abdomen and lower extremities, in emergencies, to trauma patients

who have eaten or drunk alcoholic beverages, and for those with active or unstable cardiac disease.
- (b) Complication: Sympathetic block may cause hypotension, bradycardia, nausea, and vomiting.
- (2) Nerve block
  - (a) Local anesthetic agent injected into or around a nerve supplying involved area to prevent pain
  - (b) Complications: overdose marked by excitability, twitching or convulsions, changes in pulse or blood pressure, and respiratory distress
- (3) Field block
  - (a) Regional anesthesia produced by a series of injections around the operative field; used for herniorrhaphy, dental procedures, and plastic surgery
  - (b) Complications: absorbs into bloodstream and can cause systemic cardiac depression
- (4) Local infiltration
  - (a) Injection of anesthetic agent intracutaneously and subcutaneously into tissue surrounding an incision, wound, or lesion, blocking peripheral nerve stimulation
  - (b) Used during suturing of superficial lacerations
  - (c) Complications: idiosyncratic reactions, including drowsiness, depressed respiration, hypotension, bradycardia, and weak pulse
- (5) Topical anesthesia
  - (a) Application of regional anesthesia directly to the surface of the area to be anesthetized for respiratory intubation or diagnostic procedures
  - (b) Complications: collapse or depression of the cardiovascular system after application to the respiratory tract
- 3. Patient positioning
  - a) Positioning depends on type of surgery and special needs of patient.
  - b) Dorsal recumbent, prone, and lateral positions are most frequently used.
  - c) Position should be assessed for minimal interference with circulation and respiration; protection of skeletal and neuromuscular structures; exposure of surgical site; anesthesiologist access; and patient's dignity, comfort, and safety.
- B. Essential intraoperative nursing care
  - 1. Nursing assessment: circulating nurse
    - a) Identify patient.
    - b) Assess blood pressure, pulse and respiratory rates, and level of consciousness.

c) Evaluate patient's general physical condition.

d) Review patient's chart: signed surgical consent; records for health history and physical examination; administration of preoperative medication (time, dose, and patient response); voiding, skin preparation, and other preoperative orders; lab and diagnostic tests.

e) Monitor elderly patients and those with cardiac disease for potential fluid overload.

f) Check that dentures, prostheses, jewelry, contact lenses, and wigs are removed.

2. Nursing diagnoses: circulating nurse and scrub nurse

a) Potential for infection related to entrance of microorganisms into the surgical wound, lack of strict aseptic technique

b) Potential for injury related to anesthesia, intraoperative positioning, or other hazards

c) Fluid volume excess or deficit related to inaccurate administration of IV fluids, blood, or blood products

d) Impaired gas exchange related to anesthesia

3. Nursing intervention: circulating nurse

a) Follow strict aseptic technique before and during surgery; report any break in technique to surgeon.

b) Position patient correctly for anesthesia and surgical procedures.

c) Administer IV fluids carefully; maintain accurate records and running totals of IV fluids.

d) Assess urine output every hour.

e) Assess patient for evidence of peripheral cyanosis.

f) Record pertinent observations.

g) Communicate appropriate information about surgery to recovery room personnel.

4. Nursing intervention: scrub nurse

a) Scrub for operation, prepare sutures, ligatures, and special equipment.

b) Assist surgeon and assistants during surgical procedure by anticipating required instruments, sponges, drains, and other equipment.

c) Identify all drugs or fluids both visually and verbally.

d) Check that all needles, sponges, and instruments are accounted for near end of surgery.

e) Label and send tissue and fluids to appropriate lab.

5. Nursing evaluation: circulating nurse and scrub nurse

a) Aseptic technique is observed before and during surgery.

b) Information is accurately recorded.

c) Patient is safely anesthetized and is not injured because of improper positioning.

d) All tissue and fluid samples are accurately labeled and sent to appropriate departments.

e) Information is related to recovery room personnel.

See text pages

V. Postoperative nursing management

A. Nursing assessment
  1. Respiratory system
     a) Recovery room procedures
        (1) Assess airway patency by placing hand over patient's mouth and nose to feel exhalation.
        (2) Assess rate, pattern, and depth of respiration.
     b) Clinical unit procedure: Auscultate lungs for effective expansion every 4 hours for the first 24 hours postoperatively.
     c) General care procedures
        (1) Auscultate lungs bilaterally.
        (2) Inspect chest wall for symmetric movement and use of accessory muscles.
        (3) Listen for stridor or snoring.
  2. Cardiovascular system
     a) Recovery room procedure: Assess circulation, blood pressure, pulse, and heart sounds at admission to unit and every 15 minutes until condition is stable or according to agency protocol.
     b) Clinical unit procedure: Continue to assess vital signs according to surgeon's orders and as indicated by patient's condition, using baseline data as a guide.
  3. Fluid and electrolyte balance
     a) Clinical unit procedure: Administer and closely monitor IV fluids and blood based on individual patient needs.
     b) General care procedures
        (1) Assess hydration by inspecting mucous membranes for color and moist appearance, skin for turgor, and dressings for presence and amount of drainage.
        (2) Measure nasogastric tube drainage, urinary output, and wound drainage.
  4. Neurologic system
     a) Recovery room procedures
        (1) Assess cerebral function and level of consciousness of all patients who have received any type of sedation.
        (2) Assess pupillary response to light, muscle strength, and bilateral coordination in patients who have undergone head and neck surgery.
     b) General care procedures
        (1) Assess motor function by asking patient to move extremities.
        (2) Assess strength of each limb.

5. Genitourinary system
    a) Recovery room procedures
        (1) Inspect, palpate, and percuss patient's lower abdomen for bladder distention.
        (2) Monitor urinary output.
        (3) Assess urine for color and amount (with or without indwelling catheter).
        (4) Ensure urine drainage by preventing kinks or obstruction in catheter or tube.
    b) Clinical unit procedure: Continue to monitor urinary output and assess for color and amount, especially for the first 8 hours postoperatively.
6. Gastrointestinal system
    a) Recovery room procedures
        (1) Assure nasogastric function.
        (2) Assess for nausea and prevent vomiting.
    b) General care procedures
        (1) Record amount, color, and consistency of drained material from nasogastric tube every 6 to 8 hours.
        (2) Confirm nasogastric tube placement by auscultation every 6 to 8 hours and before instilling irrigation solution or medication into the tube.
7. Integumentary system
    a) Recovery room procedures
        (1) Assess all dressings for drainage amount, color, consistency, and odor on admission to recovery room.
        (2) Assess all drains and indwelling monitoring devices for patency on admission to recovery room.
        (3) Monitor amount, color, and consistency of drainage on admission to recovery room.
    b) Clinical unit procedures
        (1) Assess dressings for drainage amount, color, consistency, and odor each time vital signs are taken.
        (2) Assess all drains for patency each time vital signs are taken.
        (3) Monitor amount, color, and consistency of drainage every 8 hours.
    c) General care procedures
        (1) Assess patient's pain and need for medication.
        (2) Assess patient after giving medication for side effects and effectiveness.
8. Complications
    a) Hemorrhage: Inspect dressings regularly for signs of bleeding; note color of blood; assess for internal bleeding.
    b) Shock: same as section II,F of this chapter
    c) Hypoxia: Assess breathing and respirations; assess for cyanosis and dyspnea, restlessness, crowing or grunting respirations, diaphoresis, bounding pulse, or rising blood pressure.

        d) Vomiting: Observe for episodes of nausea and vomiting during the postoperative phase.

        e) Wound dehiscence and/or evisceration: Monitor wound site and provide adequate support when patient coughs or vomits.

B. Nursing diagnoses

    1. Impaired gas exchange related to residual effects of anesthesia, immobility, and pain

    2. High risk for impaired skin integrity related to surgical wound healing, drains and drainage, and wound infection

    3. Pain related to surgical procedure

    4. Fluid volume deficit related to loss of blood and fluids during surgery

    5. Anxiety related to the results of surgery and to recovery from surgery

C. Nursing intervention

    1. Recovery room procedures

        a) Position patient in side-lying position; turn head to side to prevent aspiration.

        b) Insert airway to prevent obstruction and apply suction; keep head of the bed flat until patient regains voluntary gag reflex.

        c) Once airway is removed, encourage patient to cough and deep breathe.

    2. Clinical unit procedures

        a) Instruct patient to cough and deep breathe at least 5–10 times every 2 hours while awake during first 72 hours; if appropriate, encourage use of incentive spirometry 5–10 times per hour for 48–72 hours postoperatively.

        b) Prevent vomiting by administering antiemetic drugs as prescribed; if patient experiences nausea, keep emesis basin within reach of patient; if vomiting is severe or prolonged, temporarily discontinue oral feeding; observe for signs of dehydration and electrolyte imbalance.

        c) Provide information on preventing infection, care of surgical wound, diet, drug therapy, and progressive activity.

    3. General care procedures

        a) Change and care for dressing according to agency or physician protocol; assess wound for signs of infection; and empty, measure, and document characteristics of drainage.

        b) Clean edges of infected wound, loosely pack with antibiotic-saturated gauze, and cover with dry, sterile bandage.

        c) Before first dressing change, reinforce dressing if it becomes saturated with drainage.

        d) If dehiscence occurs, apply sterile saline dressing and binder and notify surgeon; if evisceration occurs, cover wound with sterile

dressing moistened with saline, monitor vital signs, assess for shock, and notify surgeon.
- e) Assess type, location, and intensity of pain and then administer narcotics as prescribed during first 24–48 hours; monitor vital signs closely after administration of narcotics.
- f) Massage stiff joints or sore back to decrease patient's discomfort; provide relaxation or distraction during acute painful procedures.
- g) Regulate IV fluids to prevent overhydration.
- h) Have oxygen and suction equipment ready for emergency use in case of hypoxia.

D. Nursing evaluation
1. Patient maintains adequate lung expansion and respiratory function as evidenced by clear breath sounds.
2. Patient describes and demonstrates care of dressings and drains.
3. Patient has complete wound healing without complications.
4. Patient states that pain is reduced or alleviated.
5. Patient understands all discharge care instructions.
6. Patient attains or maintains psychosocial well-being.

VI. Special gerontologic considerations

See text pages
_____

A. Drugs and the elderly
1. Physiology
- a) Variability in absorption, distribution, metabolism, and excretion of medications is caused by reduced capacity of liver and kidneys to metabolize and excrete drugs and by less efficient circulatory and nervous systems.
- b) Decreases in body weight, total body water, lean body mass, and plasma protein, plus an increase in body fat, also affect the metabolism of medications.
2. Nursing implications
- a) Drugs removed by renal excretion remain longer in body; overdose and drug toxicity at therapeutic dosages commonly occur. (See Client Teaching Checklist, "Adverse Drug Reactions in the Elderly.")
- b) Decline in cardiac output may increase delivery rate to target organ or storage tissue.
- c) Slower metabolism may raise drug levels in tissues and blood.
- d) Possibility of interactions between drugs is further magnified in the presence of one or more over-the-counter drugs.
- e) Unusual responses to drugs may show up as toxic reactions or complications.
- f) Medication dosages often must be reduced because of danger of overdose and drug toxicity at usual therapeutic dosages.

B. Hospital and physical care
1. Pain and fever
- a) Pain sensations may be reduced due to reduced acuity of touch, decreased speed of response, and diminished processing of sensory data.

  b) Fever may be absent or delayed in the elderly; signs of infection may be subtle (mental confusion, rapid breathing, tachycardia, and changes in facial appearance or color).

 2. Emotional response to illness

  a) Hospitalization is an imminent threat to well-being; admission is often actively avoided.

  b) Autonomy and independent decision making are important to elderly patients.

 3. Systemic response

  a) Illness places new demands on already declining organ function.

  b) Older patients may be unable to respond effectively to acute illness; response to chronic illness may decline over time.

C. Patient education

 1. Convey the idea that elderly patients can learn; encourage self-confidence.

 2. Proceed more slowly with elderly patients, speaking slowly, distinctly, and in a low-pitched tone.

 3. Use patient education materials that are large, clear, colorful, and easy to read.

✔ CLIENT TEACHING CHECKLIST ✔

Adverse Drug Reactions in the Elderly

Explain these warning signs to the client:

✔ Nausea or vomiting
✔ Anorexia
✔ Fatigue
✔ Weakness
✔ Dizziness
✔ Urinary retention
✔ Diarrhea or constipation
✔ Confusion

---

1. Because of her religious beliefs, Marie Grant, a patient with a fractured femur, refuses pain medication. Ms. Grant rates her pain as a 6 on a scale of 0 (no pain) to 10 (worst possible pain). Which is the best response the nurse can make?

   a. Ask the patient to explain why her religion does not allow pain medication.

   b. Insist that there must be some exception that allows her to have pain medication.

   c. Suggest that the patient use mental imagery and repositioning of the leg to relieve her pain.

   d. Instruct the patient about the possible complications of unrelieved pain.

2. An 87-year-old woman had abdominal surgery 6 hours ago. Which of the following assessment findings would indicate to the nurse that hypovolemic shock may be developing?

   a. Cheyne-Stokes respirations

   b. Oliguria

   c. Central cyanosis

   d. Widening pulse pressure

3. Which is the first action that the nurse would anticipate taking after hypovolemic shock has been medically diagnosed?

   a. Starting oxygen therapy

   b. Elevating the head of the bed

   c. Administering vasopressin (Pitressin)

   d. Infusing 5% dextrose in water at 150 ml per hour

4. On the morning of surgery, while the nurse is conducting the preoperative nursing assessment on an insulin-dependent diabetic who self-administers insulin every morning, the patient tells her that she has not taken her morning insulin. The nurse should first:

   a. Have the patient give herself her usual dosage of insulin.

   b. Document the fact that the patient did not take her morning insulin.

   c. Call the lab to have a fasting blood glucose sample drawn.

   d. Notify the surgeon for orders regarding insulin dosage.

5. The nurse has just finished a preoperative teaching session with Melvin Gross. Which of the following statements by Mr. Gross would indicate a need for further teaching?

   a. "I think that coughing and deep breathing are going to hurt."

   b. "I'm glad I'll be able to stay in bed for a few days after surgery."

   c. "I'm really stressed tonight. I can't wait until this operation is over."

   d. "I hope that preoperative medication will make me sleepy."

6. A patient who has been told that atropine will make his mouth dry asks why he needs to have the medication before surgery. The nurse's response would be based on which of the following facts?

   a. Atropine relaxes the vocal cords, and a dry mouth is a side effect.

   b. Some anesthetics cause tachycardia, and atropine counteracts that effect.

   c. Some anesthetics produce hypersecretion of saliva and mucus, and atropine counteracts that effect.

   d. Atropine causes retention of urine so that incontinence does not occur during surgery.

7. Which of the following assessments would be the first to indicate that a patient has recovered from spinal anesthesia?

   a. Feeling a pinprick of the toes

   b. Denying the presence of a headache

   c. Ambulating to the bathroom

   d. Complaining of incisional pain

8. When an unconscious patient is brought into the postanesthesia recovery room, the first thing the nurse should do is to:
   a. Suction the oropharynx.
   b. Take and record vital signs.
   c. Turn the patient onto his/her side.
   d. Check the dressing and drainage tubes.

9. A 22-year-old patient had surgery for a ruptured appendix 24 hours ago. Which of the following nursing diagnoses should receive the highest priority?
   a. Impaired physical mobility related to incisional pain
   b. Constipation related to decreased gastric and intestinal motility
   c. Impaired skin integrity related to surgical incision and drainage
   d. High risk for infection related to susceptibility to bacterial invasion

10. An elderly postoperative patient with limited mobility would be at highest risk for developing which of the following?
    a. Atelectasis
    b. Atrial flutter
    c. Incontinence
    d. Wound dehiscence

11. Frank Burton, who is 76 years old, had a bowel resection and colostomy 5 days ago. While the nurse is teaching him about colostomy care, Mr. Burton fumbles with the equipment to empty the colostomy bag and states that he is too old and tired to learn the procedure. The best response for the nurse is:
    a. "You may be right. Let's stop now. I'll call social service to arrange for a community health nurse to help you at home."
    b. "Let's take a break. Maybe we should have your daughter come in to learn this care so she can do it for you at home."
    c. "You're doing well. It takes some time to learn to use this equipment. It's awkward for most people at the beginning. Let's try again."
    d. "You must learn to do this for yourself, and you should practice more with the equipment. Let's try again."

ANSWERS

1. **Correct answer is c.** The patient's sociocultural and religious beliefs must be respected. Other pain relief methods should be offered if they are acceptable to the patient. Repositioning the fractured leg to decrease swelling and pressure may help. Other noninvasive pain relief measures, such as mental imagery or relaxation techniques, may cause the release of endorphins that raise the body's threshold for pain. Various distraction techniques may be used or taught to the patient in an effort to reduce the pain.

   a, b, and **d.** These responses threaten the patient for having beliefs that differ from those of the nurse. The nurse should recognize and respect religious differences and find other acceptable ways of reducing the patient's pain.

2. **Correct answer is b.** Oliguria is a decrease in urinary output below 30 ml per hour. Monitoring urinary output is a valuable indicator of vital organ perfusion. During the compensatory stage of shock, there will be reduced renal blood flow, and urinary output will be decreased.

   a. Cheyne-Stokes respirations involve alternating periods of apnea and deep breathing. In the early stages of shock, respirations are deep and rapid, with no apnea.
   c. Central cyanosis is a symptom of the late stages of shock. In the early stages, the skin is cool and pale; as shock continues, the skin becomes cold, pale, and moist.
   d. Pulse pressure narrows during shock. As the stages of shock progress, the systolic pressure of a normotensive person will be between 90 and 60 mm Hg. In the late stages, systolic pressure will drop below 60 mm Hg.

3. **Correct answer is a.** In the patient with shock, the first priority is the maintenance of adequate oxygenation to vital organs. Providing oxygen therapy is the first anticipated action.

b. The correct positioning of a patient in shock is supine, with the legs elevated 20°–30°.

c. Vasoconstricting agents such as vasopressin are ordered to reduce venous pooling, which will increase cardiac output and mean arterial pressure and improve tissue perfusion. Alternatively, some physicians order vasodilators. These drugs reduce peripheral resistance, lessening the work of the heart, increasing cardiac output, and improving tissue perfusion. Administering vasoconstrictors or vasodilators would not be the initial action taken.

d. Replacing fluids and blood with crystalloids and colloids is a priority for patients with hypovolemic shock. Crystalloids are electrolyte solutions such as Ringer's injection, not dextrose in water. Colloids include blood and bloodlike products.

4. Correct answer is d. The nurse should first notify the surgeon, who will order lab studies and insulin dosage measurements. In uncontrolled diabetes, hypoglycemia is the major risk during surgery, but controlled diabetics are at no greater risk than nondiabetics if frequent monitoring of blood glucose levels takes place.

a. This choice would put the patient at great risk for development of hypoglycemia, since she has had nothing to eat or drink for the past 8–10 hours and will not eat or drink until after surgery.

b. Documentation should be done after the surgeon is notified.

c. The surgeon must order blood glucose levels and thus should be called first. The nurse could not order lab studies.

5. Correct answer is b. Mr. Gross will not be in bed for a few days. Getting out of bed and ambulating as soon as possible after surgery decreases the risk of developing respiratory complications and thrombophlebitis. If there is a contraindication to getting out of bed, then turning and extremity exercises are initiated.

a. It is realistic to expect that coughing and deep breathing will be painful. Complete incisional pain relief usually takes a few weeks. The nurse should assure the patient that use of analgesics and proper splinting of the incision will reduce the pain level.

c. Preoperative anxiety is expected. The fact that the patient is expressing his feelings is a positive sign.

d. Preanesthetic or preoperative medication use is expected to help the patient relax and possibly feel sleepy.

6. Correct answer is c. Some anesthetics cause hypersecretion of saliva and mucus, which would promote gagging, vomiting, and regurgitation during surgery. Suction is always available during surgery to remove saliva and vomitus.

a. Atropine does not relax the vocal cords.

b. Atropine increases the heart rate and is therefore used to treat bradycardia.

d. A side effect of atropine use is urine retention, but it would not be given to prevent incontinence.

7. Correct answer is a. Feeling the pinprick is a sign that complete sensation has returned to the toes; thus, the patient has recovered from the effects of spinal anesthesia. The toes are the last part of the body to regain sensation.

b. Headache is a postoperative complication of spinal anesthesia. Keeping the patient flat, quiet, and well hydrated will increase cerebrospinal pressure and may help to prevent or relieve spinal headaches.

c. Ambulating to the bathroom would not be the first indicator of recovery. The patient should be on bed rest until the sensation in the toes has returned to prevent falls or development of a headache.

d. The patient may have incisional pain as the effects of the spinal anesthetic begin to subside, but recovery has not taken place until the toes have sensation.

8. **Correct answer is c.** The first priority is maintaining a patent airway. In the unconscious patient, the muscles of the pharynx are relaxed as a result of anesthesia, increasing the risk that the tongue will fall back and obstruct the airway. Unless contraindicated, the unconscious patient is positioned on his/her side. The side-lying position or, if this position is contraindicated, the turning of the head to one side, allows fluids to drain out the side of the mouth, preventing gagging, aspiration, or airway obstruction.

a. The oropharynx is suctioned as necessary to maintain the airway, but the first priority is to turn the patient so that fluids drain out by gravity.
b and **d.** The nurse monitors the patient's vital signs and checks the dressing and drainage tubes, but maintaining a patent airway and thus preventing hypoxemia and hypercapnia is the first priority.

9. **Correct answer is d.** The patient is at high risk for developing a wound infection due to the rupture of the appendix and probable contamination by bowel contents. The nurse should monitor WBC count and body temperature and assess the wound for redness, warmth, and edema.

a. Impaired physical mobility is an appropriate nursing diagnosis, since if there is no improvement the patient will be at risk for development of respiratory and circulatory complications. Mobility should be expected to improve because of the patient's youth and the administration of analgesics; thus, this diagnosis is not the highest priority.
b. Constipation is an appropriate nursing diagnosis but is not a priority 24 hours after surgery. Owing to irritation of and trauma to the bowel, intestinal movement may be inhibited (and not desired) for several days.

c. Impaired skin integrity is an appropriate nursing diagnosis. Aseptic technique should be used to prevent nosocomial infection of the wound, but the patient is at high risk for development of wound infection because of the ruptured appendix.

10. **Correct answer is a.** Gerontologic changes in the respiratory system include weakened respiratory muscles and loss of elasticity, resulting in a weaker cough that increases the risk of developing postoperative atelectasis.

b. Atrial flutter may be a preexisting condition that increases the risk of intraoperative myocardial infarction, but it is not a postoperative complication.
c. Incontinence is a common preexisting condition in the elderly, but it is not a postoperative complication.
d. Obesity poses a greater risk than age for development of wound dehiscence.

11. **Correct answer is c.** Urging the patient to persevere is the best response, since it offers encouragement and reflects positive thinking. The older adult should be challenged in a gentle way to be responsible and to participate in self-care activities.

a and **b.** Both these responses allow the patient to become dependent on others. Calling on the help of a community nurse or an adult child should not be done unless an exhaustive assessment of learning skills indicates that the patient does not have the physical or mental ability to do self-colostomy care.
d. Telling the patient what to do does not offer encouragement or reflect positive thinking. Thus, it is an inappropriate response to the situation.

2

Electrolytes, Fluids, Acid Balance

OVERVIEW

I. Function of electrolytes and fluids
  A. Electrolytes
  B. Fluids

II. Types of imbalances
  A. Fluid volume deficit
  B. Fluid volume excess
  C. Sodium imbalance
  D. Potassium imbalance

  E. Calcium imbalance
  F. Acid-base imbalances

III. IV therapy
  A. Osmolarity of IV fluids
  B. Types of IV fluids
  C. Complications
  D. Essential nursing care for patients undergoing IV therapy

NURSING HIGHLIGHTS

1. Nurse must understand electrolyte and fluid imbalances and acid-base disturbances and anticipate treatment strategies to provide best care.
2. Nurse should understand that because any physiologic problem can disrupt fluid and electrolyte balance to some degree, virtually every client is at some risk for these problems.
3. Nurse should explain all IV therapy procedures clearly and concisely *before* the equipment is brought into the room.
4. Nurse should allow time to answer patient's questions about IV therapy, including why it is needed, how long it may take, and what site is to be used.

GLOSSARY

atelectasis—incomplete expansion of the lungs at birth or collapse of the lungs in adulthood

diabetic ketoacidosis (DKA)—bicarbonate deficit due to accumulation of ketones in uncontrolled diabetes mellitus

hypochloremia—abnormally low levels of chlorine in the blood

hypoproteinemia—abnormally small amounts of protein in the blood

lactic acidosis—bicarbonate deficit due to accumulation of lactic acid from decreased tissue perfusion, drug reaction, or unknown cause

orthostatic hypotension—postural hypotension; low blood pressure that occurs on rising to an erect position

uremic acidosis—decreased ability to excrete acid as a result of chronic renal disease

ENHANCED OUTLINE

I. Function of electrolytes and fluids

See text pages

A. Electrolytes
   1. Present in water of cellular and extracellular spaces, they help regulate body's processes.
   2. Different electrolyte concentrations inside and outside cells create electrical potentials that develop across cell membranes.
   3. Imbalance affects transmission of impulses across nerve fibers.

B. Fluids
   1. Fluids carry nutrients and oxygen to, and remove waste from, cells.
   2. Imbalance causes severe symptoms, tissue damage, and death.

II. Types of imbalances

See text pages

A. Fluid volume deficit (FVD or hypovolemia): a decrease in the body's fluid volume
   1. Pathophysiology and etiology: decreased intake or abnormal loss of water and electrolytes due to severe diarrhea, severe vomiting, diaphoresis, rapid diuresis without replacing water and electrolytes, gastrointestinal suction, bowel obstruction, severe burns, hemorrhage, diabetes insipidus
   2. Symptoms: oliguria; concentrated urine; weak, rapid pulse; postural hypotension; acute weight loss; decreased skin turgor
   3. Diagnostic evaluation: higher than normal hematocrit, blood urea nitrogen (BUN) level elevated out of proportion to serum creatinine level
   4. Medical treatment
      a) In mild cases, orally administer fluids with water and electrolytes.
      b) In severe cases, administer IV isotonic electrolyte solution.
   5. Complications: oral infections and inadequate nutrition as a result of mouth dryness
   6. Essential nursing care for patients with fluid volume deficit
      a) Nursing assessment
         (1) Test skin turgor and elasticity by first gently pinching, then releasing skin over the back of hand, sternum, forehead; normal skin turgor is evidenced by rapid return to previous position; in patient with FVD, skin returns slowly.

          (2) Inspect oral membranes for dryness.

          (3) Inspect tongue for furrows.

     b) Nursing diagnoses

          (1) Fluid volume deficit related to diarrhea, vomiting, diuresis

          (2) Altered oral mucous membrane related to dry mouth

     c) Nursing intervention

          (1) See section II,A,4 of this chapter.

          (2) Monitor vital signs every 2–4 hours; assess skin turgor and oral mucous membranes 2–3 times daily.

          (3) Monitor intake and output closely; notify physician if patient can't consume enough fluid or if urine output decreases despite increased oral intake and IV infusion.

     d) Nursing evaluation

          (1) Fluid volume deficit is corrected.

          (2) Urine output is increased; urine color, amount, and specific gravity are normal.

          (3) Patient's vital signs, skin turgor, oral mucous membranes are normal.

          (4) Patient resumes normal intake of fluid.

B. Fluid volume excess (FVE or hypervolemia): an excess of or increase in the body's fluid volume

   1. Pathophysiology and etiology: renal failure, congestive heart failure, excessive intake of salt, corticosteroid therapy, cirrhosis, syndrome of inappropriate antidiuretic hormone (SIADH), excessive intake of sodium-containing fluids either orally or by parenteral administration

   2. Symptoms: edema, rapid weight gain, bounding pulse, distended veins, crackles, polyuria, dilute urine

   3. Diagnostic evaluation: decreased BUN and hematocrit levels, low protein intake, anemia

   4. Medical treatment

     a) In mild cases, limit oral intake or parenteral administration of fluids.

     b) In moderate to severe cases, administer diuretics as prescribed.

   5. Complications: pulmonary or cerebral edema, possibly requiring hemodialysis or ultrafiltration of the extracellular fluid (ECF), heart failure

   6. Essential nursing care for patients with fluid volume excess

     a) Nursing assessment

          (1) Examine extremities for edema, neck veins for distention, skin for general condition.

          (2) Auscultate lungs for crackles.

     b) Nursing diagnoses

          (1) Fluid volume excess related to overhydration

          (2) Impaired tissue integrity related to edema

          (3) Ineffective breathing pattern related to pulmonary edema

     c) Nursing intervention

          (1) See section II,B,4 of this chapter.

          (2) Elevate head of bed.

        (3) Change patient's position every 2 hours; check pressure points for signs of skin breakdown.

        (4) Monitor respiratory rate and pattern.

        (5) Weigh daily or as ordered; notify physician of significant weight increase.

        (6) Monitor vital signs every 1–4 hours depending on severity of condition; closely monitor input and output and notify physician of changes in urine output.

    d) Nursing evaluation

        (1) Fluid volume excess is corrected.

        (2) Patient's urine output, vital signs, and breath sounds are normal.

        (3) Patient's edema is corrected; skin turgor returns to normal.

        (4) Patient has no signs of dyspnea, orthopnea, cyanosis, or distended neck veins.

C. Sodium imbalance

   1. Hyponatremia: a deficit of sodium in the blood

    a) Etiology: profuse diaphoresis replaced only by plain water, excess administration of nonelectrolyte IV fluids, profuse diuresis, loss of gastrointestinal secretions, hyperlipidemia, Addison's disease, SIADH

    b) Symptoms: confusion, anorexia, exhaustion, muscle cramps and twitching, lethargy, hemiparesis, and eventually convulsions or coma

    c) Diagnostic evaluation: serum sodium level less than 135 mEq/L

    d) Medical treatment

        (1) In mild cases, administer sodium orally (salt water, salt tablets, or foods with a high sodium content).

        (2) In severe cases, administer IV of Ringer's lactate or isotonic saline (0.9% sodium chloride).

   2. Hypernatremia: an excess of sodium in the blood

    a) Etiology: excessive intake of salt without ingestion of water (or when excessive water is lost without an accompanying loss of sodium) caused by profuse, watery diarrhea; high fever; decreased water intake; excessive administration of parenteral sodium-containing solutions; and severe burns

    b) Symptoms: thirst; dry, sticky mucous membranes; decreased urine output; fever; dry, swollen tongue; lethargy; and (in severe cases) delusions, hallucinations, and coma

    c) Diagnostic evaluation: serum sodium levels greater than 145 mEq/L

    d) Medical treatment

        (1) In mild cases, restrict sodium intake.

        (2) In moderate to severe cases, administer plain water orally or a hypotonic sodium solution parenterally.

3. Essential nursing care for patients with sodium imbalance
    a) Nursing assessment: Weigh patient.
    b) Nursing diagnoses
        (1) Activity intolerance related to lethargy, confusion, fever
        (2) Hyperthermia related to sodium imbalance
        (3) Altered oral mucous membrane related to dry mouth
        (4) Pain related to increased cranial pressure, muscle twitching, cramps
    c) Nursing intervention
        (1) Hyponatremia
            (a) See section II,C,1,d of this chapter.
            (b) Provide information about pain; administer analgesics as prescribed.
            (c) Monitor rate of isotonic saline solution IV.
            (d) Space sodium replacement feedings (if ordered) evenly throughout waking hours.
        (2) Hypernatremia
            (a) See section II,C,2,d of this chapter.
            (b) Offer fluids at regular intervals; notify physician if output remains low.
            (c) Wet mucous membranes by offering sips of water; apply glyceride to lips.
        (3) Hyponatremia and hypernatremia
            (a) Assist with activities of daily living.
            (b) Monitor fluid intake and output; monitor vital signs every 2–4 hours.
            (c) Monitor temperature every 4 hours; report elevation.
            (d) Assess for symptom change; notify physician if symptoms worsen or lab values change.
    d) Nursing evaluation
        (1) Serum sodium returns to normal or near normal level.
        (2) Patient is alert and oriented to time, place, and person.
        (3) Urine volume, concentration, and specific gravity are normal.
        (4) Oral mucous membranes are intact.
        (5) Patient's vital signs are stable.
        (6) Patient consumes adequate amount of fluid.

D. Potassium imbalance
    1. Hypokalemia: a deficit of potassium in the blood
        a) Etiology: occurs in conjunction with use of potassium-wasting diuretics; loss of fluid from gastrointestinal tract due to severe vomiting, severe diarrhea, draining intestinal fistulas, or prolonged gastrointestinal suction; IV administration of insulin and glucose; metabolic alkalosis; prolonged administration of nonelectrolyte parenteral fluids
        b) Symptoms: fatigue, anorexia, nausea, vomiting, dysrhythmias, leg cramps, muscle weakness, paresthesias; in severe cases, hypotension, flaccid paralysis, and cardiac or respiratory arrest

       c) Diagnostic evaluation: serum potassium levels lower than 3.5 mEq/L, elevated blood pH, elevated blood glucose levels, arterial P_{CO_2} greater than 45 mm Hg

       d) Medical treatment

          (1) In mild cases, administer potassium-rich foods or potassium salt supplements.

          (2) In severe cases, administer potassium solution intravenously.

  2. Hyperkalemia: an excess of potassium in the blood

       a) Etiology: develops in conjunction with severe renal failure; severe burns; administration of potassium-sparing diuretics; overuse of potassium supplements, salt substitutes containing potassium, or potassium-rich foods; crush injuries; Addison's disease; rapid administration of parenteral potassium salts

       b) Symptoms: diarrhea, nausea, muscle weakness, paralysis, paresthesias, and dysrhythmias; in severe cases, cardiac or respiratory arrest

       c) Diagnostic evaluation: serum potassium levels greater than 5 mEq/L

       d) Medical treatment

          (1) In mild cases, decrease intake of potassium-rich foods and discontinue oral potassium supplements until lab values are normal.

          (2) In severe cases, administer cation-exchange resin, a regular insulin and glucose mixture, or sodium bicarbonate; carry out peritoneal dialysis or hemodialysis.

       e) Complication: lethal arrhythmias

  3. Essential nursing care for patients with potassium imbalance

       a) Nursing assessment: assess vital signs.

       b) Nursing diagnoses

          (1) Impaired physical mobility related to fatigue or weakness

          (2) Pain related to leg cramps

          (3) Fluid volume deficit related to vomiting

       c) Nursing intervention

          (1) Hypokalemia

             (a) See section II,D,1,d of this chapter.

             (b) Notify physician if severe muscle cramps occur; administer tranquilizers if prescribed.

          (2) Hyperkalemia

             (a) See section II,D,2,d of this chapter.

             (b) Compare recent electrocardiogram (ECG) tracings with patient's baseline tracings; ensure chest leads are always placed in same position by marking placement with pen; report and record changes in T waves, P waves, and the QRS complex, as well as changes in rate and rhythm.

(3) Hypokalemia and hyperkalemia
    (a) Monitor fluid intake and output.
    (b) Monitor vital signs closely.
    (c) Provide rest periods between activities.
d) Nursing evaluation
    (1) Serum potassium level returns to normal.
    (2) Symptoms of potassium imbalance are absent.
    (3) Heart rate and rhythm are normal.
    (4) Patient demonstrates increased mobility.
    (5) Patient states that pain is reduced or alleviated.
    (6) Fluid volume deficit is corrected.

E. Calcium imbalance
  1. Hypocalcemia: a deficit of calcium in the blood
    a) Etiology: insufficient calcium intake, vitamin D deficiency, hypoparathyroidism, burns, acute pancreatitis or intestinal malabsorption disorders, renal failure, surgical removal of parathyroid glands, alkalosis
    b) Symptoms: tingling in the extremities and mouth area, muscle and abdominal cramps, carpopedal spasms, mental changes, positive Trousseau's sign, positive Chvostek's sign, laryngeal spasms with airway obstruction, tetany, convulsions, bleeding, and dysrhythmias
    c) Diagnostic evaluation: serum calcium level less than 8 mg/dl or 4.5 mEq/L, possible decreased serum albumin level, elevated arterial pH level
    d) Medical treatment
      (1) In mild cases, administer oral calcium and vitamin D.
      (2) In severe cases, administer calcium salt intravenously.
    e) Complications: seizures
  2. Hypercalcemia: an excess of calcium in the blood
    a) Etiology: malignant neoplastic diseases, hyperparathyroidism, excessive calcium intake, renal failure, immobility
    b) Symptoms: anorexia, nausea, vomiting, constipation, abdominal pain, mental confusion, impaired memory, slurred speech, lethargy, acute psychotic behavior, polyuria, brachycardia, cardiac arrest
    c) Diagnostic evaluation: serum calcium level greater than 10.5 mg/dl or 5.5 mEq/L
    d) Medical treatment: decreasing calcium level and reversing hypercalcemia process by administering fluids, promoting renal excretion, mobilizing the patient, and restricting dietary calcium
    e) Complications
      (1) Hypercalcemic crisis results from acute rise in serum calcium to 17 mg/dl or higher, causing severe thirst, polyuria, intractable nausea, abdominal cramps, severe constipation or diarrhea, bone pain, and coma; the condition may result in cardiac arrest.
      (2) Paralytic ileus results from lack of peristalsis in at least one intestinal segment; causing buildup of intestinal contents, increased discomfort and distention, and possibly intestinal blockage.

(3) Embolus formation results from thrombus formation, which is related to decreased clotting time and impeded blood flow.

3. Essential nursing care for patients with calcium imbalance
   a) Nursing assessment: Assess vital signs and symptoms.
   b) Nursing diagnoses
      (1) Hypocalcemia
         (a) Pain related to muscle cramping and tetany
         (b) Altered nutrition, less than body requirements, related to inadequate calcium intake
      (2) Hypercalcemia
         (a) Potential for injury related to physical fractures
         (b) Constipation related to decreased intestinal motility
      (3) Hypocalcemia and hypercalcemia: knowledge deficit related to methods of preventing calcium imbalance
   c) Nursing intervention
      (1) Hypocalcemia
         (a) See section II,E,1,d of this chapter.
         (b) Closely monitor patient for neurologic signs, dysrhythmia, and airway obstruction; if severe, take seizure precautions: assess continually to determine if condition is improving or degenerating; keep emergency equipment (oxygen and suction equipment, sterile tracheostomy tray, Ambu bag) nearby in anticipation of complications; maintain side rails in up position, pad rails, keep bed in lowest position.
         (c) Check patient for bruising and bleeding.
      (2) Hypercalcemia
         (a) See section II,E,2,d of this chapter.
         (b) Assist patient when ambulating; keep upper side rails in the up position to prevent falls.
         (c) Administer prescribed laxatives, high fiber foods, fluids, and comfort measures to increase bowel motility.
      (3) Hypocalcemia and hypercalcemia
         (a) Change patient's position every 2 hours; support extremities with pillows.
         (b) Provide information about drug and diet therapy.
   d) Nursing evaluation
      (1) Serum calcium level returns to normal.
      (2) Symptoms of calcium imbalance are absent.
      (3) Patient understands symptoms and how to avoid a calcium imbalance.
      (4) Patient understands and complies with prescribed drug and diet therapy.
      (5) Patient takes oral fluids and increases activity level.

F. Acid-base imbalances
   1. Respiratory acidosis: altered respiratory function causing increase in plasma carbonic acid levels
      a) Pathophysiology and etiology
         (1) Imbalance due to inadequate excretion of carbon dioxide with inadequate ventilation, raising plasma carbon dioxide and plasma carbonic acid levels
         (2) Acute form caused by emergencies (pneumothorax, hemothorax, acute pulmonary edema, atelectasis, pneumonia); chronic form caused by chronic respiratory disorders (emphysema, bronchiectasis, bronchial asthma)
      b) Symptoms: with acute respiratory acidosis, increased pulse rate, rapid shallow breaths or hypoventilation due to hypoxia, increased blood pressure, behavioral changes, tremors, muscle twitching, flushed skin, headache, drowsiness, weakness, paralysis, stupor, and coma; with chronic respiratory acidosis, dull headache and weakness
      c) Diagnostic evaluation
         (1) Blood pH less than 7.35, a $Paco_2$ greater than 45 mm Hg
         (2) Bicarbonate, serum potassium, serum chloride, and anion gap levels vary with duration of acidosis and degree of renal compensation
      d) Medical treatment: improving ventilation (exact measures vary with cause of inadequate ventilation)
   2. Respiratory alkalosis: altered respiratory function causing decrease in plasma carbonic acid levels
      a) Pathophysiology and etiology
         (1) Imbalance due to hyperventilation, causing excessive loss of carbon dioxide and subsequently a decrease in plasma carbonic acid levels
         (2) Acute form caused by extreme anxiety, hypoxemia, gram-negative septicemia, excessive ventilation by mechanical ventilators, salicylate poisoning, fever; chronic form caused by bronchial asthma, hepatic cirrhosis, primary CNS disorders
      b) Symptoms: with acute and chronic respiratory alkalosis, light-headedness, numbness and tingling of fingers and toes, circumoral paresthesias, sweating, confusion, panic, dry mouth, nausea, vomiting, dysrhythmias, short periods of apnea, and convulsions
      c) Diagnostic evaluation
         (1) Blood pH greater than 7.45, $Paco_2$ less than 35 mm Hg
         (2) Reduced serum potassium and calcium levels, elevated serum chloride level
      d) Medical treatment: correcting hyperventilation (sedation may be required); having patient breathe into paper bag
   3. Essential nursing care for patients with respiratory acidosis or respiratory alkalosis
      a) Nursing assessment: Assess vital signs and weight.

b) Nursing diagnoses
   (1) Anxiety related to ineffective breathing pattern
   (2) Total self-care deficit related to fatigue
   (3) Ineffective breathing pattern related to impaired gas exchange
c) Nursing intervention
   (1) Respiratory acidosis
      (a) Improve ventilation.
      (b) Place patient in semi-Fowler's position to aid breathing.
      (c) Suction airway if necessary.
   (2) Respiratory alkalosis
      (a) Decrease hyperventilation by having patient concentrate on breathing, take deep breaths, and breathe into a paper bag.
      (b) Administer prescribed sedatives.
   (3) Respiratory acidosis and respiratory alkalosis
      (a) Closely monitor vital signs and lab studies.
      (b) Provide assistance with activities of daily living.
d) Nursing evaluation
   (1) Acid-base imbalance is corrected.
   (2) Normal breathing pattern is established.
   (3) Patient's anxiety is reduced.
   (4) Patient is able to resume activities of daily living.
   (5) Patient's vital signs are stable.
4. Metabolic acidosis: base bicarbonate deficit following loss in bicarbonate or gain in acid other than carbonic acid
   a) Pathophysiology and etiology: overproduction or underelimination of hydrogen ions, or underproduction or overelimination of bicarbonate ions (from diarrhea, intestinal fistulas, lactic acidosis, uremia, diabetic ketoacidosis, shock, or starvation)
   b) Symptoms: anorexia, nausea, vomiting, diarrhea, abdominal pain, dehydration, increased respiratory rate and depth, headache, confusion, flushing, lethargy, drowsiness, weakness, disorientation, bradycardia, peripheral vasodilation; severe metabolic acidosis may result in stupor, coma, and death
   c) Diagnostic evaluation
      (1) Blood pH less than 7.35, bicarbonate levels less than 22 mEq/L
      (2) Elevated serum potassium and serum chloride levels; elevated anion gap
   d) Medical treatment: eliminating cause of imbalance, replacing lost fluids and electrolytes; administering bicarbonate
5. Metabolic alkalosis: base bicarbonate excess following gain in bicarbonate or loss in acid other than carbonic acid
   a) Pathophysiology and etiology: excessive oral or parenteral use of bicarbonate-containing drugs or other alkaline salts, rapid decrease

in extracellular fluid volume, vomiting, prolonged gastric suctioning, hypokalemia
- b) Symptoms: anorexia, dizziness, nausea, vomiting, circumoral paresthesias, confusion, tingling of fingers and toes, carpopedal spasm, hypertonic reflexes, tetany, and decreased respiratory rate
- c) Diagnostic evaluation
  - (1) Blood pH greater than 7.45, bicarbonate level greater than 26 mEq/L, elevated Pa_{CO_2}
  - (2) Reduced serum potassium, serum calcium, and serum chloride levels
- d) Medical treatment: eliminating cause of imbalance, administering potassium salt (if accompanied by hypokalemia), administering sodium chloride fluids to correct fluid volume depletion (if accompanied by rapid decrease in extracellular fluid volume)
6. Essential nursing care for patients with metabolic acidosis or metabolic alkalosis
   - a) Nursing assessment
     - (1) Evaluate mental status.
     - (2) Assess vital signs and weight.
     - (3) Determine fluid loss (if vomiting).
     - (4) Determine neurologic symptoms.
   - b) Nursing diagnoses
     - (1) Anxiety related to discomfort, respiratory distress, nausea, and vomiting
     - (2) Fluid volume deficit related to nausea and vomiting
     - (3) Altered nutrition, less than body requirements, related to nausea and vomiting
     - (4) Sensory or perceptual alterations (tactile) related to metabolic acid-base imbalance
   - c) Nursing intervention
     - (1) Metabolic acidosis: Administer bicarbonate.
     - (2) Metabolic alkalosis: Administer sodium chloride.
     - (3) Metabolic acidosis and metabolic alkalosis
       - (a) Monitor fluid intake and output and report significant changes to physician.
       - (b) Resume foods and fluids in small amounts following episodes of nausea or vomiting.
       - (c) Monitor patient's mental state and sensory perceptions.
       - (d) Monitor patient's vital signs every 4 hours or as ordered.
   - d) Nursing evaluation
     - (1) Acid-base imbalance is corrected.
     - (2) Patient's anxiety is reduced.
     - (3) Normal fluid balance is attained and maintained.
     - (4) Patient's nutritional deficits are corrected.
     - (5) Patient's vital signs are stable.

See text pages

_____

III. IV therapy

A. Osmolarity of IV fluids
1. Isotonic solutions: those with the same osmotic pressure as the body's ECF
2. Hypotonic solutions: those with lower osmotic pressure than the body's ECF
3. Hypertonic solutions: those with greater osmotic pressure than the body's ECF

B. Types of IV fluids
1. Dextrose (D-glucose) in water
a) Supplies carbohydrates in a readily usable form
b) Available in various concentrations
(1) 2.5%, 5%, and 10% solutions for peripheral vein infusion
(2) 10%, 20%, 30%, 38.5%, 40%, 50%, 60%, and 70% solutions for central venous infusion

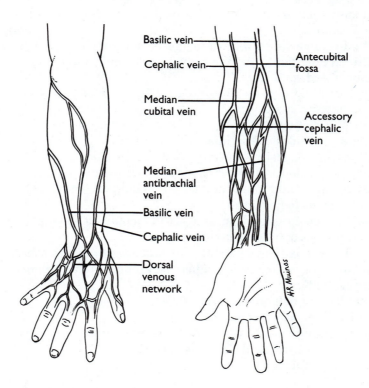

Figure 2–1
Venipuncture Sites for Administration of Fluids

      (3) 20% solution for supplying calories in minimal amount of solution

      (4) 25% and 50% solutions for treating acute hypoglycemia

2. Dextrose in sodium chloride (saline)
   a) Supplies carbohydrates and sodium chloride in a readily usable form
   b) Available in various concentrations
      (1) Dextrose 2.5% in 0.45% sodium chloride
      (2) Dextrose 5% in 0.2%, 0.33%, 0.45%, and 0.9% sodium chloride
      (3) Dextrose 10% in 0.45% and 0.9% sodium chloride

3. Alcohol in dextrose solutions
   a) Increase caloric intake
   b) Replace fluids
   c) Available in two concentrations
      (1) 5% alcohol and 5% dextrose in water supplies 450 cal/L.
      (2) 10% alcohol and 5% dextrose in water supplies 720 cal/L.

4. Combined electrolyte solutions: electrolytes and various concentrations of dextrose or fructose

5. Sodium chloride solutions
   a) Provide fluid replacement
   b) Available in four concentrations
      (1) 0.45% solution provides fluid replacement when fluid loss exceeds electrolyte depletion.
      (2) 0.9% solution (normal saline) supplies fluid and sodium chloride.
      (3) 3% and 5% solutions provide sodium and chloride for hyponatremia and hypochloremia caused by electrolyte losses, drastic dilution of body water after excessive water intake, and emergency treatment of severe salt depletion.

6. IV fat emulsion
   a) Prevents and treats essential fatty acid deficiency
   b) Provides nonprotein calories for patients who do not obtain sufficient calories from glucose

7. Amino acid solutions
   a) Promote protein synthesis
   b) Reduce protein breakdown rate
   c) Promote wound healing
   d) Used for debilitated patients and those receiving long-term parenteral nutrition

8. Blood products
   a) Plasma expanders
      (1) Substitute for whole blood and plasma
      (2) Maintain volume of circulating blood and treat shock
   b) Whole blood: supplies blood cells and plasma when red blood cells are needed with minimal amount of fluid replacement
   c) Platelets: may be administered to those with hemorrhagic disorders
   d) Plasma: may be used to replace coagulation factors that are deficient in bleeding disorders
   e) Serum albumin: treats shock, burns, hypoproteinemia, acute liver failure, and acute nephrosis

C. Complications
  1. Extravasation: escape of fluid from blood vessel into surrounding tissues while needle or catheter is in the vein
  2. Infiltration: collection of fluid into tissues (usually subcutaneous) when needle or catheter is out of vein
  3. Phlebitis, thrombophlebitis, and thrombosis: caused by local irritation of vein wall by needle or catheter, chemicals, or infection
  4. Fluid or circulatory overload: excess amount of fluid in body; may cause high blood pressure, congestive heart failure, and pulmonary edema
  5. Clots: may form in needle or catheter when flow of a solution is stopped
  6. Infection: caused by contamination of IV solution, needle, catheter IV tube, or contaminated drugs added to IV solution
  7. Embolism: caused by air entering IV system (air embolism) or from breaking away of thrombus formed in vein wall (thromboembolism)

D. Essential nursing care for patients undergoing IV therapy
  1. Nursing assessment
     a) Assess patient's hydration by measuring fluid intake and output.
     b) Assess diameter of patient's vein and appropriate gauge of needle.
  2. Nursing diagnoses
     a) Anxiety related to need for IV therapy
     b) Fluid volume excess related to excessive IV fluid intake
     c) Impaired physical mobility related to IV therapy
     d) Potential for infection related to contamination of IV line, skin site, or IV solution
  3. Nursing intervention
     a) Explain all procedures of IV insertion to patient before beginning (See Nurse Alert, "Starting IV Fluids").
     b) Monitor infusion rate every 15 minutes and adjust as necessary.
     c) Monitor patient for signs of fluid overload.
     d) Assist patient with activities of daily living.
     e) Follow asepsis procedures when IV therapy is started, when additional IV solution is added, when medications are administered by IV, and when dressings are changed.
     f) Change dressings to venipuncture site every 48–72 hours or according to hospital policy or physician's orders.
     g) Examine venipuncture site regularly for symptoms of infection (e.g., inflammation, redness, or streaking).
  4. Nursing evaluation
     a) Patient shows little or no anxiety about IV therapy.
     b) Fluid volume excess is prevented.

c) Patient performs activities of daily living within limits of immobility related to IV therapy.

d) No signs of systemic or local infection are present.

e) Hospital procedures are followed regarding administration of IV therapy.

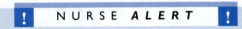

NURSE ALERT

Starting IV Fluids

1. Verify IV order, solution label, and patient.
2. Discuss process with patient.
3. Choose site: Use most distal site of arm or hand first so subsequent IVs can be moved progressively upward.
4. Connect infusion bag and tubing, run solution through tubing to remove air, and cover end of tubing.
5. Position patient, apply tourniquet 5 to 15 cm above injection site, and check for radial pulse below tourniquet.
6. Scrub injection site for 60 seconds with 70% alcohol pledget, moving outward from injection site.
7. Pull skin taut over vein; pierce skin to reach but not penetrate vein with needle bevel at 45° angle.
8. Decrease needle angle until nearly parallel with skin, then enter vein directly above or from side.
9. If blood backflow is visible, straighten angle and advance needle.
10. Release tourniquet and attach infusion tubing; open clamp enough to allow drip.
11. Anchor needle firmly in place with tape.
12. Apply antimicrobial ointment over site, cover with sterile gauze pad, and tape in place.

1. Ms. Williams, a 75-year-old nursing home resident, is admitted to the hospital with a 3-day history of vomiting and diarrhea. Which assessment is a priority for the nurse?

   a. Palpating the bladder for distention
   b. Weighing the patient
   c. Inspecting the oral membranes and tongue
   d. Pinching the skin on the abdomen

2. Ms. Williams's lab results include: sodium 132 mEq/L, potassium 3.0 mEq/L, BUN 30 mg/dl, creatinine 2.2 mg/dl, calcium 7.5 mg/dl, blood pH 7.48, and bicarbonate 29. These results and the patient's history of vomiting and diarrhea indicate to the nurse that the patient has a:

   a. Fluid volume deficit and is in metabolic alkalosis.
   b. Fluid volume excess and is in metabolic acidosis.
   c. Fluid volume deficit and is in respiratory alkalosis.
   d. Fluid volume excess and is in metabolic alkalosis.

3. The physician orders an IV drip for Ms. Williams of 1000 ml of 5% dextrose in normal saline with 40 mEq of potassium chloride to run at 100 ml per hour. The nurse's first action is to:

   a. Choose an IV site on the most distal site of the arm.
   b. Question the physician's ordering of normal saline.
   c. Discuss the IV insertion and therapy with the patient.
   d. Bring all necessary IV equipment into the patient's room.

4. On assessment, a patient who was admitted with congestive heart failure is found to have edema of the feet and legs, respiratory crackles, dyspnea, and neck vein distention. The nurse's first action is to:

   a. Instruct the patient about following a low-sodium diet.
   b. Elevate the head of the bed.
   c. Administer IV fluids.
   d. Allow the patient to rest.

5. The best way for the nurse to monitor accurately for fluid volume excess in a patient with renal failure is to:

   a. Check the ankles for pitting edema.
   b. Measure all fluid intake.
   c. Assess breath sounds daily.
   d. Weigh the patient daily.

6. Ms. Torres, who has been taking potassium supplements at home, has been admitted with a potassium level of 6.8 mEq/L. Based on this information, the nurse monitors the patient for:

   a. Muscular weakness and cardiac dysrhythmias.
   b. Dry tongue, fever, and lethargy.
   c. Muscle cramps and convulsions.
   d. Vomiting and abdominal pain.

7. Three days after admission, Ms. Torres's potassium level is 3.5 mEq/L. Her physician has written discharge orders that include a potassium supplement. Which of the following will the nurse include in Ms. Torres's discharge teaching plan?

   a. A list of potassium-rich foods to be avoided or taken in limited amounts
   b. A review of the signs and symptoms of hypercalcemia
   c. Instructions not to take her potassium supplement
   d. Instructions on how to administer a Kayexalate (cation-exchange resin) enema

8. A 21-year-old male is admitted with a spontaneous pneumothorax. The nurse knows that this patient is at risk for respiratory acidosis if:

   a. His blood pH is less than 7.35.
   b. He continues having difficulty breathing.
   c. His $Paco_2$ is less than 35 mm Hg.
   d. He remains anxious and is not sedated.

9. Ms. Martin had a thyroidectomy yesterday. Because of this surgery, the nurse should be alert for which of the following findings?

   a. Tingling around the mouth
   b. Calcium level of 9 mg/dl
   c. Urinary output of 30–40 ml per hour
   d. Arterial blood pH of 7.35

10. Ms. Carroll has been receiving intravenous therapy. Which of the following would indicate to the nurse that the IV cannula should be removed immediately?

    a. The cannula has not been changed in the past 48 hours.
    b. The tape has loosened around the IV site.
    c. The infusion stops with arm movement.
    d. The IV site is swollen and red.

11. After the nurse has inserted Mr. Jones's IV cannula and started the IV infusion, the patient asks many questions repeatedly and states that he does not like being "hooked up to this thing." He is sweating and flushed. Based on this behavior, which of the following nursing diagnoses is most appropriate?

    a. Activity intolerance related to IV therapy
    b. Pain related to IV therapy
    c. Altered thought processes related to the need for IV therapy
    d. Anxiety related to the need for IV therapy

12. An IV site is slightly swollen, but the fluid continues to infuse. The patient denies discomfort. The most appropriate nursing action is to:

    a. Remove the cannula and insert a new one.
    b. Stop the IV fluid infusion for 2 hours and then restart it.

    c. Restrict the venous flow proximal to the site and check the drip rate.
    d. Apply a warm compress and document the assessment and nursing actions.

ANSWERS

1. **Correct answer is c.** Of the choices given, inspecting the oral membranes for dryness and tongue turgor is the most reliable method of assessing for fluid volume deficit (FVD) in the elderly. FVD would be anticipated in a patient who has had vomiting and diarrhea for 3 days.

   a and **b.** Palpating the bladder and weighing the patient are assessments that can be made, but they are not the priority. A low urine output would be expected in FVD. Weighing the patient would provide a baseline for later comparison.

   d. Testing skin turgor and elasticity is not reliable as a sign of FVD in elderly patients. In addition, the abdomen is not a recommended site to test.

2. **Correct answer is a.** The history of vomiting and diarrhea for 3 days indicates a loss of fluid without any replacement, and the lab results indicate fluid volume deficit (FVD) and metabolic alkalosis. The low sodium and potassium levels, the high BUN and creatinine levels, and the patient's history indicate FVD. The elevated pH and bicarbonate levels, along with the low potassium and calcium levels, indicate alkalosis. The history of vomiting and diarrhea indicates a metabolic cause for the alkalosis.

   b, c, and **d.** All are incorrect, since the given values and history do not support these conclusions.

3. **Correct answer is c.** The nurse should first explain all IV therapy procedures to the patient before equipment (**d**) is brought into the room or an IV site is chosen (**a**).

   b. The physician's order for normal saline is acceptable, based on Ms. Williams's lab values and history. She needs fluids, sodium chloride (saline), and potassium chloride to correct her fluid and electrolyte imbalances.

4. **Correct answer is b.** The assessment indicates that this patient has a fluid volume excess (FVE) and dyspnea. Elevating the head of the bed will promote lung expansion and is the first nursing action to be taken.

a. Checking for pitting edema is not the first action for this acutely ill patient but would be appropriate later, as the patient's condition improves.
c. Administering IV fluids is not a first nursing action because the patient has too much fluid. An IV cannula may be inserted for administration of medication, especially diuretics. Oral and parenteral fluids should be limited.
d. The patient does need rest, but first this acutely ill patient requires immediate nursing and medical care.

5. **Correct answer is d.** Weighing the patient is the most accurate assessment. An acute weight gain of 0.9 kg or 2 lb indicates accumulation of approximately 1 liter of fluid. Weight should be taken at the same time each day on the same scale and can be compared from day to day.

a. Pitting edema is indicative of FVE, but it is not as accurate as weighing the patient daily. It may be difficult to assess small differences in the amount of edema.
b. Measuring fluid intake is indicated for a patient with renal failure. In addition, output must be measured. Together, they are one method of monitoring for FVE.
c. Assessing breath sounds at regular intervals, not just daily, is a way to monitor for FVE, but it is not the most accurate method.

6. **Correct answer is a.** Muscular weakness and cardiac dysrhythmias are the signs and symptoms of hyperkalemia.

b. Dry tongue, fever, and lethargy are among the signs and symptoms of hypernatremia.
c. Muscle cramps and convulsions are among the signs and symptoms of hypocalcemia.

d. Vomiting and abdominal pain are among the signs and symptoms of hypercalcemia.

7. **Correct answer is a.** Since she will be taking a potassium supplement, Ms. Torres needs to have dietary information on foods high in potassium to prevent potential overdosing on the potassium found in foods.

b. Ms. Torres had hyperkalemia, and hypercalcemia symptoms are not involved.
c. The physician has ordered the potassium supplement. This is an appropriate order, and the patient needs further information about the dietary sources of potassium to prevent overdosing.
d. Administering a Kayexalate enema would be an inappropriate order for home care. Kayexalate is appropriate in the treatment of hyperkalemia, but this patient's potassium is now in the normal range.

8. **Correct answer is b.** A patient with an ineffective breathing pattern is at risk for respiratory acidosis.

a. A pH <7.35 indicates that acidosis has already developed.
c. A $Paco_2$ <35 mm Hg indicates alkalosis.
d. Although anxiety may contribute to respiratory acidosis, there is not enough information given to warrant the conclusion that he needs sedation.

9. **Correct answer is a.** Hypocalcemia is associated with thyroidectomy. Tingling around the mouth is indicative of hypocalcemia. Hypocalcemia may occur 24–48 hours after thyroid or parathyroid surgery.

b, c, and **d.** These are normal assessment findings.

10. **Correct answer is d.** These symptoms indicate inflammation caused by thrombophlebitis. Therefore, immediate removal of the IV cannula is indicated to prevent further inflammation or dislodging of the clot.

a. The IV cannula is usually changed every 48 hours to prevent complications. This is a routine nursing action, not an immediate action.

b. Loosening of the tape alone would not indicate dislodgement of the cannula. Retaping and further assessment would be the proper steps.

c. Infusion that stops with arm movement indicates a positional IV problem. Further assessment and immobilization of the arm would be the correct steps to take.

11. **Correct answer is d.** Mr. Jones is exhibiting symptoms of anxiety by sweating, having a flushed face, repeating questions, and making a negative statement about the IV equipment.

a. Mr. Jones should be able to continue most activities. He will be able to ambulate by pushing the IV pole.

b. The patient has not complained of pain. After insertion of the cannula, the IV site should not be painful.

c. Mr. Jones's reaction is common and is not a sign of an altered thought process. His repeated questions indicate anxiety.

12. **Correct answer is c.** Restricting the venous flow and checking the drip rate are the first actions to take, since the patient has no pain and the IV fluid is dripping. If the IV line is infiltrated, it will continue to drip even if venous flow is restricted, since it is dripping into surrounding body tissues and not into the vein.

a. Removing the cannula would be premature, since further assessment needs to be done.

b. Temporarily stopping the infusion is not an appropriate nursing action. It will not allow further assessment and is not a solution to the problem. Such a delay in IV therapy could cause more harm.

d. Applying a warm compress is not an appropriate nursing action. Further assessment must be done to check for infiltration, thrombophlebitis, or other complications.

3

Immune System Function

OVERVIEW

I. Structure and function of immune system
A. Definition
B. Types of immunity
C. Function of immune system
D. Factors affecting immune system functioning
E. Types of diseases of immune system

II. Types of immune response
A. Antibody-mediated (humoral) immune response
B. Cell-mediated immune response

III. Selected disorders
A. Hypersensitivity reaction
B. AIDS

NURSING HIGHLIGHTS

1. Nurses should always be aware of the possibility of anaphylaxis, especially during allergy tests, diagnostic procedures requiring the use of a contrast medium, and the period following an organ transplant.
2. Nurses are responsible for protecting the AIDS patient's privacy by safeguarding confidential information; inadvertent disclosure of confidential patient information may cause personal, financial, and emotional hardships for infected individuals.
3. Nurses caring for AIDS patients need expert assessment, communication, and interpersonal skills; the ability to deal with a wide range of physical problems and psychologic reactions; and a commitment to and respect for the dignity of patients from all walks of life.

GLOSSARY

eosinophil—a cell that makes up a small percentage of the total white blood cell count except during an allergic reaction

IgE antibodies—immunoglobulin E antibodies; produced by cells in the lining of the respiratory and intestinal tracts and important in forming antibodies

retrovirus—an RNA-containing tumor virus that contains the enzyme reverse transcriptase

I. Structure and function of immune system

See text pages
_____

A. Definition: collection of cells and proteins that protect the body from foreign substances, especially such potentially harmful infectious microorganisms as bacteria, viruses, and fungi

B. Types of immunity
   1. Naturally acquired active immunity: immunity to specific microorganism as a result of a previous invasion
   2. Artificially acquired active immunity: immunity to specific microorganism as a result of the administration of a killed or attenuated antigen or toxoid
   3. Passive immunity: short-term immunity as a result of the injection of antibodies from another organism (such as an antitoxin used to treat botulism or tetanus, antivenin used to treat snakebite, and human immune serum used for passive immunization against measles, pertussis, etc.)

C. Function of immune system
   1. Foreign substances (called antigens) entering the body stimulate the formation of antibodies.
   2. T cell and B cell lymphocytes fight antigens; B cell response forms antibodies (immunoglobulins) that destroy antigens.
   3. T cell response releases several types of sensitized T cells that become memory cells, reacting to a later invasion by the same antigens.
   4. Some T cells become killer T cells that directly attack antigens; in organ transplants, killer T cells attack the transplant as foreign.

D. Factors affecting immune system functioning
   1. Age: The elderly are more likely to experience immunosuppression due to impaired production and function of T and B cell lymphocytes as well as increased incidence of autoimmune diseases.
   2. Nutrition: Insufficient protein intake results in atrophy of lymphoid tissues, depression of antibody response, reduction in the number of T cells, and impairment of phagocytic function.
   3. Concurrent injury or illness: Burns, trauma, infection, surgery, and chronic illness may suppress the functioning of the immune system.
   4. Cancer: Tumors release antigens and may suppress the immune system's defenses.
   5. Medications: Antibiotics, corticosteroids, nonsteroidal anti-inflammatory drugs (NSAIDs), and cytotoxic drugs may alter the functioning of the immune system.
   6. Radiation: Radiation destroys lymphocytes and decreases the population of cells required to replace them.

E. Types of diseases of immune system
   1. Immunopathology
      a) Immunopathology occurs when body fails to differentiate between self and nonself.

        b) If the antigen is foreign, the body is protected; if not, autoimmune disease and tissue damage result.

        c) An example is a hypersensitivity reaction.

  2. Immunodeficiencies

        a) Regardless of underlying problem, immunodeficiency causes recurrent, severe infections, often involving unusual organisms.

        b) Immunodeficiencies may be either primary (deficiency with no known cause) or secondary (deficiency that occurs in the course of underlying disease).

        c) An example of secondary deficiency is AIDS.

II. Types of immune response

See text pages
_____

A. Antibody-mediated (humoral) immune response: characterized by the production of antibodies, or immunoglobulins (Ig), by B cell lymphocytes in response to an antigen

B. Cell-mediated immune response: characterized by the presence of T cell lymphocytes, which attack antigens directly rather than through the production of antibodies

III. Selected disorders

See text pages
_____

A. Hypersensitivity reaction (type I, immediate or anaphylactic hypersensitivity): a state of altered immunologic response to a substance the body recognizes as foreign

  1. Pathophysiology and etiology

        a) Hypersensitivity reaction follows a reexposure to an allergen after sensitization.

        b) Within minutes of exposure to allergen, plasma cells produce IgE antibodies, triggering the release of chemical mediators that cause allergic symptoms.

        c) Clinical symptoms are determined by the amount of allergen and the amount of mediator that are released.

  2. Symptoms

        a) Allergic rhinitis (hay fever): sneezing, itchy nose, nasal congestion, itchy, watery eyes; sore throat, frontal headache, wheezing

        b) Drug allergy: in dermatitis medicamentosa, sudden rash that may be bright red and itchy, usually generalized but may appear on one area; other reactions include anaphylaxis, drug fever, lymph node enlargement, pulmonary reactions, hepatic syndromes, and lupus syndromes

        c) Food allergy: nausea, vomiting, diarrhea, abdominal cramps, itching, rash, wheezing, coughing

d) Urticaria (hives): itching, swelling, redness, wheals
e) Angioedema: swelling extending deep into skin tissues or mucous membranes, usually in the head and neck; may end in respiratory arrest
f) Anaphylaxis
    (1) Immediate, possibly fatal reaction occurring after exposure to an allergen to which a person is extremely sensitive
    (2) Symptoms: urticaria; angioedema; itching and swelling in nose, mouth, throat, and bronchi causing moderate to severe upper airway obstruction; may progress to anaphylactic shock
3. Diagnostic evaluation
  a) Blood tests
    (1) White blood cell count: During infective states, high levels of eosinophils may be present.
    (2) Total serum IgE levels: High levels may reveal a hypersensitivity reaction.
    (3) Radioallergosorbent test (RAST): After patient's blood is exposed to a variety of suspected allergen particle complexes, antibodies combine with radiolabeled allergens.
  b) Skin tests
    (1) Scratch test: Allergen is applied to scratch on skin; a raised wheal or localized erythema indicates a hypersensitivity reaction.
    (2) Intradermal injection: Diluted allergen solution is injected intradermally; a raised wheal or localized erythema indicates a hypersensitivity reaction.
  c) Smear tests: Conjunctival secretions, nasal secretions, and sputum may contain eosinophils and indicate a hypersensitivity reaction.
  d) Provocative tests: Allergen is administered directly to respiratory mucosa, and target organ response is observed.
4. Medical treatment
  a) Treatment of allergy symptoms
    (1) Allergen avoidance and environment modification (see Client Teaching Checklist, "Minimizing Exposure to Allergens")
    (2) Drug therapy
        (a) Antihistamines: oral, topical, IV, or intramuscular preparations that relieve allergy symptoms
        (b) Nasal decongestants: topical drops or sprays to relieve nasal congestion
        (c) Immunotherapy: regular injections of diluted allergen to stimulate antibody formation
        (d) Corticosteroids: medications to treat inflammatory response
        (e) Epinephrine: Injection used to treat serious allergic reactions (such as anaphylaxis); also included in some topical nasal decongestants

      b) Emergency treatment of anaphylactic shock
- (1) Administer epinephrine IV.
- (2) Establish IV saline immediately.
- (3) Administer other vasopressors (such as dopamine) to treat hypotension.
- (4) Provide oxygen and mechanical ventilation as needed.
- (5) Perform cardiopulmonary resuscitation.

5. Essential nursing care for patients with type I hypersensitivity reaction
    a) Nursing assessment
- (1) Obtain history (except for anaphylaxis, which is an emergency situation): medical, surgical, food, family allergy, drug.
- (2) Record symptoms in detail with factors that increase or decrease symptoms.
- (3) Examine and describe in detail any skin lesions.

    b) Nursing diagnoses
- (1) Altered oral mucous membrane related to angioedema of oral cavity
- (2) Ineffective airway clearance related to chronic allergy

---

✔ CLIENT TEACHING CHECKLIST ✔

Minimizing Exposure to Allergens

There are several ways for clients with allergies to decrease their exposure to allergens. Explain to clients the following measures they can take:

If you are sensitive to dust:

✔ Remove from your home all carpets, curtains, venetian blinds, stuffed furniture, feather pillows, and other items that collect dust. Instead, replace them with wooden or linoleum flooring, pull shades, wooden furniture, and cotton coverings that can be cleaned or laundered frequently.

✔ Use an air conditioner in the summer and a steam or hot water heat system in the winter. An electrostatic air cleaner may also be effective in removing airborne allergens.

If you are sensitive to pollen or mold:

✔ On days when the pollen count is high, stay indoors with the air conditioner on.
✔ Close your windows at night, and keep your car windows closed when you drive.
✔ Do not mow lawns, rake leaves, work in a garden, or keep houseplants.
✔ Do not hang bed linens or clothes on a line to dry.
✔ Wear a mask when you may encounter increased concentrations of allergens.

          (3) Ineffective breathing pattern related to allergic reaction

          (4) Knowledge deficit related to treatment modalities

    c) Nursing intervention

          (1) Reexamine drug history before any new drug is added.

          (2) Closely observe patient with known drug allergy; assess respiratory rate and oral cavity frequently and whenever a new drug is ordered.

          (3) Instruct patient to maintain patent respiratory system by avoiding exposure to persons with upper respiratory infections.

          (4) Explain treatment modalities in detail: Allow time for patient to read and ask questions; explain medical regimen, environmental recommendations, new diets, drug therapies, immunotherapy requirements; caution against overuse of drugs and nose drops or sprays; thoroughly explain symptoms and self-treatment for anaphylaxis.

          (5) If anaphylaxis occurs: Apply tourniquet above area (if allergen has been injected), inject epinephrine immediately; if necessary, repeat dose 2 more times at 20- to 30-minute intervals; bring emergency equipment to the patient and summon help immediately.

    d) Nursing evaluation

          (1) Patient exhibits normal breathing patterns.

          (2) Patient states awareness of what must be done and what to expect once treatment begins.

          (3) Patient states understanding of treatment modalities necessary to reduce or eliminate symptoms.

          (4) Patient states understanding of hypoallergenic diet, demonstrates understanding of anaphylaxis symptoms, and shows ability to self-administer emergency epinephrine.

B. AIDS: the most severe form of a continuum of illnesses associated with HIV infection

  1. Pathophysiology and etiology

    a) HIV is one of the retroviruses, carrying its genetic material in RNA instead of DNA.

    b) HIV reprograms genetic materials of invaded cells, using the cell to reproduce the virus instead of itself; rate of HIV reproduction is related to individual's health.

    c) HIV is transmitted by entry of contaminated body secretions (semen, vaginal secretions, blood) into recipients' bloodstreams through certain types of sexual behaviors, IV drug use, and transfusions of contaminated blood.

  2. Symptoms: range from mild abnormalities in immune response without overt symptoms to profound immunosuppression associated with a variety of life-threatening infections and malignancies that are rare in non-HIV-infected people; may include coughing, shortness of breath, fever, night sweats, weight loss, fatigue, lymph node disease, diarrhea, memory loss, confusion, headache, visual changes, personality changes, seizures, rashes, dry skin, skin lesions, pain, and discomfort

3. Diagnostic evaluation
   a) Enzyme-linked immunosorbent assay (ELISA) test determines presence of HIV antibodies and documents exposure to HIV, but it is *not* a diagnosis of AIDS.
   b) Western blot analysis identifies presence of HIV antibodies and confirms seropositivity as identified by ELISA test.
4. Medical treatment
   a) HIV-related infections
      (1) *Pneumocystitis* pneumonia: antibacterial drug trimethoprim-sulfamethoxazole (TMP/SMZ) or antiprotozoal drug pentamidine
      (2) Cryptococcal meningitis: IV administration of amphotericin B for at least 4–6 weeks; oral administration of the antifungal agent fluconazole as maintenance therapy
      (3) Retinitis caused by cytomegalovirus: lifetime administration of ganciclovir (Cytovene)

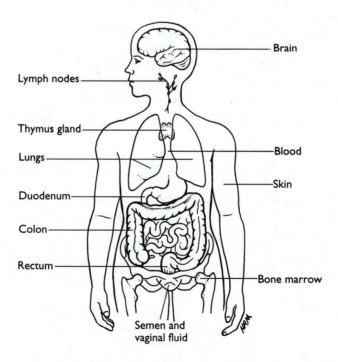

Figure 3–1
Places Where HIV May Be Harbored

        (4) Other infections: a number of antimicrobial drugs currently being investigated
  b) Malignancies
        (1) Kaposi's sarcoma (KS): interferon, various chemotherapeutic agents, radiation therapy
        (2) AIDS-related lymphomas: combined chemotherapy and radiation therapy
  c) Other
        (1) Reproduction of HIV: zidovudine (AZT)
        (2) Immune system damage: interferon, interleukin-2
5. Essential nursing care for patients with AIDS
  a) Nursing assessment
        (1) Assess nutritional status by noting dietary history, weight, triceps skin fold measures, blood urea nitrogen, serum protein, albumin, and transferrin levels.
        (2) Inspect skin and mucous membranes for evidence of breakdown, ulceration, or infection.
        (3) Monitor respiratory status by noting cough, sputum production, shortness of breath, orthopnea, tachypnea, and chest pain.
        (4) Assess neurologic status by checking orientation to person, place, and time; consciousness level; and memory.
        (5) Assess fluid and electrolyte status by examining skin and mucous membranes for turgor and dryness and by monitoring fluid intake and output, blood pressure, and pulse.
        (6) Evaluate patient's knowledge about the disease and its transmission.
  b) Nursing diagnoses
        (1) Impaired skin integrity related to cutaneous manifestations of HIV infection or diarrhea
        (2) High risk for infection related to immunodeficiency
        (3) Ineffective airway clearance related to increased bronchial secretions and decreased ability to cough
        (4) Knowledge deficit related to prevention of HIV transmission
        (5) Fear related to terminal illness
  c) Nursing intervention
        (1) Assess skin and oral mucosa routinely for changes in appearance, location, and size of lesions and for signs of infection.
        (2) Provide egg crates, air mattresses, or water mattresses to eliminate excess pressure on skin.
        (3) Apply medicated lotions, ointments, and dressings to affected skin surfaces as prescribed; avoid using excess tape; administer antipruritics, antibiotics, and analgesics as prescribed.
        (4) Provide education about how to prevent infection: Maintain good personal hygiene, disinfect bathroom and kitchen surfaces with dilution of 1:10 ratio of bleach and water, avoid exposure to the sick, avoid smoking, maintain good diet, exercise.

      (5) Provide pulmonary measures every 2 hours to clear airway: coughing, deep breathing, postural drainage, percussion, and vibration.

      (6) Provide information about AIDS transmission to patients, friends, and family (see Client Teaching Checklist, "Safer Sex Guidelines for Persons with HIV Seropositivity"); thoroughly discuss all fears and misconceptions.

      (7) Encourage patients to express anxiety and fear, explore resources for support and coping mechanisms, encourage social interaction.

   d) Nursing evaluation

      (1) Patient maintains skin integrity.

      (2) Patient experiences no infections.

      (3) Patient maintains effective airway clearance.

      (4) Patient understands means of preventing disease transmission.

      (5) Patient expresses fears and develops coping strategies and support system.

✔ CLIENT TEACHING CHECKLIST ✔

Safer Sex Guidelines for Persons with HIV Seropositivity

Explain to clients who have tested positive for HIV antibody the following safer sex procedures:

✔ If possible, avoid sexual intercourse, especially practices that may injure tissue (anal intercourse); avoid oral-genital contact.

✔ Inform potential sexual partners of your HIV-positive status.

✔ Reduce your number of partners, preferably to one.

✔ Always use a latex condom; animal skin condoms will not protect you from HIV; nonoxynol-9 spermicide may provide added protection from HIV.

✔ Women should avoid pregnancy.

1. Mr. Butler, an adult who has recently been exposed to chickenpox (varicella zoster), asks if it is possible for him to "catch the disease." He says that he had chickenpox as a child. The nurse can best answer the question by explaining which of the following types of immunity?

   a. Active acquired
   b. Passive acquired
   c. Artificially acquired
   d. Natural passive acquired

2. On the third day after kidney transplantation, Marie Jasko is experiencing acute rejection of the new kidney. In caring for her, the nurse will anticipate the need to:

   a. Seek another kidney.
   b. Increase the IV fluid rate.
   c. Increase the immunosuppressive medications.
   d. Maintain complete bed rest.

3. Thirty seconds after an IV antibiotic is started, a patient begins to exhibit dyspnea, wheezing, and apprehension. The nurse should first:

   a. Call for medical assistance.
   b. Continue to assess the patient.
   c. Obtain IV epinephrine.
   d. Turn off the IV antibiotic.

4. The mother of a 2-year-old child brings her daughter to the hospital. The child has urticaria on the face and neck, watering eyes, copious watery discharge from the nose, and wheezing. An allergy to peanut butter is diagnosed as the cause of the symptoms. Which of the following statements by the mother would indicate that she needs further teaching?

   a. "I'll need to read food labels to check for peanuts."

   b. "I'll wait 6 months before I give her peanut butter."
   c. "I'll introduce new foods one at a time."
   d. "I'll buy this drug (antihistamine) on the way home."

5. Before administering an allergen intradermal test to Roger Bradley, the nurse should recommend which of the following to him?

   a. Discontinue antihistamines after testing.
   b. Stay for 20 minutes after testing.
   c. Be transported to the hospital for wheal development.
   d. Take epinephrine before testing.

6. The home health nurse visits Joe Manetta, who has multiple allergies to dust, pollens, and molds. Which of the following would indicate to the nurse that Mr. Manetta is trying to minimize his exposure to allergens?

   a. Cutting the grass with a handkerchief over his mouth
   b. Hanging bed linens outside to dry
   c. Dusting wooden furniture with a damp cloth
   d. Placing fans in the windows to cool the house

7. Which one of the following patients would the nurse expect to be at greatest risk for infection with the human immunodeficiency virus (HIV)?

   a. A 50-year-old monogamous woman whose husband has sexual affairs
   b. A 19-year-old sexually active male who always uses condoms
   c. A 5-year-old girl whose mother is currently an IV drug user
   d. A 45-year-old homosexual male who has a 15-year monogamous relationship

8. A 35-year-old male is admitted with *Pneumocystis carinii* pneumonia secondary to acquired immunodeficiency syndrome (AIDS). On initial assessment, he is disoriented and emaciated and has several skin lesions. Which of the following would the nurse do first?

   a. Orient the patient to time, place, and person.
   b. Provide a high-calorie, high-nutrition snack.
   c. Apply gauze dressings to cover the skin lesions.
   d. Elevate the head of the bed.

9. While the nurse is caring for Grace Miller, a 29-year-old woman with AIDS, Ms. Miller states, "I've lost everything since I got AIDS: my family, my home, and most of all, my health." The best response for the nurse to make is:

   a. "You feel like you've lost everything?" as the nurse stops and sits down beside the patient.
   b. "I'll call the social worker as soon as I have a chance," as the nurse continues care.
   c. "You're just saying that because you're not feeling well. Things will look better tomorrow," as the nurse leaves the room.
   d. "You should call your family. I know they would come," as the nurse finishes care.

ANSWERS

1. **Correct answer is a.** When Mr. Butler had varicella as a child, the varicella antigen entered the body, and the body made antibodies against the varicella. His body developed an immune response that will probably protect him from contracting chickenpox for the rest of his life.

   b. Passive acquired immunity is a temporary immunization obtained by injecting antibodies from another organism into the body. Mr. Butler's body developed its own varicella antibodies.

   c. Artificially acquired immunity is obtained by administering a killed or attenuated antigen or toxoid that causes the body to develop antibodies and prevents it from contracting a specific disease. Mr. Butler's body developed its own antibodies.

   d. Natural passive immunity is present at birth and consists of antibodies that are passed from the mother to the fetus or infant and that will protect the child from certain antigens. Mr. Butler's body developed varicella antibodies when he had chickenpox as a child.

2. **Correct answer is c.** Acute rejection is a type IV hypersensitivity reaction. The recipient's mature T lymphocytes recognize the donor cells (kidney) as foreign materials, triggering the destruction of the new kidney cells by killer (cytotoxic) T cells. This process usually occurs a few hours to a few days after the transplant. Increasing the amount of medication can stop this rejection process.

   a. Increasing the IV fluid rate would be more appropriate for hyperacute rejection, in which cytotoxic antibodies in the recipient quickly destroy the donor cells (kidney). This process can occur before the surgery is completed and might require another donor kidney. Hyperacute rejection can usually be avoided by pretransplant cell crossmatching.

   b. The amount of fluid entering the body for kidney filtration will not affect the rejection process and may put the patient into fluid overload, especially if the kidney is not filtering properly.

   d. Bed rest will not have any effect on acute rejection. The patient should be out of bed and ambulating to prevent other postoperative complications.

3. **Correct answer is d.** The patient is exhibiting symptoms of anaphylaxis, a type I hypersensitivity reaction. The first action is to discontinue immediately the source (IV) of the allergen (antibiotic).

   a. The nurse should call for medical assistance, but discontinuing the antibiotic is the first action to be taken.

b. Assessment of the patient would continue, but immediate action must be taken to prevent further reaction and possible death.

c. IV epinephrine is the drug of choice in treating anaphylaxis, but turning off the source of the allergen is the first action.

4. **Correct answer is b.** Especially in children, food allergies may disappear if the food is avoided, but 6 months is not long enough. Avoiding the substance for 1 or 2 years is necessary.

   a. Reading food labels demonstrates an understanding of the need to avoid hidden sources of the allergen.

   c. Introducing new foods one at a time demonstrates an understanding that the child may have other food allergies. If several foods are introduced at one time, it will be difficult to identify the allergen.

   d. Purchasing the antihistamine demonstrates that the mother understands that the allergic reaction may recur. Antihistamines, usually diphenhydramine (Benadryl), are the drugs of choice for preventing further allergic reactions.

5. **Correct answer is b.** After allergen intradermal testing, the patient is at risk for developing anaphylaxis. Therefore, Mr. Bradley needs to be assessed for signs of anaphylaxis, and emergency drugs and treatment must be immediately available.

   a. Antihistamines are discontinued 48 hours before testing so that they will not mask a reaction to an offending allergen. Longer-lasting antihistamines may need to be stopped 5–7 days before testing.

   c. Wheals develop about 15 minutes after the allergen injection, indicating a positive skin test. This is expected and is not an emergency situation.

   d. It would not be appropriate to take epinephrine before testing. Epinephrine is usually the drug of choice if an anaphylactic reaction develops after testing.

6. **Correct answer is c.** Using a damp cloth for dusting prevents the dust (allergen) from becoming airborne, being inhaled, and causing allergic symptoms.

   a. Cutting the grass should be avoided, but if it must be done, a mask should be worn over the mouth and nose. A handkerchief would not filter allergens as well as a mask or fit as tightly.

   b. Pollens and molds will gather on damp fabric and remain there when it is placed on the bed, causing allergic symptoms.

   c. Window fans will draw pollens and molds into the house and circulate the dust that is already in the house, causing allergic symptoms. Air conditioning is recommended for cooling.

7. **Correct answer is a.** This woman is most at risk because her husband's sexual history puts him at high risk for becoming infected with HIV and transmitting it to her via sexual relations.

   b. This teenager is at risk, but using a condom decreases the risk. An intact latex condom is impermeable to HIV.

   c. This 5-year-old is at low risk. IV drug users are at high risk for HIV infection and, if pregnant, can infect the fetus. When a person is infected with HIV, antibodies usually develop 1–14 months after exposure. This child is unlikely to develop antibodies 5 years after birth. If her mother is currently infected, the child should not become infected unless contaminated body secretions enter her bloodstream.

   d. This man is at low risk. A large percentage of HIV cases have occurred in the male homosexual population, but being involved in a monogamous relationship lowers the risk. Because it takes 1–14 months to develop antibodies and the couple has been monogamous for 15 years, it is unlikely that either partner has HIV.

8. **Correct answer is d.** The pneumonia will impair respiratory function. Elevating the head will improve oxygenation, which is the first priority. It may also make the patient more comfortable.

a. The patient is disoriented, which may be related to neurologic changes that occur in patients with AIDS. The disorientation may also be related to poor oxygenation due to his pneumonia. Therefore, improving oxygenation is the priority.

b. The patient is emaciated, which often results from the anorexia, nausea, diarrhea, and wasting syndrome that occur in AIDS. However, improving oxygenation is the priority.

c. Patients with AIDS are prone to develop Kaposi's sarcoma and herpes simplex skin lesions. Skin care, although important, would not be the first priority for this patient.

9. **Correct answer is a.** This statement allows Ms. Miller to verbalize her feelings of grief and isolation associated with having AIDS.

Sitting down signals to her that the nurse wants to listen; thus, it encourages verbalization and therapeutic communication.

b. Promising to call the social worker and continuing care signal to the patient that the nurse does not want to listen or communicate. Although Ms. Miller should have a referral to social service, this is an opportunity for the nurse to listen and communicate with the patient.

c. Denying the legitimacy of the patient's feelings is demeaning. In addition, leaving may stop verbalization. The nurse may not return later, or the patient may not want to talk at another time.

d. The nurse is telling Ms. Miller what to do, and calling the family may not be appropriate for her. The patient is expressing the need to verbalize feelings of loss and isolation.

4

Care of Patient with Infectious Disease

OVERVIEW

I. **Process of infection**
   A. Infectious organisms
   B. Source of infection
   C. Method of contamination

II. **Defense against infection**
   A. Skin and mucous membranes
   B. Immunoglobulins
   C. Gastric juices and lysozyme
   D. Cilia
   E. Interferon
   F. Reticuloendothelial system
   G. Inflammatory response

III. **Diagnosis of infection**
   A. Bacteriologic studies
   B. Immunologic tests
   C. Skin tests

IV. **Types of infections**
   A. Community-acquired infections
   B. Nosocomial infections

V. **Selected sexually transmitted diseases (STDs)**
   A. Ulcerative conditions
   B. Infections of epithelial surfaces
   C. Pelvic inflammatory disease
   D. Essential nursing care for patients with sexually transmitted diseases

NURSING HIGHLIGHTS

1. Nurse must listen to the fears and possible misconceptions of some patients regarding vaccinations and inform them of the benefits of accepting this type of preventive care.
2. Nurse must assume increasing responsibility for prevention of infection, understand the routes of transmission of infection, and use the appropriate methods to prevent the spread of microorganisms.
3. Nurse should assume a professional, understanding, and nonjudgmental attitude toward patient during assessment for STD.
4. Nurse should allow patients with STDs to express fears, anxieties, and emotions and show understanding about the problems of informing the uninfected spouse.

GLOSSARY

aerobic—requires oxygen for survival

anaerobic—does not require oxygen for survival

chancre—a skin lesion marking the first sign of syphilis

nosocomial infection—infection acquired in a hospital

phagocytosis—process whereby bacteria and particles are ingested and digested by cells called phagocytes

reticuloendothelial system—those cells throughout the body that perform phagocytosis

tabes dorsalis—sclerosis of the posterior column of the spinal cord caused by syphilis

ENHANCED OUTLINE

See text pages
_____

I. Process of infection

A. Infectious organisms
1. Bacteria
a) Single-celled microorganisms that are round (cocci), rod-shaped (bacilli), or spiral (spirochetes); may be aerobic or anaerobic
b) Examples: staphylococcal infections, typhoid fever, tetanus, pulmonary tuberculosis
2. Viruses
a) Microorganisms that occur in two types, depending on nucleic acid composition (DNA or RNA); can only multiply with invaded cell or tissue's metabolic and reproductive materials
b) Examples: influenza, rabies, poliomyelitis, viral hepatitis, herpes simplex
3. Fungi
a) Yeasts or molds; divided into three types
(1) Superficial mycotic infections (dermatophytoses) that affect skin and hair
(2) Intermediate mycotic infections that affect subcutaneous tissues
(3) Systemic mycotic infections that affect deep tissues and organs
b) Examples: histoplasmosis, ringworm
4. Helminths
a) Intestinal parasites in three main groups: roundworms (nematodes), tapeworms (cestodes), and flukes (trematodes) that mate and reproduce in the host
b) Examples: trichinosis, hookworm disease

5. Rickettsiae
   a) Microorganisms that resemble bacteria and are transmitted by fleas, ticks, lice, or mites
   b) Examples: Rocky Mountain spotted fever, typhus
6. Protozoans
   a) Single-celled animals classified according to motility
   b) Examples: amebic dysentery, malaria
7. Mycoplasmas
   a) Single-celled microorganisms that lack a cell wall and can assume various shapes
   b) Examples: pneumonitis, pharyngitis

B. Source of infection
   1. Environment (community-acquired infection)
   2. Hospital (nosocomial infection)

C. Method of contamination
   1. Direct contact: body contact with infected excreta, secretions, or drainage (see Nurse Alert, "Universal Blood and Body Fluids Precautions")
   2. Indirect contact
      a) Contact with object or substance contaminated by an infected person
      b) Contact with air contaminated by infected droplets from an infected person's cough or sneeze
   3. Vectors: contact with insects or animals that carry an infectious disease
   4. Airborne transmission: contact with airborne infected particles that have traveled over 1 meter through the air

---

! NURSE ALERT !

Universal Blood and Body Fluids Precautions

Nurses should follow these precautions with all patients to protect themselves from blood-borne communicable diseases.

- Always wear gloves when in contact with any patient's blood and body fluids, broken skin, or mucous membranes; when handling surfaces or items soiled with blood and body fluids; and when performing vascular access procedures. Wash hands and change gloves after each patient contact.
- Wear a mask, goggles, and gown during procedures likely to cause splashes of blood and body fluids.
- Wash hands immediately after contact with blood and body fluids; always wash hands as soon as gloves are removed.
- All sharp items should be considered potentially infective and handled with extreme care. Place needles and sharp instruments in puncture-resistant containers for disposal; needles should never be bent, recapped, or removed from syringe.
- Use mouthpieces or other ventilation devices when performing mouth-to-mouth resuscitation.

See text pages
_____

II. Defense against infection

A. Skin and mucous membranes
   1. Unbroken skin is a mechanical barrier against infection.
   2. Skin's acidic balance creates undesirable medium for pathogenic microorganisms.
   3. Vaginal mucous membrane secretions favor growth of nonpathogenic, acid-producing bacteria that create a hostile environment to pathogenic microorganisms.

B. Immunoglobulins: present in body fluids

C. Gastric juices and lysozyme
   1. Acidic gastric juices destroy many microorganisms in the gastrointestinal tract.
   2. Lysozyme, present in many body secretions, destroys bacteria.

D. Cilia
   1. Hairlike projections from the mucous membrane lining the upper respiratory tract trap microorganisms, dust, and foreign particles.
   2. Mucus in the respiratory tract traps microorganisms and foreign particles; cilia move them up toward the pharynx to be swallowed or spit out.

E. Interferon
   1. White blood cells produce this protein substance in response to viral infections.
   2. Once released, interferon triggers the manufacture of antiviral protein.

F. Reticuloendothelial system
   1. Phagocytosis
      a) Infection triggers phagocytic response that engulfs and digests invading organisms and prevents infection.
      b) Two types of phagocytes, macrophages (large) and microphages (small), are capable of phagocytosis; phagocytes may be stationary or may move throughout body.
   2. Immune response: same as section II of Chapter 3

G. Inflammatory response
   1. Vascular response
      a) Following invasion by a microorganism, vasoconstriction occurs; release of histamines then causes vasodilation.
      b) Heat and redness appear as early signs of inflammation.
   2. Fluid exudation (inflammatory exudate)
      a) Capillary walls become permeable, allowing molecules of water, colloids, and ions to pass into the intercellular tissues of the injured area.
      b) Swelling and pain appear at injury site as fluid collects between cells.

3. Cellular exudation
   a) White blood cells destroy microorganisms and any toxins they have produced at injury site.
   b) White blood cells remove debris and dead bacteria produced by phagocytosis.

III. Diagnosis of infection

See text pages
_____

A. Bacteriologic studies
   1. Microscopic examination: Specimen is placed on slide and examined; gram staining identifies colorless bacteria (those that absorb dye are gram-positive; those that do not are gram-negative).
   2. Cultured exam: Specimen is placed in growth medium and examined microscopically in 24–48 hours to identify causative agent.
   3. Sensitivity study: Specimen is exposed to various antibiotics to determine which type is effective against identified microorganism.

B. Immunologic tests
   1. Agglutination (clumping) tests: diagnose cirrhosis, lymphatic leukemia, atypical pneumonia
   2. Precipitation tests: determine severity of some inflammatory diseases and diagnose coccidioidomycosis
   3. Complement-fixation test: diagnoses histoplasmosis, blastomycosis, and rickettsial diseases
   4. Immunofluorescence tests: identify immunoglobulins (such as for Epstein-Barr virus and toxoplasmosis)

C. Skin tests: Specimen is injected intradermally; site is then examined for a reaction.

IV. Types of infections

See text pages
_____

A. Community-acquired infections
   1. General principles of prevention and control
      a) Effective immunization program
      b) Sanitary food and water procedures, proper waste disposal
      c) Education on personal cleanliness
      d) Early detection and treatment of infectious diseases through screening programs and outbreak investigation
   2. Essential nursing care for community-acquired infections
      a) Nursing assessment
         (1) Take comprehensive history.
            (a) Symptoms: types, onset, severity, order, and progression
            (b) Direct contacts: people with infection or illness, sexual contact, large crowds, animal contact, and animal or insect bites
            (c) Indirect contacts: skin injury, recent food and water intake, recent blood donations or transfusions, dental procedures, and parenteral injections
            (d) Drugs: prescription, nonprescription, and illegal

(e) Travel: foreign and domestic
(f) Immunizations: active and passive
(g) Diseases: past and current
(2) Perform physical assessment.
    (a) General: fever, fatigue, malaise, muscle pain, joint pain, swollen glands, headache
    (b) Skin: rash, lesions, redness, warmth, swelling, drainage, pain
    (c) Gastrointestinal tract: nausea, vomiting, diarrhea, abdominal distention, fever
    (d) Respiratory tract: cough, congestion, sore throat, rhinitis, sputum, chest pain, fever
    (e) Genitourinary tract: dysuria, purulent discharge, urgency, frequency, hematuria, pelvic or flank pain, fever

b) Nursing diagnoses
  (1) Ineffective breathing pattern related to infection and inflammation
  (2) Hyperthermia related to infectious process
  (3) Diarrhea related to infection of gastrointestinal tract and antibiotic therapy
  (4) Fluid volume deficit related to fever, diarrhea, diaphoresis, and failure to drink fluids

c) Nursing intervention
  (1) Monitor for shortness of breath, coughing, use of accessory muscles; monitor respiratory rate, depth, pattern, and chest expansion.
  (2) Turn patient at least every 2 hours; encourage patient to cough, yawn, and take deep breaths every 2–4 hours.
  (3) Encourage increased oral intake of fluids.
  (4) If patient's temperature is extremely high (over 104°F), give tepid water sponge baths or apply cool compresses.
  (5) Monitor vital signs every 4 hours; notify physician if fever does not respond to treatment.
  (6) Monitor severity and intensity of diarrhea: instruct patient to clean perineal area after each bowel movement and to administer ointments to relieve pain and aid healing.
  (7) Offer oral fluids and monitor vital signs every 2–4 hours; monitor fluid intake and output; administer fluid and electrolyte replacement as ordered; observe for signs of potassium, sodium, or chloride deficiency.

d) Nursing evaluation
  (1) Patient's breathing pattern returns to normal.
  (2) Patient attains normal body temperature.

       (3) Patient attains normal defecation pattern.

       (4) Patient maintains adequate fluid balance.

  3. Discharge planning (patient education)

    a) Provide brief, focused explanations about infectious organisms, how they are spread, how to avoid their spread, and how the illness is treated.

    b) Provide information about the control of environmental contaminants (insects, rodents, and other animal vectors and reservoirs of human infections) and about the importance of nutrition, immunizations, personal hygiene, home cleanliness, and prompt health care.

B. Nosocomial infections

  1. General principles of prevention and control

    a) Isolation and precautions

      (1) Precautions depending on type of infection

      (2) Appropriate barriers worn by nurses who come in contact with patient's blood, body fluids, or excretions (see Nurse Alert, "Universal Blood and Body Fluids Precautions")

      (3) Isolation for patients with specific infectious diseases (private rooms, masks, gloves, and gowns)

    b) Surveillance: detecting, reporting, and recording of nosocomial infections

    c) Disposal of contaminated materials: should be placed in a nonpenetrable bag that is sealed and has contents marked

    d) Hand washing: before and after each patient contact, 60 seconds of washing with a cleansing agent using friction and running water

    e) Personal grooming: daily changing of uniforms; having clean, short hair and fingernails; not wearing jewelry

    f) Sterilization: washing and sterilizing all reusable instruments, equipment, and linens

  2. Essential nursing care for nosocomial infections

    a) Nursing assessment

      (1) Take comprehensive history.

        (a) Symptoms

        (b) Patient contacts with visitors, hospital staff

        (c) Places visited by patient (x-ray, operating room, physical therapy, lounges, shower and tub rooms)

        (d) Food history: hospital diet, food brought by visitors

      (2) Perform physical assessment (same as IV,A,2,a,2 of this chapter).

    b) Nursing diagnoses

      (1) Same as section IV,A,2,b of this chapter

      (2) Potential for infection related to failure of hospital staff to observe proper techniques

      (3) Social isolation related to restriction of visitors

    c) Nursing intervention

      (1) See section IV,A,2,c of this chapter.

      (2) Wash hands; follow hospital isolation and precaution procedures.

      (3) Encourage family to visit; interact with patient often.

      d) Nursing evaluation

        (1) See section IV,A,2,d of this chapter.

        (2) Patient does not experience spread of infection; nor is it spread to others.

        (3) Patient understands and accepts a temporary change in social interaction.

  3. Discharge planning (patient education)

    a) See section IV,A,3,a of this chapter.

    b) Explain to patient with streptococcal infection the importance of completing the entire course of antibiotics to prevent complications; advise patient to monitor temperature and to use warm saline gargle to relieve sore throat.

    c) Ensure that patient has access to proper storage facilities if medications must be refrigerated.

V. Selected sexually transmitted diseases (STDs)

See text pages

A. Ulcerative conditions

  1. Syphilis

    a) Definition: a sexually transmitted disease that results in chancres, rash, tissue destruction, heart damage, and brain damage

    b) Pathophysiology and etiology: caused by the spirochete *Treponema pallidum,* which penetrates broken skin or mucous membranes in the genitalia, rectum, or mouth during sexual intercourse; may also be acquired by kissing or intimate bodily contact; may be passed from mother to fetus through the placenta

    c) Symptoms

      (1) Primary stage: Chancre appears on the genitals, anus, cervix, or other body part; if untreated, chancre heals in several weeks.

      (2) Secondary stage: Fever, malaise, rash, headache, sore throat, and lymph node enlargement occur.

      (3) Tertiary stage: tabes dorsalis, joint changes, incontinence, cardiovascular problems, and impotence occur; patient is not infectious now, since spirochetes have invaded central nervous system and body organs.

  2. Genital herpes

    a) Definition: a sexually transmitted disease that produces painful and itchy blisters on the genitals

    b) Pathophysiology and etiology

      (1) Genital herpes is caused by the herpes simplex virus type 2 (HSV-2) transmitted by sexual intercourse with an infected person; herpes simplex virus type 1 (HSV-1) causes cold sores

but may also produce genital lesions following oral-genital contact with an infected person.

    (2) Either virus may be introduced into the eye, mouth, genital area, or skin site; HSV-2 may be transmitted from mother to infant during vaginal birth.

  c) Symptoms

    (1) HSV-1: oral lesions, low grade fever, malaise, enlarged lymph nodes in neck; pharyngitis, keratoconjunctivitis, chills, muscle soreness, and difficulty swallowing

    (2) HSV-2: painful vesicular lesions on buttocks, penis, perineum, vulva, cervix, and vagina; malaise, fever, chills, and headache

B. Infections of epithelial surfaces

  1. Genital warts

    a) Definition: soft warts that grow in and around the entrance of the vagina, cervix, anus, and penis and that are transmitted by sexual contact

    b) Pathophysiology and etiology: caused by human papillomavirus infection after sexual contact with an infected person

    c) Symptoms: painless, soft, fleshy wartlike growths on genitalia or cervix or in vagina

  2. Chlamydia

    a) Definition: a sexually transmitted disease causing genital infections and in many cases infertility in men and women

    b) Pathophysiology and etiology: caused by a strain of *Chlamydia trachomatis;* transmitted through sexual contact or from mother to infant during vaginal birth

    c) Symptoms: inflammation of urethra and epididymis in men and of cervix in women; women may also experience mucopurulent discharge, pain, and pelvic infection.

  3. Gonorrhea

    a) Definition: sexually transmitted disease that causes infection of mucosal surface of the genitourinary tract, rectum, and pharynx

    b) Pathophysiology and etiology: caused by the organism *Neisseria gonorrhoeae;* transmitted through sexual contact and from mother to infant during vaginal birth

    c) Symptoms

      (1) Total lack of symptoms occurs in about half the women and some men who contract gonorrhea.

      (2) Symptoms appear between 2 and 6 days after infection, including urethritis with a purulent discharge and painful urination (men); women may experience vaginal discharge, abnormal menstrual bleeding, and painful urination.

      (3) Untreated infections may spread to prostate, seminal vesicles, and epididymis in men; to cervix, endometrium, and fallopian tubes in women.

C. Pelvic inflammatory disease (PID)
  1. Definition: inflammatory disorder in women in which organisms travel from vagina or cervix to pelvic organs (except uterus)
  2. Pathophysiology and etiology
    a) PID is usually caused by *Neisseria gonorrhoeae* or *Chlamydia trachomatis,* but other organisms may be responsible.
    b) Bacteria enter the body through vagina, peritoneum, lymphatics, or bloodstream.
  3. Symptoms
    a) Infectious vaginal discharge (should be handled with care by patient and nurse to prevent spread of infection)
    b) Backache, lower abdominal or pelvic pain (especially during intercourse or during pelvic exam), chills, fever, nausea, vomiting, dysuria, tachycardia, menorrhagia, and dysmenorrhea

D. Essential nursing care for patients with sexually transmitted diseases
  1. Nursing assessment
    a) Take thorough history, including symptoms, recent sexual contacts, date of exposure, any history of STDs.
    b) Assessment depends on symptoms; gloves must be worn while performing physical assessment and disposed of as potentially infected materials.
  2. Nursing diagnoses
    a) Pain related to STD
    b) Anxiety related to embarrassment and fear
    c) Potential for infection transmission related to presence of infectious agent
    d) Altered sexuality patterns related to presence of infection
  3. Nursing intervention
    a) Reassure patient that pain is relieved when infection heals; report severe discomfort and fever to physician; administer analgesics as ordered.
    b) Follow universal precautions when coming into contact with blood and/or body fluids of *all* patients (see Nurse Alert, "Universal Blood and Body Fluids Precautions").
    c) Provide emotional support, comfort, and privacy and allow patient to express feelings.
    d) Advise patients about how to avoid transmitting infection, including information about chancroid, sexually transmitted enteric infection, hepatitis B, and delta hepatitis.
    e) Emphasize importance of changing sexual patterns to promote health.
    f) Inform patients of risk and dangers of certain sexual practices and repeated STD infections.

4. Nursing evaluation
   a) Patient states that pain is alleviated.
   b) Patient states that anxiety is reduced or eliminated.
   c) Infection is not spread to others.
   d) Patient expresses desire to prevent future infections by eliminating unsafe sexual behaviors.

1. Harold Robinson has been admitted to the hospital unit to rule out a diagnosis of tuberculosis. The nurse places him in acid-fast bacteria isolation, understanding that this technique is based on which of the following links in the infection chain?

   a. Pathogen
   b. Mode of transmission
   c. Host
   d. Portal of entry

2. Herman Potarski, a 64-year-old patient, has had a transurethral resection of the prostate. When the nurse irrigates his urinary bladder catheter, the type of aseptic technique to be used is the same as that used for irrigation of the:

   a. Vagina.
   b. Upper GI tract.
   c. Eye.
   d. Lower GI tract.

3. Rosemary Cross, R.N., the circulating nurse in the operating room, accidentally brushes her sleeve against the waist area of the scrub nurse's gown during a surgical procedure. Subsequent actions by the nurses should be based on which of the following?

   a. Because both nurses are sterile, no further action is warranted.
   b. Minor breaks in sterile technique should not disrupt surgical procedures.
   c. The circulating nurse wears clean scrub attire, which contains microorganisms.
   d. The gowns should be changed if there is blood or body fluid on the circulator's sleeve.

4. Kyle Hoskins, a 6-year-old boy with a sore throat, difficulty in swallowing, and a fever of 102°, is seen at the pediatrician's office. He is diagnosed with possible pharyngitis. It is necessary to obtain a throat culture on Kyle to:

   a. Evaluate whether medical treatment has been effective.

   b. Determine whether the symptoms are the result of a causative organism.
   c. Assess whether his tonsils are inflamed.
   d. Monitor the spread of the organism to other family members.

5. The nurse notes the sign, "Strict Isolation," on a patient's door. Which of the following patients would be placed in this type of category-specific isolation?

   a. A 5-month-old who has never had chickenpox.
   b. A 70-year-old with positive acid-fast bacillus culture results who is coughing.
   c. A 64-year-old with herpes zoster (shingles).
   d. A 54-year-old with staphylococcal cellulitis of the left leg.

6. A nurse is practicing meticulous hygiene by washing her hands between patients. What is the most important purpose of this activity?

   a. To prevent spread of infection in the patient's body
   b. To decrease the number of organisms on the patient's skin
   c. To reduce smells in the patient's room
   d. To avoid spread of infection between patients

7. David Swift, a 32-year-old homosexual, is concerned about the transmission of sexually transmitted diseases (STDs). He asks the nurse how he could alter his sexual practices to prevent himself from acquiring an STD. The best response would be:

   a. "Abstinence from all sexual contact is the most effective method of preventing these diseases."
   b. "Some STDs are transmitted through the use of contaminated needles, as in intravenous drug use."
   c. "Decreasing your number of sexual partners will have minimal effect on your risk of acquiring an STD."
   d. "STDs are curable as long as you have frequent examinations."

8. Which of the following test results would be included in the definitive diagnosis of Ms. McGuire's pelvic inflammatory disease (PID)?

a. Positive pregnancy test for human chorionic gonadotropin
b. Elevated white blood cell (WBC) count
c. Positive endocervical cultures
d. Elevated erythrocyte sedimentation rate (ESR)

9. When counseling a female patient about the long-term complications of genital herpes (HSV-2), the nurse would discuss the future risk of:

a. Gonorrheal infections.
b. Cervical cancer.
c. Pelvic inflammatory disease.
d. Chlamydial infections.

ANSWERS

1. **Correct answer is b.** CDC isolation guidelines are based on the transmission of infectious organisms. Category-specific isolation precautions are related to the disease's exact mode of transmission. All the other links in the chain affect whether or not infection occurs but are not a consideration when determining the isolation category.

a. How the pathogen is transmitted determines the isolation category. The pathogen may have several modes of transmission.
c. The host's susceptibility will play a role in whether infection occurs but has no relation to the isolation category.
d. The portal of entry indicates only the bodily tract by which the organisms enter the body, not the method by which they are transported from the infected source to the susceptible host.

2. **Correct answer is c.** Although not normally regarded as a sterile body area, the eye is considered a sterile area for purposes of irrigation. Solutions or medications instilled into the eye should be sterile, and the technique used should be surgical asepsis.

a, b, and d. The vagina and upper and lower GI tracts are not considered sterile bodily areas for purposes of irrigation.

3. **Correct answer is c.** The circulating nurse is a member of the surgical team who is wearing clean, not sterile, scrub attire. Therefore, microorganisms are present on her gown as well as on the sleeves of her jacket. The gown of the scrub nurse should be changed immediately.

a. Only the scrub nurse is considered to be sterile.
b. There is no such thing as a minor break in sterile technique. Any break in technique is significant.
d. Even if there is no blood or body fluid on the sleeve, the circulating nurse is not considered to be a sterile member of the surgical team.

4. **Correct answer is b.** A throat culture is necessary to determine whether bacterial pharyngitis is present. Group A hemolytic streptococci are the most common causative organisms in bacterial pharyngitis. If the culture is positive for streptococci, subsequent antibiotic therapy would be initiated to prevent rheumatic fever and other complications.

a. It is premature to evaluate medical treatment, since treatment of symptoms has not yet been initiated.
c. Inflammation of the tonsils may accompany pharyngitis, but that is not the reason for performing a throat culture.
d. A throat culture taken from the boy will not indicate whether other family members have the causative organism.

5. **Correct answer is c.** Herpes zoster (shingles) is caused by reactivation of the latent varicella-zoster virus in patients who have previously had chickenpox. Its mode of transmission can be either by direct contact or by the airborne route.

a. If the infant does not currently have the varicella-zoster virus at a contagious stage, there is no need for isolation precautions.

b. A patient with positive acid-fast bacillus culture results who is coughing should be placed in "acid-fast bacteria isolation."
d. A staphylococcal wound infection would require "drainage and secretion isolation."

6. **Correct answer is d.** Transmission of organisms from one patient to another is a major cause of nosocomial infections. Hand washing between patients is the single most effective method of preventing the spread of infection.

   a and b. Preventing contamination among patients, not curbing the spread of infection in a single patient, is the main purpose of hand washing.
   c. Reducing odorous smells is not a goal of hand washing.

7. **Correct answer is a.** Abstinence from sexual contact is the only sure way to prevent STD.

   b. Although it is true that some STDs are transmitted through the use of contaminated needles, the patient is asking the nurse about sexual practices.

c. Decreasing the number of sexual contacts does reduce the risk of contracting a STD.
d. Some STDs are not curable, such as acquired immunodeficiency syndrome (AIDS) and the late stages of some other STDs.

8. **Correct answer is c.** If the gram-stained endocervical secretions are positive for *N. gonorrhoeae,* the diagnosis of PID is confirmed.

   a. The presence of human chorionic gonadotropin in a patient with acute pelvic pain could indicate an ectopic pregnancy rather than PID.
   b and d. Elevated WBC count and ESR levels may be present in PID but do not constitute a diagnosis.

9. **Correct answer is b.** Female patients with genital herpes are at risk for developing cervical cancer as well as HIV infection.

   a, c, and **d.** Clients with HSV-2 are not known to be at increased risk for gonorrhea, chlamydia, or PID.

5

Care of Cancer Patient

OVERVIEW

I. Prevention and detection
    A. Prevention methods
    B. Detection methods

II. Management of cancer
    A. Surgery
    B. Radiation therapy
    C. Chemotherapy
    D. Biologic response modifiers
    E. Hospice care

III. Selected oncologic emergencies
    A. Superior vena cava syndrome
    B. Spinal cord compression
    C. Hypercalcemia
    D. Pericardial effusion and cardiac tamponade
    E. Disseminated intravascular coagulopathy
    F. Syndrome of inappropriate antidiuretic hormone
    G. Septicemia

NURSING HIGHLIGHTS

1. Nurse should remember that psychosocial and sexual needs of the cancer patient are as important as the physiologic needs and require skill and attention.
2. Nurse must be aware of the risk for cancer complications and oncologic emergencies and should be knowledgeable and skilled in assessing their occurrence, because early detection increases the chance of successful treatment.
3. Community-based hospice nurses must possess advanced skill in assessment and management of pain, nutrition, bowel dysfunction, and skin impairments.

GLOSSARY

carcinoembryonic antigen (CEA) test—detects elevated CEA levels often found with colon or breast cancer
cytokines—chemicals involved in growth regulation
fibrinolysis—dissolution of fibrin, the protein that causes blood to clot
intravenous pyelogram—radiograph of the ureter and pelvis after radiopaque material has been injected intravenously

lymphokines—chemicals secreted by sensitized lymphocytes that produce cellular immunity

pulsus paradoxus—suppressed pulse at the beginning of each full inspiration

tomography—noninvasive radiographic procedure that shows a precise image of structures in one plane of tissue by blurring images in all other planes

xeroradiography—method of photoreproduction used in radiography

ENHANCED OUTLINE

See text pages

I. Prevention and detection

A. Prevention methods
   1. Periodic physical exams
   2. Cancer screening programs
   3. Self-exam of breasts, testicles, and all skin surfaces
   4. Avoidance of risk factors

B. Detection methods
   1. Lab tests: acid phosphatase test, CEA test, tumor-specific antigen test, serum alkaline test, serum and urine calcium tests, complete blood cell count
   2. Radiographs: studies with contrast media (upper GI series, barium enemas, intravenous pyelograms), tomography, xeroradiography, computed tomographic (CT) scan, radioisotope studies
   3. Emission computer tomography: positron emission tomography (PET) and single photon emission computerized tomography (SPECT)
   4. Other: cytology (Pap smear), biopsy, endoscopic exam, ultrasound, magnetic resonance imaging (MRI), bone scan

See text pages

II. Management of cancer

A. Surgery
   1. Types
      a) Diagnostic
         (1) Performed to obtain biopsy
         (2) Includes excisional method, incisional method, needle biopsy
      b) Prophylactic
         (1) Performed to remove lesions likely to turn into cancer
         (2) Includes prophylactic mastectomies and colectomies for high-risk patients

c) Palliative
   (1) Performed to relieve complications of cancer (ulcerations, obstructions, hemorrhage, pain, or infection)
   (2) Includes nerve blocks, tumor resection, simple mastectomies for ulcerative breast disease, surgical removal of hormone-producing glands that might enhance tumor growth
d) Reconstructive
   (1) Performed to produce better function or appearance after curative or radical surgery
   (2) Includes breast reconstruction, ostomy revision, prosthesis implant

2. Nursing considerations
   a) See sections III, IV, and V of Chapter 1 for discussions of preoperative, intraoperative, and postoperative nursing management.
   b) Education and support: Assess patient and family needs; explore fears and coping mechanisms; act as liaison between patient, family, and physician when discussing surgical options.
   c) Complications: Assess for infection, bleeding, thrombophlebitis, wound dehiscence, organ dysfunction.
   d) Discharge and follow-up care
      (1) Providing postoperative education about wound care, activity, nutrition, and medications
      (2) Providing follow-up care and treatment plans as early as possible to ensure continuity of care

B. Radiation therapy
   1. Types
      a) External: delivered over a period of several weeks on an outpatient basis
      b) Internal: delivered through implants that give a high dose of radiation to a specific area
   2. Dosage: depends on size of tumor and sensitivity of target tissues to radiation
   3. Toxicity: depends on region receiving radiation
      a) General: fatigue, malaise, nausea, vomiting, headache
      b) Gastrointestinal system: anorexia, nausea, vomiting, diarrhea
      c) Bone marrow: anemia, leukopenia, thrombocytopenia
      d) Skin: erythema, desquamation (skin shedding), alopecia (hair loss)
   4. Nursing considerations
      a) Education and support
         (1) Explain entire radiation procedure to patient and answer questions.
         (2) Advise patient to report any discomfort during radiation procedure to nurse and radiologist.
         (3) Advise patient to avoid use of unprescribed ointments and creams, to avoid extremes of heat and cold, to wear loose clothing over site, and to avoid shampooing, tinting, and permanent waving if scalp is being irradiated.

  b) Skin care

   (1) Keep skin over treated area clean and dry; avoid exposure to sunlight; check daily for signs of redness, ulceration, and infection.

   (2) Administer steroid cream or aerosol spray for itching, if prescribed.

   (3) Advise patient to bathe carefully and to avoid soap and friction over treated skin; remind patient not to wash off skin markings.

   (4) Apply cornstarch over irradiated areas where 2 skin surfaces are in contact, provided skin has not broken down.

   (5) Help patient hide pigment changes on exposed areas with makeup or clothing once therapy is completed and skin has healed.

  c) Oral hygiene and nutrition

   (1) Inspect mouth and lips for stomatitis daily; apply anesthetic ointment for pain if prescribed.

   (2) Administer frequent mouth rinses with a solution of warm water, salt, and baking soda; use soft toothbrush or toothpaste on cotton swab.

   (3) Do not serve food for at least 1 hour before or after therapy; administer antiemetic if prescribed; weigh patient regularly; check meal tray for amount of food consumed; record intake and output.

   (4) Consult dietitian for special supplements.

  d) Special care of radioactive implant patients

   (1) Prepare room with essential items before treatment (bags and tissues, water glass, reading materials).

   (2) Follow rules of time, distance, and shielding when caring for patient (see Nurse Alert, "Safety Principles for Patients with Radioisotopes in Situ").

 C. Chemotherapy

  1. Types

   a) Cell cycle–specific drugs

    (1) Antimetabolites

    (2) Plant alkaloids

   b) Cell cycle–nonspecific drugs

    (1) Alkylating agents

    (2) Antitumor antibiotics

    (3) Hormonal agents

    (4) Nitrosoureas

Safety Principles for Patients with Radioisotopes in Situ

Always keep these safety principles in mind when radioisotopes are used to treat cancer.
- The less time a person spends near a radioactive substance, the less radiation she/he will receive.
- Rate of exposure varies inversely to the square of distance from patient. Nurses standing 4 feet away from radiation source receive 25% of radiation they would receive if standing 2 feet away from source. Prepare patient to receive a limited amount of nursing time and plan carefully so less time will be spent at bedside.
- Wear radiation film badge (measures whole-body exposure); do not share film badge.
- Use lead shield or apron for prolonged contact.
- Patient should be in a private room.
- Pregnant women (staff and visitors) and children should avoid exposure.
- Limit each visitor to one-half hour per day and ensure that visitors are kept a minimum of 6 feet away from the patient.
- Radiation overexposure produces no immediate symptoms; radiation injury can occur without your awareness.

2. Administration
   a) Routes of administration: oral, topical, intravenous, intramuscular, subcutaneous, arterial, intracavitary, and intrathecal
   b) Dosage: based on patient's total body surface area, previous reaction to chemotherapy or radiation therapy, and physical performance status
3. Toxicity
   a) General: alopecia, fatigue, easy bruising
   b) Gastrointestinal system: nausea, vomiting, altered taste, stomatitis, esophagitis, anorexia, mucositis, diarrhea
   c) Hematopoietic system: increased risk of infection, bleeding, anemia; reduced bone marrow activity, red blood cells, white blood cells
   d) Renal system: kidney damage, hemorrhagic cystitis
   e) Cardiopulmonary system: irreversible cardiac toxicity, irreversible lung damage, pulmonary fibrosis
   f) Reproductive system: possible sterility, possible chromosomal damage
   g) Neurologic system: neurologic damage (with plant alkaloids), peripheral neuropathies, loss of deep tendon reflexes, paralytic ileus (usually reversible)
4. Nursing considerations
   a) Education and support
      (1) Explain entire chemotherapy procedure and answer questions at patient's level of comprehension.
      (2) Discuss strategies for pain relief; reassure and encourage patient.

    b) Skin and hair care
       (1) Maintain skin integrity by avoiding friction, shaving, heat, cold, ointments, and creams.
       (2) Discuss potential hair loss; advise patient to avoid excess shampooing, combing, and brushing as well as tints, permanents, styling tools, and hair sprays; instruct patient to wear sunscreen or hat when outdoors.
    c) Nutrition
       (1) Limit nausea and vomiting by distracting and relaxing patient, adjusting diet, preventing unpleasant odors and sounds, and administering prescribed antiemetics or sedatives.
       (2) Monitor fluid and electrolyte levels often and encourage adequate fluid intake.
    d) Prevention of infection: Lessen risk for infection by using asepsis procedures, handling patient gently, monitoring lab tests, and reporting changes promptly.

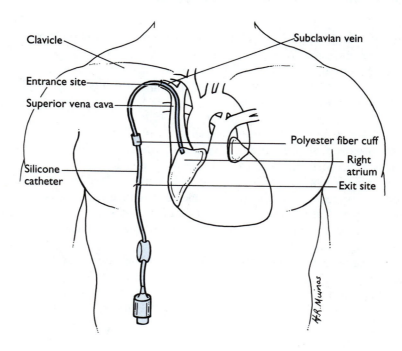

Figure 5–1
Right Atrial Catheter

D. Biologic response modifiers (BRMs)
  1. Types
    a) Interferons: may stimulate immune system or inhibit tumor growth; also enhance lymphocyte and antibody production and inhibit cell multiplication
    b) Monoclonal antibodies: may help destroy tumors when combined with radioactive materials, chemotherapy, hormones, lymphokines, interferons
    c) Lymphokines and cytokines
      (1) Interleukin-2 (IL-2 [e.g., Proleukin]): stimulates production and activation of several different types of T cell lymphocytes; combines with null lymphocyte to become a lymphokine-activated killer cell able to destroy cancer cells
      (2) Colony-stimulating factors (CSFs [e.g., Filgrastim]): stimulate production of all blood cells; may help reverse bone marrow suppression
      (3) Tumor necrosis factor (TNF): causes cell lysis
  2. Administration
    a) Treatment takes place in research setting because of experimental nature of BRMs.
    b) Treatment focuses on restoring, stimulating, or augmenting natural immune defenses.

E. Hospice care
  1. Comprehensive multidisciplinary program focuses on relief of symptoms and pain when a cure or remission is no longer possible.
  2. Nurse provides psychosocial support, spiritual support, and respite care for patient and family and helps them to cope with changes in role, changes in family structure, grief, and loss for up to a year after the patient's death.

III. Selected oncologic emergencies (paraneoplastic syndromes)

See text pages
_____

A. Superior vena cava syndrome
  1. Definition: symptoms resulting from compressed superior vena cava
  2. Pathophysiology and etiology
    a) Caused by compression of superior vena cava by a tumor or enlarged lymph nodes
    b) Usually a result of lung cancer or metastatic disease
  3. Symptoms
    a) Progressive shortness of breath, dyspnea, cough
    b) Edema of face, neck, arms, hands, and thorax; skin tightness, problems swallowing
    c) Engorged jugular, temporal, and arm veins; venous patterns visible on chest wall
    d) If prolonged, may cause increased intracranial pressure, visual disturbances, headache, and altered mental status; and eventually, cerebral anoxia, laryngeal edema, bronchial obstruction, and death

    4. Nursing intervention
- a) Ease patient's breathing by elevating head of bed, administering oxygen and diuretics as ordered, and reducing anxiety.
- b) Monitor patient's fluid volume and administer fluids with caution.
- c) Prevent increase in intracranial pressure (bending, lifting, straining, Valsalva maneuver).

B. Spinal cord compression
1. Pathophysiology and etiology
- a) Caused by metastatic tumors invading spinal canal and compressing cord
- b) Usually a result of lung, colon, breast, or prostate cancers; lymphoma; or multiple myeloma
2. Symptoms
- a) Constant back pain exacerbated by movement, coughing, or sneezing
- b) Neurologic symptoms including numbness; tingling; loss of sensation in urethra, vagina, and rectum; incontinence; motor weakness; paralysis
3. Nursing intervention
- a) Administer pain medication as prescribed.
- b) Maintain patient's muscle tone by assisting with range of motion exercises.
- c) Provide intermittent urinary catheterization and bowel training programs.

C. Hypercalcemia (see sections II,E,2–3 of Chapter 2)

D. Pericardial effusion and cardiac tamponade
1. Definition: cardiovascular disorder that occurs when fluid accumulates in the pericardial space and compresses the heart
2. Pathophysiology and etiology
- a) Fluid accumulation caused by invasive tumor, metastatic lesion, or response of pericardial tissue to malignancy
- b) Pressure on myocardium, causing drop in ventricular volume and cardiac output; cardiac pump failure and circulatory collapse
- c) Usually a result of breast, lung, or esophagus cancer; lymphoma; leukemia; or melanoma
3. Symptoms
- a) High central venous pressure, arterial hypotension, and distant heart sounds
- b) Pulsus paradoxus, shortness of breath with normal breath sounds, weakness, diaphoresis, compensatory tachycardia
- c) Chest pain, orthopnea, anxiety, lethargy, altered consciousness, and eventually circulatory collapse and cardiac arrest

4. Nursing intervention
    a) Elevate head of bed, minimize physical activity, and provide supplemental oxygen as prescribed.
    b) Turn patient frequently and encourage patient to cough and take deep breaths every 2 hours.
    c) Monitor drainage of pericardial drainage tube (if left after a pericardiocentesis).

E. Disseminated intravascular coagulopathy (DIC)
    1. Definition: abnormal activation of coagulation and fibrinolysis causing destruction of coagulation factors and platelets
    2. Pathophysiology and etiology
        a) Caused by clots forming when normal coagulation mechanisms are triggered by malignant tumors
        b) Usually a result of lung, gastrointestinal, prostate cancers; melanoma; leukemia; multiple blood transfusions; septicemia; and some chemotherapy drugs
    3. Symptoms
        a) General: easy bruising, prolonged bleeding from multiple sites, gingival bleeding, slow gastrointestinal bleeding, pain, neurologic alterations, tachycardia, dyspnea, oliguria
        b) Acute DIC: may produce life-threatening hemorrhage and infarction
        c) Chronic DIC: may produce no symptoms
    4. Nursing intervention
        a) Minimize physical activity to decrease risk of injury.
        b) Minimize invasive procedures; monitor and prevent bleeding.
        c) Maintain adequate oral hygiene.
        d) Turn patient frequently and encourage patient to cough and take deep breaths every 2 hours.

F. Syndrome of inappropriate antidiuretic hormone (SIADH)
    1. Definition: uncontrolled, continuous secretion of antidiuretic hormone
    2. Pathophysiology and etiology: caused by small cell lung cancer; cancers of brain, larynx, nasopharynx, esophagus, duodenum, pancreas, colon, ovary, and prostate; Hodgkin's disease; thymomas; lymphosarcomas; and certain chemotherapy drugs
    3. Symptoms
        a) Hyponatremia, water retention, personality changes, irritability, anorexia, nausea, vomiting, weight gain, fatigue, myalgia, headache, lethargy, muscle cramps, and confusion
        b) Sodium levels below 110 mEq/L: seizure, papilledema, abnormal reflexes, coma, and death
    4. Nursing intervention
        a) Minimize physical activity.
        b) Restrict fluid intake as ordered.
        c) Monitor fluid intake and output and weigh patient daily.

G. Septicemia
    1. Definition: Often fatal condition in which microorganisms enter bloodstream of cancer patients.

2. Pathophysiology and etiology
    a) Caused by chemotherapy, which impairs immunity and allows microorganisms to flourish
    b) Usually a result of granulocytopenia, altered hematopoietic function, and impaired immune functioning in cancer patients
3. Symptoms: altered mental status, cool and clammy skin, high or low temperature, hypotension, decreased urinary output, dysrhythmias, and disorientation
4. Nursing intervention
    a) Monitor all immunosuppressed patients for septic shock.
    b) Administer antibiotics as prescribed; closely monitor response.
    c) Avoid invasive procedures.

1. The nurse is planning a lecture on cancer for a community group. Which of the following would she include as a primary cancer prevention measure?

   a. Performing monthly breast self-exams
   b. Increasing amounts of vitamins A and C in the diet
   c. Avoiding high-fiber diets
   d. Having an annual Pap smear

2. Ms. Murphy, who is scheduled to have a mastectomy after a positive biopsy for cancer, discusses with the nurse her decision to have breast reconstruction done at the same time. The nurse:

   a. Discourages the patient, since this will require a longer operation.
   b. Supports the patient, since undergoing 1 operation would be easier on her.
   c. Supports the patient, because it would focus her attention away from the disfigurement caused by the mastectomy.
   d. Discourages the patient, because she should cope with the cancer first.

3. Nathan Green is receiving radiation therapy for a malignant oral lesion. The nurse should instruct the patient to:

   a. Wait 1 hour after the treatment before eating.
   b. Avoid drinking hot fluids and eating hot foods.
   c. Vigorously brush the teeth and gums after every meal.
   d. Rinse the mouth with a commercial mouthwash containing alcohol every 2 hours.

4. The nurse may most expect which of the following changes in the laboratory values of a patient who is receiving cancer chemotherapy drugs?

   a. Elevated white blood cell count
   b. Elevated platelet count
   c. Increased blood urea nitrogen
   d. Decreased red blood cell count

5. Rita Fleming, who has malignant melanoma, is admitted for a treatment protocol involving interleukin-2 (IL-2), a biologic response modifier (BRM). The patient asks how a BRM works. The nurse's explanation would include which of the following?

   a. The BRM helps the immune system to fight the cancer.
   b. The BRM is a chemical that kills all the cancer cells.
   c. The BRM destroys the immune system so that chemotherapy can fight the cancer.
   d. The BRM alters the cancer cells, but this treatment has not been proven to work.

6. The nurse would expect which of the following patients to be at highest risk for developing superior vena cava syndrome?

   a. A patient with a brain tumor
   b. A patient with a lung tumor
   c. A patient with leukemia
   d. A patient with breast cancer

7. The nurse is admitting Marie Burns to the hospice program. Ms. Burns has breast cancer with metastasis to the spine and is receiving radiation therapy for spinal cord compression. Which of the following would the hospice nurse do first?

   a. Insert an indwelling catheter.
   b. Ambulate the patient.
   c. Offer pain medication.
   d. Offer a nutritional snack.

8. Frank Gullo, who has metastasis from colon cancer, is being treated for sepsis. He has developed bruising during the past 24 hours, and his prothrombin and partial thromboplastin times are prolonged. Which of the following actions would be appropriate for the nurse?

   a. Discontinue and restart a positional IV.
   b. Apply pressure for 30 seconds to venipuncture sites.
   c. Brush and floss the patient's teeth after every meal.
   d. Minimize the client's physical activities.

9. Ms. Martinez, a cancer patient who has had a total uterectomy with salpingo-oophorectomy, has just completed a chemotherapy regimen that has caused fatigue and alopecia. During a discussion with the nurse, she states, "I don't know how my husband can stand to look at me." The best response for the nurse to make is:

   a. "Have you and your husband discussed how your body has changed?"
   b. "When you get a wig, it will make a big difference in your appearance."
   c. "You should call your husband and tell him how you feel about this."
   d. "You've been through so much that I'm sure he's very proud of you."

ANSWERS

1. **Correct answer is b.** Primary prevention measures are those that may prevent or reduce the risk of cancer in healthy people. Increasing the amount of dietary vitamin A has been shown to reduce the risk of cancer of the esophagus, larynx, and lungs. Increasing vitamin C intake may protect against cancer of the stomach and esophagus.

   a and d. Breast self-exams and Pap smears are secondary prevention measures aimed at diagnosing cancers early and allowing prompt intervention.
   c. High-fiber diets are recommended to reduce the risk of breast, prostate, and colon cancers.

2. **Correct answer is c.** Reconstructive surgery is done to produce better function or appearance, which gives the patient a positive focus when disfigurement and death are a concern.

   a and d. The patient should not be discouraged from having the reconstruction, since this is her decision.
   b. It is not necessarily true that a single operation will be easier on her. Like any surgical patient, she may have complications.

3. **Correct answer is a.** Radiation to the oral cavity may cause a transitory loss of or change in the sense of taste. The patient may have a better appetite and improved nutrition if he waits until the food can be tasted.

   b. There is no contraindication to ingesting hot food or liquids during radiation therapy. Consuming a variety of fluids and foods should be encouraged.
   c. Mr. Green should perform gentle care of the mucous membranes and teeth. Because he is at risk for developing stomatitis, a soft toothbrush or cotton swabs should be used carefully.
   d. Most commercial mouthwashes that contain alcohol should be avoided, since they may dry and irritate the oral mucous membranes. Warm water or saline rinses of the mouth are recommended.

4. **Correct answer is d.** Most cancer chemotherapy drugs cause depression of bone marrow function (myelosuppression), decreasing the number of blood cells produced. A decrease in number of red blood cells (anemia) can be expected.

   a and b. Myelosuppression would result in a decreased number of white blood cells (leukopenia) and platelets (thrombocytopenia).
   c. Increased blood urea nitrogen (BUN) level can occur with the increased lysis of cells by chemotherapeutic drugs, but this is not as common as decreased red blood cell count.

5. **Correct answer is a.** BRM treatment restores, stimulates, or augments the natural defenses of the immune system.

   b. The BRM may not be a chemical and may not kill all cancer cells, so this would be a misleading statement.
   c. BRMs do not destroy the immune system, so this would be a false statement.
   d. It is not accurate to say that the BRM alters cancer cells; instead, it acts on the immune system. Although BRM treatment is considered investigational, there have been positive outcomes in many patients.

6. **Correct answer is b.** Superior vena cava syndrome occurs most often in patients with lung cancer, since the tumor compresses the superior vena cava.

   a, c, and **d.** Patients with a brain tumor, leukemia, or breast cancer would be at less risk because of the location or type of cancer.

7. **Correct answer is c.** Patients with spinal cord compression usually have pain that may be constant or caused by movement. Since hospice care focuses on relief of symptoms and pain, giving pain medication would be the priority.

   a. Patients with spinal cord compression may be at risk for development of urinary stasis and incontinence. Indwelling or intermittent catheterization may be required but would not be the nurse's first action.
   b and **d.** Ms. Burns may be at risk for development of immobility and inadequate nutrition, but these are not the first actions to be taken by the hospice nurse.

8. **Correct answer is d.** Mr. Gullo may be at risk for development of disseminated intravascular coagulopathy (DIC). Physical activity should be minimized to decrease the risk of bleeding and injury.

   a. Invasive procedures should be kept to a minimum, since the patient may have excessive bleeding from the venipuncture sites. Thus, a positional IV should not be discontinued or restarted. The arm can be positioned to improve the flow of the IV fluid.
   b. Pressure should be applied to venipuncture sites for 1–5 minutes or longer, depending on clotting time.
   c. Since the patient is at risk for development of bleeding gums, gentle oral care, such as rinsing the mouth or gentle use of toothettes, should be provided.

9. **Correct answer is a.** Asking Ms. Martinez whether she and her husband have discussed the changes in her body allows for further communication and provides more assessment information. It is an opportunity to encourage the patient to have a discussion with her husband to share concerns about physical changes in her body and about the couple's altered sexuality.

   b. The patient should have a wig if she chooses, but this superficial communication is not the best response.
   c. Telling the patient what to do, in this case to call her husband, is an inappropriate response.
   d. Saying that Mr. Martinez must be proud of his wife is a superficial statement that assumes too much. The patient and her husband should be encouraged to discuss their concerns.

6

Respiratory Function

OVERVIEW

I. Structure and function of respiratory system
  A. Upper respiratory system
  B. Lower respiratory system
  C. Gas exchange

II. General diagnostic tests
  A. Endoscopy procedures
  B. Radiography
  C. Radioisotope procedures
  D. Sputum studies
  E. Magnetic resonance imaging
  F. Thoracentesis
  G. Skin tests
  H. Pulmonary function tests
  I. Blood gas studies

III. General nursing assessments
  A. History
  B. Observation and physical exam
  C. Diagnostic tests

IV. Nursing considerations with selected therapies and techniques
  A. Endotracheal intubation
  B. Tracheostomy
  C. Laryngectomy
  D. Thoracic surgery
  E. Mechanical ventilation
  F. Oxygen administration
  G. Postural drainage

V. Selected disorders of upper respiratory system
  A. Upper airway infection
  B. Pharyngitis
  C. Laryngeal obstruction
  D. Cancer of the larynx

VI. Selected disorders of lower respiratory system
  A. Cancer of the lung and bronchus
  B. Chronic obstructive pulmonary disease
  C. Respiratory failure
  D. Pulmonary embolism
  E. Pleural effusion
  F. Chest trauma
  G. Pneumonia
  H. Influenza
  I. Tuberculosis

NURSING HIGHLIGHTS

1. Nurse should provide support and psychologic preparation for patients undergoing diagnostic evaluation tests for respiratory disorders; these patients are often short of breath, fatigued, and anxious about the results.

2. Nurse should focus on respiratory patient's reactions and responses to treatment; education is an essential aspect of nursing care when ventilators and oxygen delivery systems are part of the patient's management.

GLOSSARY

dysphagia—difficulty in swallowing
Homans' sign—pain in calf when toe is passively dorsiflexed
impedance plethysmography—diagnostic test to detect deep venous thrombosis
laryngography—radiography of larynx after application of radiopaque dye
mediastinoscopy—endoscopic examination of the mediastinum

ENHANCED OUTLINE

I. Structure and function of respiratory system

See text pages
_____

A. Upper respiratory system
  1. Nose: filters, warms, and humidifies air
  2. Paranasal sinuses: reduce weight of skull, give resonance to voice
  3. Pharynx: carries air into bronchi and lungs and food and liquids into esophagus
  4. Tonsils and adenoids: protect body against invasion by microorganisms
  5. Larynx: permits vocalization, protects lower airway from foreign substances, aids in coughing

B. Lower respiratory system
  1. Trachea: carries air from laryngeal pharynx into bronchi and lungs
  2. Bronchi: carry air from trachea to lungs
  3. Bronchioles: carry air from bronchi to alveoli
  4. Alveoli: exchange oxygen for carbon dioxide with capillaries

C. Gas exchange
  1. Cells obtain energy from oxidation of carbohydrates, fats, and proteins; circulating blood supplies necessary oxygen and removes carbon dioxide.
  2. Oxygen diffuses through capillary wall to interstitial fluid and then through cell tissue membrane; carbon dioxide proceeds in opposite direction.
  3. After tissue capillary exchange, venous blood travels to lungs; oxygen diffuses from alveoli to blood while carbon dioxide diffuses from blood to alveoli.
  4. Air moving in and out of airways replenishes oxygen and removes carbon dioxide from air spaces in lungs.

See text pages

_____

II. General diagnostic tests

A. Endoscopy procedures: direct visual examination with an endoscope (biopsy specimen may be obtained)
1. Laryngoscopy
   a) Direct laryngoscopy: observation of larynx using laryngoscope
   b) Indirect laryngoscopy: observation of vocal cords using a light and laryngeal mirror
2. Bronchoscopy: direct examination of larynx, trachea, and bronchi using fiberoptic bronchoscope

B. Radiography
1. X-ray: reveals only extensive pathologic process and major contrast between bones, soft tissues, and air
2. Computed tomography (CT): scans in successive layers by narrow beam x-ray to provide cross-section view and fine tissue density
3. Tomography (planigraphy): provides films of sections of lungs at different planes, showing cavities

C. Radioisotope procedures
1. Perfusion lung scan: intravenous injection of radioisotope to evaluate pulmonary blood flow and to diagnose and locate pulmonary emboli
2. Ventilation scan: inhalation of radioactive gas and oxygen to assess air movement in lungs
3. Inhalation scan: administration of droplets of radioactive material by positive-pressure ventilator to visualize trachea and major airways

D. Sputum studies: identification of abnormal cell formation or pathogenic microorganisms

E. Magnetic resonance imaging (MRI): imaging of tissues along any plane inside the body

F. Thoracentesis: aspiration of air or fluid from pleural space to diagnose or treat respiratory conditions

G. Skin tests: used with other data to diagnose infectious, viral, and fungal diseases

H. Pulmonary function tests: identification of respiratory function abnormalities and evaluation of status of respiratory patient

I. Blood gas studies: measurement of oxygen, carbon dioxide, and hydrogen (as pH), usually on arterial blood

III. General nursing assessments

See text pages
_____

A. History
   1. Ask patient about smoking, including passive exposure to smoke.
   2. Ask patient about family history of lung disease or allergies and exposure to pollutants and allergens.

B. Observation and physical exam
   1. Upper respiratory system: Inspect and palpate nose and sinuses; inspect pharynx for color, symmetry, and evidence of exudate, ulceration, or enlargement.
   2. Lower respiratory system: Palpate trachea gently for position and mobility; inspect and palpate thorax for color, turgor, loss of subcutaneous tissue, and symmetry; assess respiratory signs and symptoms; percuss and auscultate for breath sounds; assess breathing pattern.

C. Diagnostic tests: nursing responsibilities
   1. Bronchoscopy
      a) Preprocedure care
         (1) Explain procedure at patient's level of comprehension.
         (2) Withhold food and fluids 6 hours before procedure.
         (3) Administer preoperative medications as prescribed. (Caution: Giving sedatives to patients with respiratory insufficiency may cause respiratory arrest.)
         (4) Remove contact lenses, dentures, and prostheses.
      b) Postprocedure care
         (1) Give nothing by mouth until cough reflex returns; once cough returns, give ice chips and then water.
         (2) Observe for breathing problems, cyanosis, hypotension, tachycardia, dysrhythmias, hemoptysis, and dyspnea.
         (3) Record color and amount of sputum raised.
   2. Thoracentesis
      a) Preoperative care
         (1) Explain procedure to patient; reassure patient that local anesthetic will be used.
         (2) Bring all necessary supplies to patient's room and leave them covered.
      b) Postoperative care
         (1) Apply pressure dressing to wound and inspect every 2 hours.
         (2) Observe for breathing problems, severe coughing, severe chest pain, tachycardia, and light-headedness.
         (3) Record color and amount of sputum raised.

IV. Nursing considerations with selected therapies and techniques

See text pages
_____

A. Endotracheal intubation
   1. Before intubation, establish strategies for communication to be used until patient is able to speak.

2. Tape tube to patient's face and mark proximal end for position maintenance.
3. Auscultate lungs every 30–60 minutes; if breath sounds are not present bilaterally, notify physician.
4. Maintain high humidity; check T-piece for mist.
5. Hyperinflate every hour (volume ventilators have built-in sigh mechanisms).
6. Maintain airway patency by suctioning oropharynx and mouth with catheter as needed.
7. Reposition patient every 2 hours and as needed.

B. Tracheostomy
   1. Maintain airway patency by suctioning with catheter; clear inner cannula as needed and wipe clean when patient coughs; clean skin around stoma every 4 hours, applying bacteriostatic ointment around stoma if crusting occurs.
   2. Administer heated mist to prevent excess coughing and crusting.
   3. Place patient in semi-Fowler's position.
   4. Check vital signs at least every 4 hours; measure fluid intake and output.
   5. Keep extra tracheostomy set, call light, and writing materials by patient's bedside.
   6. Keep cuffed tracheostomy tube *deflated* except during and after eating or tube feeding, during intermittent positive pressure breathing treatments, when patient cannot swallow oral secretions, and when mechanical ventilation is used.
   7. Reassure patient about anxieties.

C. Laryngectomy (total)
   1. Preoperative care
      a) Allow patient to verbalize fears about cancer and loss of voice; explain details about surgery and prognosis.
      b) Review equipment, treatment, and speech rehabilitation plans that will be part of postoperative care.
      c) Establish means of communication for postoperative period.
   2. Postoperative care
      a) Care for tracheostomy (same as section IV,B of this chapter).
      b) Auscultate chest; perform tracheal suctioning as needed; clean area around stoma every 4 hours or as needed.
      c) Administer analgesics as prescribed; avoid extreme movement of the head; place small pillow or folded towel under the head to relieve suture line tension.
      d) Encourage patient to turn and deep breathe every 2 hours; monitor vital signs every 4 hours; report fever or purulent drainage.

e) Teach patient care of tracheostomy.
f) Refer patient to community resources for support.

D. Thoracic surgery
  1. Preoperative care
     a) Encourage increased intake of fluids, use of humidifier, and avoidance of bronchial irritants.
     b) Teach patient diaphragmatic breathing.
     c) Clear airways of secretions with bronchodilators (as prescribed) followed by chest percussion, humidification, and postural drainage.
     d) Explain postoperative period, emphasizing importance of turning and coughing (see Client Teaching Checklist, "Coughing and Huffing Techniques").
  2. Postoperative care
     a) Assess for such complications as infection, hemorrhage, shock, dysrhythmias, mediastinal shift, atelectasis, bronchopulmonary fistula, pneumothorax, pleural effusion, and gastric distention.
     b) Monitor IV fluids to prevent pulmonary edema by overinfusion; symptoms include crackles, bubbling chest sounds, dyspnea, frothy pink sputum, and tachycardia.
     c) Measure blood pressure, pulse, and respirations every 15 minutes for first 1–2 hours.
     d) Maintain airway patency by performing endotracheal suctioning if endotracheal tube is present.
     e) Elevate head of bed 30°–40° once patient is oriented and stabilized.

✔ CLIENT TEACHING CHECKLIST ✔

Coughing and Huffing Techniques

Explain to postoperative patients the following methods to promote clearance of secretions:

Coughing

✔ Sit upright with knees flexed and body bent slightly forward.
✔ Splint incision with firm hand pressure or support with pillow while coughing.
✔ Take 3 deep breaths followed by a deep, slow inhalation through the nose.
✔ Contract abdominal muscles and cough twice forcefully, with mouth open and tongue out.
✔ If sitting is impossible, lie on side with hips and knees bent.

Huffing

✔ Take a deep breath from the diaphragm.
✔ Exhale forcefully against your hand in a quick, distinct pant (or "huff").
✔ Practice doing small huffs, working up to one strong huff during exhalation.

f) Have patient perform diaphragmatic and pursed lip breathing every 2 hours.

g) Care for chest tubes (see section IV,A).

E. Mechanical ventilation (in hospital and home)
1. Administer pain medications as prescribed.
2. Auscultate lungs every 2–4 hours; assure bilateral expansion and clear airways.
3. Perform sterile suction of lower airway with chest percussion, vibration, and lavage as needed; change patient position frequently.
4. Check arterial blood gases.
5. Decrease risk for infection by maintaining good oral hygiene and by elevating head above stomach.
6. Explain all procedures; encourage patient to participate in self-care; and provide stress-reduction techniques.

F. Oxygen administration
1. Types
   a) Venturi mask (24%–40% oxygen concentration at 4–8 L/min)
   b) Nasal cannula (23%–42% oxygen concentration at 1–6 L/min)
   c) Simple masks (40%–60% oxygen concentration at 6–8 L/min)
   d) Partial rebreathing masks (50%–75% oxygen concentration at 8–11 L/min)
   e) Aerosol masks, tracheostomy collars and face tents (30%–100% oxygen concentration at 8–10 L/min)
2. Interventions
   a) Assess frequently for inadequate oxygenation; symptoms include confusion, restlessness progressing to lethargy, diaphoresis, pallor, tachycardia, tachypnea, and hypertension; perform pulse oximetry as needed.
   b) Deliver low-flow, low-concentration oxygen unless ordered otherwise by a physician, since a high concentration of oxygen can depress respiration.
   c) Change tubing frequently to guard against cross-infection.
   d) Observe strict fire safety rules and post "No Smoking" signs.
   e) When oxygen is administered at home, teach family proper techniques, the importance of humidity, and safety rules; ensure that physician's order includes the disorder, prescribed oxygen flow and concentration, and conditions for use.

G. Postural drainage
1. Auscultate chest before and after procedure to identify areas needing drainage and effectiveness of treatment; perform postural drainage before meals and at bedtime.

2. Administer nebulized bronchodilators, water, or saline if prescribed; provide emesis basin, sputum cup, and paper tissues.
3. Keep patient in each position for 10–15 minutes; instruct patient to breathe in slowly through the nose and out through the lips to keep airway open; when changing position, patient should cough and bring up secretions.
4. Suction secretions mechanically if patient cannot cough; use chest percussion or vibration to loosen secretions if necessary.
5. Note amount, color, viscosity, and character of sputum after procedure; evaluate patient's color and pulse.

V. Selected disorders of upper respiratory system

See text pages
_____

A. Upper airway infection
   1. Definition: common acute or chronic condition affecting upper respiratory airway; terms (rhinitis, sinusitis, laryngitis, chest cold) related to site of major symptoms
   2. Pathophysiology and etiology: caused by infection spread through upper respiratory airway; highly contagious
   3. Symptoms: headache, fever, pain, sneezing, nasal congestion, sore throat, malaise, cough; may last 5 days to 2 weeks
   4. Medical treatment
      a) Common cold: rest, increased fluid intake, prevention of chilling, decongestants, vitamin C, expectorants, warm salt water gargles, and aspirin or acetaminophen
      b) Sinusitis: antibiotics, saline irrigation, heated mist, and oral or topical decongestants
   5. Essential nursing care for patients with upper airway infection
      a) Nursing assessment
         (1) Examine upper respiratory airway passages with flashlight and nasal speculum or tongue blade; note appearance of mucous membranes, swelling or enlargement, and drainage.
         (2) Palpate sinuses, trachea, and neck lymph nodes for tenderness or enlargement.
      b) Nursing diagnoses
         (1) Pain related to upper airway irritation
         (2) Ineffective airway clearance related to excessive secretions
         (3) Fluid volume deficit related to hyperthermia or inability to swallow liquids
         (4) Knowledge deficit related to prevention of upper respiratory infections
      c) Nursing intervention
         (1) Administer analgesics or topical anesthetics.
         (2) Recommend hot compresses to relieve sinus congestion and warm water gargles to relieve sore throat.
         (3) Encourage patient to rest as much as possible.

        (4) Humidify environment with vaporizers to help loosen secretions.

        (5) Offer ice chips or ice water often (2–3 L of fluid per day).

        (6) Instruct patient on hygienic measures to reduce susceptibility to upper airway infection (see Client Teaching Checklist, "How to Avoid Respiratory Infections").

    d) Nursing evaluation

        (1) Patient's pain or discomfort is lessened or relieved.

        (2) Patient's airway is effectively cleared of secretions.

        (3) Patient maintains an adequate fluid balance.

        (4) Patient understands the importance of correct health habits to prevent or control the disorder.

B. Pharyngitis

  1. Definition

    a) Acute: a febrile inflammatory disorder of the throat

    b) Chronic: persistent problems with inflammation of throat

  2. Pathophysiology and etiology

    a) Acute: caused by virus or bacteria

    b) Chronic: caused by prolonged exposure to environmental dust particles; vocal strain; smoking; or upper respiratory, pulmonary, or cardiac conditions

---

✔ CLIENT TEACHING CHECKLIST ✔

How to Avoid Respiratory Infections

Describe to clients the following ways to lessen one's risk of contracting respiratory infections:

✔ Eat a well-balanced diet and get appropriate exercise, rest, and sleep.

✔ Wash hands frequently and thoroughly.

✔ Avoid excessive use of alcohol and cigarettes.

✔ Correct air dryness with home humidification (especially during winter).

✔ Avoid irritants (dust, chemicals, tobacco, and smoke) and allergens whenever possible.

✔ Avoid unnecessary chilling of the skin (especially feet), since chilling lowers resistance.

✔ Obtain influenza vaccination if advised by a physician (usually recommended for the elderly and for those with chronic illnesses).

✔ Avoid crowds during flu season.

✔ Maintain adequate dental hygiene.

---

3. Symptoms
   a) Acute: fever, sore throat, malaise, inflamed pharyngeal area, enlarged cervical lymph nodes and tonsils
   b) Chronic: difficulty swallowing, throat irritation, excessive mucus production
4. Diagnostic evaluation
   a) Acute: throat culture with sensitivity studies
   b) Chronic: history and visual exam of pharynx
5. Medical treatment
   a) Acute: if caused by virulent bacteria (such as group A streptococcal infection), treated with penicillin; bed rest, fluids, analgesic and antipyretic, and soft or liquid diet
   b) Chronic: avoiding cause of condition (rest voice, give up smoking); treating any upper respiratory, pulmonary, or cardiac condition
6. Essential nursing care for patients with pharyngitis
   a) Nursing assessment: see section V,A,5,a of this chapter
   b) Nursing diagnoses
      (1) See sections V,A,5,b,1,3–4 of this chapter
      (2) Potential for infection transmission related to pharyngitis
   c) Nursing intervention
      (1) See sections V,A,5,c,1–3,5–6 of this chapter.
      (2) Explain importance of completing full course of antibiotic therapy to control infection, prevent complications, and prevent spread of infection.
      (3) Instruct patient to avoid contact with others until infection is eliminated.
   d) Nursing evaluation
      (1) See section V,A,5,d in this chapter.
      (2) Patient's infection is controlled and is not transmitted to others.

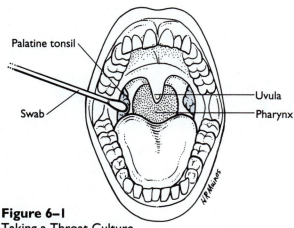

Figure 6–1
Taking a Throat Culture

C. Laryngeal obstruction
   1. Definition: life-threatening emergency due to blocked larynx
   2. Pathophysiology and etiology: caused by edema of larynx due to allergic reaction, severe throat inflammation or edema, or aspiration of foreign bodies
   3. Symptoms
      a) Partial obstruction: breathing problems
      b) Total obstruction: respiratory arrest
   4. Diagnostic evaluation: observing respiratory distress
   5. Medical treatment
      a) Allergic reaction or edema: epinephrine or corticosteroid, application of ice pack to back of neck, cricothyroidotomy, or tracheotomy
      b) Aspiration of foreign body: Heimlich maneuver
   6. Essential nursing care for patients with laryngeal obstruction
      a) Nursing assessment: evaluating patient's ability to breathe and possible cause (such as aspiration of food)
      b) Nursing diagnoses
         (1) Anxiety related to inability to breathe
         (2) Ineffective breathing pattern related to edema

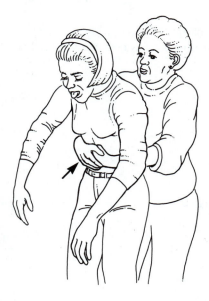

Figure 6–2
Heimlich Maneuver

c) Nursing intervention
   (1) Reassure patient and begin treatment immediately.
   (2) For allergic reactions or edema, administer prescribed drug and closely monitor; if drug fails, physician may need to perform emergency tracheotomy.
   (3) For object in pharynx, try to remove with finger; for object in larynx or trachea, attempt Heimlich maneuver; if Heimlich maneuver fails, physician may need to perform emergency tracheotomy.
d) Nursing evaluation
   (1) Patient's anxiety is reduced or eliminated.
   (2) Foreign object is removed, patient's airway is clear, and patient's breathing pattern returns to normal.

D. Cancer of the larynx
   1. Definition: potentially curable form of cancer located on vocal cords or other part of larynx
   2. Pathophysiology and etiology: cause unknown, but risk increased by chronic laryngitis, irritants (alcohol, cigarette smoke, and industrial pollutants), vocal strain, and heredity
   3. Symptoms: persistent hoarseness, difficulty swallowing, swelling or lump in throat, foul breath, dyspnea, dysphagia, pain when talking, weakness, weight loss, and anemia
   4. Diagnostic evaluation
      a) Laryngoscopy under general anesthesia; laryngeal biopsy for microscopic exam of lesion
      b) MRI, CT scan, and laryngography to detect extent of tumor growth
   5. Medical treatment
      a) Surgery
         (1) Early cases: laryngofissure (partial laryngectomy) or supraglottic (horizontal) laryngectomy
         (2) Advanced cases: total laryngectomy, radical neck dissection
      b) Radiation therapy
      c) Chemotherapy
   6. Essential nursing care for patients with cancer of the larynx
      a) Nursing assessment
         (1) Ask patient about risk factors that may predispose her/him to cancer of the larynx, such as smoking, alcohol consumption, vocal strain, chronic respiratory conditions, and exposure to pollutants or dust.
         (2) Inspect and palpate patient's neck area for masses indicating tumor growth or node enlargement.
      b) Nursing diagnoses
         (1) Anxiety related to diagnosis and treatment
         (2) Body image disturbance related to surgery

(3) Impaired verbal communication related to tumor growth and metastasis to other structures

(4) Altered nutrition, less than body requirements, related to anxiety, dysphagia, or metastatic process

c) Nursing intervention

(1) Provide information to the patient and family regarding cancer of the larynx and the various methods of treatment.

(2) Offer reassurance and provide emotional support.

(3) Involve patient in self-care activities.

(4) Suggest loose-fitting, high-collared clothing to help cover stoma, neck, and shoulder area after surgery.

(5) Assist patient with alternative methods of communication.

(6) Monitor patient's food intake and offer soft foods or liquids if dysphagia is present.

(7) Refer patient to self-help support groups such as the American Laryngectomee Association.

d) Nursing evaluation

(1) Patient's anxiety is reduced and she/he demonstrates an understanding of the disorder and the various methods of treatment.

(2) Patient accepts changes in body image and shows willingness to perform self-care activities.

(3) Patient is able to communicate with others.

(4) Patient consumes an adequate amount of food and fluids and has no nutritional deficiency.

VI. Selected disorders of lower respiratory system

See text pages
_____

A. Cancer of the lung and bronchus

1. Definition

a) Bronchogenic carcinoma: malignant tumor arising from the bronchial epithelium

b) Lung cancer: malignant tumor of lung tissue

2. Pathophysiology and etiology: caused by cigarette smoke (active and passive), air pollution, arsenic, asbestos, and radioactive dust

3. Symptoms

a) Bronchogenic carcinoma: cough with bloody sputum, fatigue, weight loss, anorexia; dyspnea and chest pain late in disease

b) Lung cancer: vague early symptoms include anorexia, weight loss, fatigue, and chronic cough; pain only in late stage

4. Diagnostic evaluation: chest radiography, bronchoscopy with bronchial washings and tissue biopsy, lung and bone scans, CT scan, MRI, cytologic analysis of sputum, lymph node biopsy, and mediastinoscopy

5. Medical treatment
   a) Surgical removal of tumor (lobectomy or pneumonectomy depending on size and location); lymph node dissection
   b) Radiation therapy (usually palliative)
   c) Chemotherapy
6. Essential nursing care for patients with cancer of the lung and bronchus
   a) Nursing assessment
      (1) Assess sputum production, breathing patterns, weight, and mental status.
      (2) Assess patient's cardiac status for murmurs or arrhythmias.
      (3) Palpate and percuss chest wall for changes in tactile fremitus and areas of dullness; auscultate lungs for adventitious or absent breath sounds.
      (4) Examine patient's skin for cyanotic or ecchymotic areas.
   b) Nursing diagnoses
      (1) Ineffective airway clearance related to tumor obstruction
      (2) Pain related to tumor pressure
      (3) Impaired gas exchange related to tissue destruction
      (4) Fear related to diagnosis and treatment regimen
   c) Nursing intervention
      (1) Provide humidifiers or vaporizers to help loosen secretions.
      (2) Place patient in semi-Fowler's position or in a reclining chair.
      (3) Administer analgesics as prescribed.
      (4) Monitor hypoxemic patient every 2 hours, noting color of skin, lips, and nail beds and performing pulse oximetry; evaluate for signs of respiratory difficulty marked by dyspnea or use of accessory muscles for breathing.
      (5) Explain treatment to patient and answer questions.
      (6) Provide emotional support.
   d) Nursing evaluation
      (1) Patient maintains a patent airway.
      (2) Patient reports that pain is reduced or eliminated.
      (3) Patient breathes without severe dyspnea and shows no signs of cyanosis.
      (4) Patient understands the diagnosis and treatment plan and reports that anxiety is reduced.

B. Chronic obstructive pulmonary disease (COPD)
   1. Definition: group of disorders including chronic bronchitis, bronchiectasis, emphysema, and asthma
   2. Pathophysiology and etiology: caused by interaction of genetics and environment (cigarette smoking, air pollution, and occupational exposure)
   3. Symptoms
      a) Chronic bronchitis: persistent, productive cough; dyspnea; bronchospasm; expectoration of thick, white mucus

  b) Bronchiectasis: chronic cough, expectoration of purulent sputum (upon standing, sputum separates into 3 layers), hemoptysis, clubbing of fingers, fatigue, anorexia, weight loss

  c) Emphysema: exertional dyspnea, chronic cough, expectoration of mucopurulent sputum, anorexia, weight loss, weakness, distention of neck veins during expiration

  d) Asthma: cough, dyspnea, wheezing, production of thick sputum

4. Diagnostic evaluation: pulmonary function studies, chest radiography, arterial blood gas studies, sputum studies

5. Medical treatment

  a) Chronic bronchitis and bronchiectasis: prescription of bronchodilators and/or antibiotics; cessation of smoking, postural drainage, chest percussion, increased intake of fluids, steroid therapy

  b) Emphysema: prescription of bronchodilators, aerosol therapy, antibiotics, corticosteroids, oxygen therapy

  c) Asthma: prescription of beta agonists, methylxanthines, anticholinergics, corticosteroids, or mast cell inhibitors

6. Essential nursing care for patients with chronic obstructive pulmonary disease

  a) Nursing assessment

   (1) Assess symptoms, pulse (rate and quality), and respiration.

   (2) Auscultate lungs for normal and abnormal breath sounds.

   (3) Check for cyanosis, engorged neck veins, peripheral edema, clubbing of fingers, mental changes.

   (4) Assess color, amount, and consistency of sputum.

  b) Nursing diagnoses

   (1) Impaired gas exchange related to airflow limitation, mucus production, and respiratory muscle fatigue

   (2) Ineffective airway clearance related to bronchoconstriction, mucus production, and ineffective cough

   (3) Ineffective breathing pattern related to shortness of breath, mucus production, bronchoconstriction, and airway irritants

   (4) Activity intolerance related to fatigue, hypoxemia, and ineffective breathing pattern

   (5) Knowledge deficit related to treatment

  c) Nursing intervention

   (1) Monitor levels of dyspnea and hypoxia; administer bronchodilators as prescribed.

   (2) Monitor effectiveness of oxygen therapy; instruct patient about oxygen use (see section IV,F of this chapter).

   (3) Perform postural drainage with percussion and vibration; instruct patient in effective breathing and coughing to help raise secretions; encourage high fluid intake.

(4) Encourage patient to report sputum changes or any worsening of symptoms that could indicate infection.

(5) Teach diaphragmatic, pursed lip breathing.

(6) Encourage exercise to improve respiratory fitness; encourage patient to remain active up to tolerance level; emphasize symptom control and sense of mastery.

(7) Share goals and treatment expectations with patient; explain that all lung irritations, including smoking, are harmful.

d) Nursing evaluation

(1) Patient has improved gas exchange.

(2) Patient achieves airway clearance.

(3) Patient's breathing pattern is improved.

(4) Patient achieves activity tolerance.

(5) Patient acquires effective coping mechanisms.

(6) Patient adheres to therapeutic program.

C. Respiratory failure

1. Definitions

a) Acute respiratory failure: life-threatening condition in which alveolar ventilation cannot maintain the body's need for oxygen and removal of carbon dioxide

b) Chronic respiratory failure: same as acute respiratory failure, except there is progressive, irreversible loss of lung function

c) Adult respiratory distress syndrome (ARDS): severe respiratory distress in patients who do not respond to treatment for acute respiratory failure

2. Pathophysiology and etiology

a) Acute respiratory failure: may be caused by oversedation, anesthesia administration, head injury, chest trauma, upper abdominal surgery, hemothorax, pneumothorax, pneumonia, and neurologic diseases (myasthenia gravis, multiple sclerosis, and amyotrophic lateral sclerosis)

b) Chronic respiratory failure: seen in patients with such chronic respiratory disorders as emphysema and chronic bronchitis

c) ARDS: may be caused by pneumonia, shock, trauma, fat or air embolism, drug overdose, pneumonitis, aspiration of gastric contents, major surgery, drowning, uremia, severe pancreatitis, and smoke inhalation

3. Symptoms

a) Acute respiratory failure: apprehension, dyspnea, wheezing, and cyanosis; if untreated, cardiac dysrhythmias, hypotension, congestive heart failure, respiratory acidosis, and ARDS

b) Chronic respiratory failure: same as symptoms of underlying disease

c) ARDS: 8–48 hours after onset of illness or injury, rise in respiratory rate; shallow, labored breathing; cyanosis; mental confusion; agitation; drowsiness; may result in death if untreated

4. Diagnostic evaluation: symptoms, patient history, arterial blood gas studies
5. Medical treatment
   a) Acute respiratory failure: establishment of patent airway (if airway is obstructed); administration of humidified oxygen by nasal cannula, Venturi, or reservoir mask; providing mechanical ventilation
   b) Chronic respiratory failure: long-term treatment of underlying cause
   c) ARDS: treatment of initial cause; intubation and mechanical ventilation
6. Essential nursing care for patients with respiratory failure
   a) Nursing assessment: evaluation of respiratory status
   b) Nursing diagnoses
      (1) Anxiety related to inability to breathe
      (2) Ineffective airway clearance related to thick secretions, inability to cough
      (3) Activity intolerance related to dyspnea, decreased respiratory function
      (4) Potential for infection related to chronic respiratory disease
   c) Nursing intervention
      (1) Perform tracheal suctioning as necessary; explain reason for oxygen by mask or nasal cannula; stay with patient when severe respiratory distress occurs; listen to concerns and provide a way to signal for help.
      (2) Keep airways patent; administer humidified oxygen and bronchodilators; encourage patient to take deep breaths.
      (3) Teach breathing exercises (blowing out candles, diaphragm breathing, blowing small objects along a table top, and pursed lip breathing).
      (4) Allow patient to perform easy tasks at her/his own pace.
      (5) Thoroughly clean all inhalation therapy equipment; protect patient from allergens and visitors with upper respiratory infections; notify physician if patient shows signs or symptoms of respiratory infection.
   d) Nursing evaluation
      (1) Patient's anxiety is reduced.
      (2) Patient maintains a clear airway by effective coughing and deep breathing.
      (3) Patient's breathing pattern is normal.
      (4) Patient's activity intolerance shows improvement.
      (5) Patient shows no evidence of infection; patient's temperature is normal.

D. Pulmonary embolism
  1. Definition: obstruction of one or more pulmonary arteries by a thrombus or thrombi such as blood, air, or fat originating in the venous system or right side of the heart
  2. Pathophysiology and etiology
     a) After embolic obstruction, alveolar dead space increases because of decreased blood flow to area.
     b) Pulmonary vascular resistance increases due to reduction in size of pulmonary vascular bed, increasing pulmonary arterial pressure and increasing right ventricle work to maintain blood flow.
     c) When the right ventricle fails, cardiac output and systemic blood pressure decrease; shock follows.
  3. Symptoms
     a) Most common symptom is sudden chest pain; other symptoms include dyspnea, tachypnea, fever, tachycardia, apprehension, cough, blood-streaked sputum, diaphoresis, hemoptysis, and syncope.
     b) Massive embolism can cause sudden death; multiple small emboli can lodge in terminal pulmonary arterioles producing multiple small lung infarctions.
  4. Diagnostic evaluation: chest radiography, electrocardiogram, radiofibrinogen leg scan, impedance plethysmography, arterial blood gas studies, ventilation-perfusion scan, and pulmonary angiography
  5. Medical treatment
     a) Anticoagulation therapy to prevent recurrence of emboli
     b) Thrombolytic therapy to resolve emboli more rapidly
     c) Surgical intervention to remove emboli or prevent their passage
     d) Hyperbaric oxygen chamber, oxygen therapy
        (1) Thoracotomy with cardiopulmonary bypass
        (2) Interruption of inferior vena cava
        (3) Transvenous catheter embolectomy
  6. Essential nursing care for patients with pulmonary embolism
     a) Nursing assessment
        (1) Assess patient for Homans' sign.
        (2) Auscultate lungs for rales and adventitious breath sounds.
        (3) Assess patient for cyanosis, dyspnea, coughing, blood-tinged sputum, tachycardia, shallow respirations, and distended neck veins.
        (4) Assess patient for signs and symptoms of fat embolism: irritability, confusion, pallor, tachycardia, tachypnea, dyspnea, cough, crackles, wheezes, production of thick white sputum.
     b) Nursing diagnoses
        (1) Pain related to pulmonary embolism
        (2) Knowledge deficit related to treatment or prevention of infection
        (3) Anxiety related to possible recurrence of pulmonary embolism

         c) Nursing intervention

            (1) Place patient in semi-Fowler's position; administer narcotic analgesics as prescribed.

            (2) Monitor thrombolytic and anticoagulant therapy; monitor vital signs every 2 hours.

            (3) Encourage ambulation and active and passive leg exercises; elevate foot of bed; instruct patient to avoid prolonged sitting, immobility, constricting clothing, and crossing legs

            (4) Use antiembolism stocking, CPM machine.

            (5) Provide emotional support; encourage patient to discuss anxieties; instruct patient how to prevent recurrence; discuss signs and symptoms of pulmonary embolism (see Client Teaching Checklist, "Preventing Emboli").

            (6) Postoperatively, measure pulmonary arterial pressure and urinary output; monitor arterial catheter insertion site for hematoma formation and infection.

         d) Nursing evaluation

            (1) Patient's pain is reduced or eliminated.

            (2) Patient understands treatment, prevention of infection.

            (3) Patient's anxiety is reduced or eliminated.

     E. Pleural effusion

       1. Definition: collection of fluid in the pleural space; usually a complication of another disease

       2. Pathophysiology and etiology

         a) Fluid may be a clear transudate or exudate, or it may be blood, pus, or chyle.

         b) Transudate is caused by changes in pleural fluid formation and reabsorption; exudate is caused by inflammation from bacterial products or tumors.

✔ CLIENT TEACHING CHECKLIST ✔

Preventing Emboli

Describe the following recommendations to patients at risk for developing emboli:

✔ Wear antiembolism stockings as directed.

✔ Avoid sitting for long periods.

✔ Do not cross legs when sitting.

✔ When traveling: change position often, walk occasionally, exercise legs and ankles while sitting.

✔ Drink plenty of fluids.

---

    c) Pleural effusion may be a complication of tuberculosis, pneumonia, congestive heart failure, pulmonary embolism, pulmonary viral infections, and lung cancer.

3. Symptoms: fever, dyspnea, and pain; large amount of effusion indicated by dullness or flatness to percussion over areas of fluid with minimal or absent breath sounds

4. Diagnostic evaluation
    a) Fluid confirmed by chest radiography, ultrasound, CT scan, and thoracentesis
    b) Fluid analyzed by bacterial cultures, gram stain, acid-fast bacillus stain, CBC, blood chemistry studies, and pH

5. Medical treatment
    a) Thoracentesis to remove fluid, collect specimen for analysis, relieve dyspnea
    b) Chest tube drain connected to water-seal drainage system or suction to evacuate pleural space and reexpand lung
    c) Drugs instilled in pleural space to prevent fluid collection
    d) Other treatments: chest wall irradiation, surgical pleurectomy, diuretic therapy

6. Nursing interventions for patients with pleural effusion
    a) Prepare and position patient for thoracentesis and offer support during procedure.
    b) Help patient assume least painful position during thoracentesis.
    c) Administer pain medication as prescribed.
    d) Monitor chest tube drainage and record amount every 8 hours.
    e) Provide essential nursing care specific to underlying cause of pleural effusion.

F. Chest trauma
1. Definition: serious injury to the chest, most often from auto accidents, crushing chest injuries, falls, gunshot wounds, blast wounds, and stab wounds

2. Pathophysiology and etiology
    a) Chest injuries can cause loss of patent airway, altered intrathoracic pressure, chest wall and rib cage destruction, altered central nervous system, insufficient myocardial function.
    b) Pathologic mechanisms lead to impaired ventilation and perfusion, acute respiratory failure, hypovolemic shock, and death.

3. Diagnostic evaluation: chest radiography, CBC, urinalysis, arterial blood gas studies, electrocardiogram

4. Medical treatment
    a) Restore, maintain patent airway and cardiopulmonary function
    b) Chest tube, fluids

6. Essential nursing care for patients with chest trauma
    a) Nursing assessment
        (1) Identify type and extent of injury, estimated blood loss, and presence of drugs or alcohol.

        (2) Assess respiratory status by observing skin color, respiratory rate, and respiratory pattern; auscultate lungs for abnormal or absent breath sounds.

        (3) Examine airway, thorax, neck veins; palpate throat.

        (4) Assess for presence of mediastinal shift.

    b) Nursing diagnoses

        (1) Fear related to injury or inability to breathe

        (2) Ineffective breathing pattern related to hemothorax, pneumothorax, or pain

        (3) Pain related to injury

    c) Nursing intervention

        (1) Remain with patient and offer reassurance and emotional support.

        (2) Explain treatment to patient.

        (3) Monitor administration of oxygen, blood, plasma expanders, and blood products.

        (4) Monitor patient for changes in respiratory status; immediately report any changes to physician.

        (5) If narcotic analgesics are ordered by physician, count respiratory rate before administering and again in 30–45 minutes; notify physician if analgesics do not relieve pain.

    d) Nursing evaluation

        (1) Patient's fear is reduced or eliminated.

        (2) Patient's breathing pattern returns to normal.

        (3) Patient's pain is reduced or eliminated.

G. Pneumonia

  1. Definition

    a) Acute illness caused by lung inflammation or infection

    b) Types

        (1) Lobar pneumonia: confined to one or more lobes of the lung

        (2) Bronchopneumonia: patchy and diffuse infection throughout both lungs

        (3) Hypostatic pneumonia: caused by hypoventilation of lung tissue over prolonged period

        (4) Chemical pneumonia: caused by inhalation of toxic chemicals

  2. Pathophysiology and etiology

    a) Caused by microorganisms (bacteria, viruses, Rickettsiae, or fungi)

    b) Atypical pneumonia caused by mycoplasmas, viruses, psittacosis, and *Legionella pneumophila*

    c) Viral pneumonia: while less serious, takes longer to resolve and leaves patients weaker than bacterial pneumonia

3. Symptoms
   a) Bacterial pneumonia: sudden symptoms, sharp chest pain, rapid prostration, shaking chills, fever as high as 106°F, painful cough and breathing, rusty sputum; without treatment, patient may die of heart failure or asphyxia
   b) Viral pneumonia: copious sputum, sterile blood cultures, less frequent chills, slow pulse and respirations; low mortality
4. Diagnostic evaluation: sputum culture, sensitivity studies, chest radiography, and CBC
5. Medical treatment
   a) Antibiotics
   b) Supportive treatment (bed rest, oral or intravenous fluids)
   c) Cool mist vaporizer
   d) Supplementary oxygenation
   e) Endotracheal intubation or tracheotomy for severe infection with thick, abundant secretions
6. Essential nursing care for patients with pneumonia
   a) Nursing assessment
      (1) Assess for fever, chest pain, rapid or bounding pulse, tachypnea, dyspnea, coughing, sputum production, use of accessory muscles, pain, cyanosis, flushing, and mental status.
      (2) Auscultate chest for breath sounds and passage of air throughout lung fields.
   b) Nursing diagnoses
      (1) Activity intolerance related to altered respiratory function
      (2) Hyperthermia related to infection
      (3) Pain related to pneumonia
      (4) Fluid volume deficit related to decreased oral intake and abnormal fluid loss
      (5) Potential for infection transmission related to coughing
      (6) Ineffective breathing pattern related to infectious process and pain while breathing
   c) Nursing intervention
      (1) Plan activities so patient can rest.
      (2) Monitor vital signs every 4 hours; administer antipyretic agent; notify physician if fever remains or if pulse rate increases or decreases sharply.
      (3) Monitor often for pain; support chest with both hands and use firm pressure to splint chest wall as patient coughs.
      (4) Administer fluids every 2 hours; measure intake and output; administer fluids intravenously as necessary.
      (5) Maintain good hand washing techniques to prevent spread of infection; administer antibiotics as ordered.
      (6) Encourage patient to cough and take deep breaths every 2 hours; place patient in semi-Fowler's position; perform postural drainage if required.
      (7) Observe for cyanosis; administer oxygen as necessary.

d) Nursing evaluation
   (1) Patient is able to carry out activities of daily living with minimal assistance.
   (2) Patient attains and maintains normal body temperature.
   (3) Patient's pain is eliminated or controlled.
   (4) Patient's fluid volume deficit is corrected; patient maintains adequate fluid intake.
   (5) Infection is not spread to others.
   (6) Patient attains and maintains clear airway by effective coughing and deep breathing.
   (7) Patient's breathing pattern is normal.

H. Influenza
   1. Definition: acute respiratory disease of relatively short duration
   2. Pathophysiology and etiology
      a) Caused by one of three major strains of virus: A, B, or C; these mutate and produce variants (subtypes).
      b) Flu viruses are transmitted through the respiratory tract; flu occurs mainly in epidemics.
      c) Because the virus changes, antibodies against it are not effective against a new subtype.
   3. Symptoms
      a) Incubation is 2–3 days; onset is abrupt, with chills, headache, muscular aches, fever, anorexia, weakness, respiratory symptoms, sneezing, sore throat, dry cough, nasal discharge, and cold sores.
      b) Gastrointestinal form usually begins with abdominal pain, nausea, vomiting, and diarrhea.
      c) Fever of 100°–103°F may persist for three days; other symptoms continue for up to 10 days; cough may persist longer.
   4. Diagnostic evaluation: assessment of symptoms; possible chest radiography, sputum culture, or sensitivity test to rule out other diseases
   5. Medical treatment
      a) Hospitalization only in severe cases
      b) Copious fluid intake, aspirin or acetaminophen, cool vapor inhalation, bed rest
      c) Patient observation for sign or symptom changes (fever, pulse rate, breathing problems, etc.)
   6. Essential nursing care for patients with influenza: see sections VI,G,6,a–d of this chapter

I. Tuberculosis (TB)
   1. Definition: a highly communicable infectious disease usually involving the lungs, although it can spread to almost any part of the body

2. Pathophysiology and etiology
   a) *Mycobacterium tuberculosis* (tubercle bacillus) causes pulmonary tuberculosis, especially in presence of lowered resistance, overcrowding, poor hygiene, or alcoholism.
   b) Distinguishing feature is rust-colored sputum.
   c) TB is transmitted by direct contact with a person who has the active disease, through inhalation of droplets from coughing, sneezing, and spitting.
   d) Organisms multiply slowly; they are killed by heat, sunshine, drying, and ultraviolet light.
   e) TB bacillus remains in the body years after immune system has controlled original infection; if immunity is diminished, organisms begin to multiply.
3. Symptoms
   a) Onset is insidious; symptoms often do not appear until disease is advanced.
   b) Patient may have fatigue, anorexia, weight loss, nonproductive cough, high temperature, night sweats, bloody cough, weakness, wasting, dyspnea, and chest pain.
4. Diagnostic evaluation
   a) Intracutaneous test (Mantoux test), chest radiography, sputum exam
   b) Gastric lavage or gastric aspiration sometimes used to determine the presence of organisms
5. Medical treatment
   a) Combination antituberculosis drugs
   b) Surgery
      (1) Segmental or wedge resection (when disease is located primarily in one lung section)
      (2) Lobectomy (if diseased area is large)
      (3) Pneumonectomy (if entire lung is diseased)
6. Essential nursing care for patients with tuberculosis
   a) Nursing assessment
      (1) Inquire about patient's past exposure to TB or bacille Calmette-Guérin (BCG) vaccine.
      (2) Assess for anorexia, nausea, weight loss, low-grade fever, fatigue, irregular menses, fever, night sweats, cough, and sputum production.
   b) Nursing diagnoses
      (1) Altered nutrition, less than body requirements, related to nausea and infection
      (2) Potential for infection transmission related to tuberculosis
      (3) Anxiety related to diagnosis
   c) Nursing intervention
      (1) Instruct patient to increase her or his intake of foods rich in protein, vitamin C, and iron and to maintain a balanced diet.
      (2) Inform patient and family members about prescribed drug therapy regimen.

(3) Instruct patient to cover mouth while coughing or sneezing.

(4) Advise patient to avoid exposure to dust or silicone particles.

(5) Instruct patient to return for examinations of sputum every 2–4 weeks until 2 sputum cultures are negative; until that time, patient is to be considered infectious, and precautions should be taken to prevent spread of TB.

(6) Offer reassurance and emotional support.

1. Mr. Early receives oxygen therapy via nasal cannula at a rate of 2 L/minute. When the patient asks why the flow rate is so low, the nurse's best response would be:

   a. "Your oxygen intake must be precisely monitored because of the carbon dioxide your body has become accustomed to retaining."

   b. "I will gradually increase the flow rate of the oxygen to accommodate your comfort level when breathing."

   c. "Your respiratory status depends on the ability of your body to adapt to high levels of oxygen in your blood."

   d. "You will need to receive a high concentration of oxygen until your color becomes more pink."

2. Further assessment of Mr. Early reveals signs of cor pulmonale. The nurse understands that the pathophysiology underlying this condition results from:

   a. Chronic dilatation of the bronchi and bronchioles, causing an increase in pulmonary artery pressures.

   b. Increased peripheral vascular resistance, which causes left ventricular hypertrophy.

   c. Increased pulmonary blood flow, causing increased pulmonary artery pressures.

   d. Increased arterial oxygen tension and decreased carbon dioxide content in the blood.

3. Jennifer McCook, who is 14 years old, is having an acute asthma attack that has been minimally responsive to therapy for the past 24 hours. When she suddenly stops wheezing, which of the following interventions should the nurse initiate?

   a. Pulmonary assessment, with close observation of vital signs

   b. Stat paging of the physician and preparing for respiratory arrest

   c. Providing assurance to the patient that the attack is abating

   d. Asking the patient to verbalize her feelings about the attack

4. Mr. Ralph DeCarlo had a total laryngectomy 3 days ago. Which of the following assessments indicates a life-threatening postsurgical complication?

   a. Drainage from the wound drain of 20 ml in 8 hours

   b. Inability to utilize esophageal speech

   c. The need to suction mucoid secretions from the laryngectomy tube

   d. Continuous pulsations of the laryngectomy tube

5. Which of the following would be a priority nursing diagnosis for Mr. DeCarlo 7 days after his total laryngectomy?

   a. Body image disturbance related to presence of tracheostomy tube

   b. Impaired verbal communication related to inability to master esophageal speech

   c. Altered nutrition, less than body requirements, related to NPO status

   d. Knowledge deficit related to tracheostomy and stoma care

6. Six-year-old Rita Finley has had a tonsillectomy. When discussing the nursing diagnosis of potential fluid volume deficit related to bleeding and hemorrhage, the nurse would inform the parents that:

   a. It is easiest for Rita to drink fluids through straws.

   b. Ear pain should be reported to a physician immediately.

   c. Excessive coughing should be avoided.

   d. Nonpharmacologic analgesic is the preferred method of pain control.

7. Which of the following persons would be at greatest risk for developing an influenza virus infection?

   a. An 85-year-old woman with chronic renal failure who lives in Venezuela

   b. A 67-year-old man who lives in an extended care facility in New York City

c. A 70-year-old woman with a history of congestive heart failure who lives in a personal-care home in Michigan

d. A 65-year-old man with emphysema who lives with his daughter in Arizona

8. Ms. Carol Helmstatter, who is 72 years old, is diagnosed with streptococcal pneumonia. When assessing her upon admission to the hospital unit, you would expect to find which of the following signs and symptoms?

a. Severe headache, myalgia, dyspnea, and nonproductive cough

b. Fever, headache, nausea, vomiting, and diarrhea

c. Fever, dyspnea, nonproductive cough, and recent weight loss

d. Sudden onset of fever, severe shaking chills, and productive cough

9. The nurse is assessing the tuberculin skin test of Mr. James Bauer 60 hours after the injection. Which of the following would be interpreted as a significant finding?

a. Formation of a wheal >10 mm in diameter

b. Itching around the injection site

c. Erythema measuring 9 mm in diameter

d. An area of induration 10 mm in diameter

10. A follow-up chest x-ray reveals a calcified nodule in Mr. Bauer's right middle lung lobe. The nurse may infer that which process has taken place?

a. Liquefaction necrosis

b. Bronchogenous dissemination

c. Formation of Ghon's tubercle

d. Lymphogenous dissemination

11. Mr. Bauer's physician uses a multiple-drug regimen to treat him for tuberculosis. What instructions should the nurse give the patient when teaching him about this therapy?

a. The course of drug therapy may last 9 months or more.

b. Once treatment has started, people in close contact with the patient are no longer at risk of developing tuberculosis.

c. Medications will be discontinued when acid-fast bacillus sputum cultures are negative.

d. Following effective treatment with medication, the patient will be immune to tuberculosis.

ANSWERS

1. **Correct answer is a.** Oxygen therapy must be closely monitored in patients with chronic obstructive pulmonary disease, since their respiratory centers have become insensitive to the use of an elevated $PaCO_2$ level as a respiratory stimulant. In these patients, hypoxemia is the major stimulus for respiration, and the peripheral chemoreceptors in the carotid and aortic arch bodies become the major stimulus for breathing. Excessive oxygenation removes the stimulus of hypoxemia. The patient then develops carbon dioxide narcosis and may become apneic. "Pinking up" is a sign of hypoventilation that is related to high arterial PO_2 levels; it occurs prior to apnea.

b, c, and **d.** All are incorrect, based on the data given in correct answer **a.**

2. **Correct answer is c.** In pulmonary emphysema, the alveoli are destroyed by abnormalities of lung enzymes. A decrease in alveolar capillary surface causes impaired oxygen diffusion, leading to hypoxemia. Later, impaired carbon dioxide elimination leads to respiratory acidosis. The alveolar walls continue to rupture, and the pulmonary capillary bed is reduced in size. Pulmonary blood flow is increased, and the right ventricle is forced to maintain a higher blood pressure in the pulmonary artery. As hypertrophy of the right ventricle progresses, cor pulmonale, or right-sided heart failure, takes place.

a. Chronic dilatation of the bronchioles occurs in bronchiectasis.

b and **d.** Both are incorrect based on the information given in correct answer **c.**

3. **Correct answer is a.** In status asthmaticus, which is severe asthma that lasts >24 hours and is unresponsive to conventional therapy, there is no correlation between the severity of the attack and the intensity of the patient's wheezing. In fact, sudden disappearance of wheezing may indicate greater obstruction and impending respiratory failure. Thus, the patient should be carefully monitored.

   b. The patient should be thoroughly assessed before the physician is paged.
   c. The patient's condition may be worsening, not improving.
   d. During an asthma attack, the patient should speak minimally, and the nurse should ask questions that require only 1- or 2-word answers to conserve the patient's energy.

4. **Correct answer is d.** Pulsations of the laryngectomy tube indicate that the tube is placing pressure on the carotid artery. This pressure could rupture the artery, especially if a wound infection is present. The physician should be notified immediately.

   a. After laryngectomy, use of wound drains is discontinued when the drainage is <50–60 ml/day. Thus, drainage of 20 ml in 8 hours would not be considered excessive.
   b. Esophageal speech is taught to the patient 1 week after surgery, or when he/she begins oral feedings. If the patient cannot master this type of communication, it is not considered to be a complication of the surgery, nor is it life threatening. Other methods of communication are available.
   c. Mucous secretions are normal during the immediate postoperative period.

5. **Correct answer is c.** In determining a priority nursing diagnosis, physiologic considerations are foremost. Postoperatively, the patient who has had a laryngectomy is NPO for approximately 10–14 days, receiving enteral nutrition by nasogastric tube.

Alternative sources of nutrition and hydration are important for maintaining fluid and electrolyte balance and providing for optimal wound healing and metabolic needs.

   a, b, and **d.** These are all pertinent nursing diagnoses but do not have the highest priority.

6. **Correct answer is c.** The patient who has had a tonsillectomy should be discouraged from coughing, since this may place stress on the suture line, precipitating bleeding and hemorrhage.

   a. Fluids should not be given via straws, since the straw may also place stress on the suture line.
   b. Ear pain following a tonsillectomy is expected.
   d. Normally there would be no contraindication to pharmacologic therapy for pain control.

7. **Correct answer is b.** The influenza vaccine is recommended for patients in high-risk groups: the elderly, cardiac and pulmonary patients, and others with chronic conditions. Persons living in close quarters and those living in the Northern Hemisphere are also considered at high risk. The patient who lives in an extended-care facility in Michigan is at the highest risk.

   a, c, and **d.** None of these patients is at the highest risk of infection.

8. **Correct answer is d.** Streptococcal pneumonia is a type of bacterial pneumonia. Accordingly, the patient will exhibit shaking chills, productive cough, and high fever.

   a. These symptoms indicate a viral pneumonia.
   b. These symptoms indicate legionnaires' disease, another type of pneumonia.
   c. These symptoms indicate *Pneumocystis carinii* pneumonia, which is caused by protozoa.

9. **Correct answer is d.** When assessing the site of a tuberculin skin test, one would interpret as significant an area of induration measuring 10 mm or more in diameter.

a. A wheal is the round elevation of the skin that is formed when the tuberculin bacillus extract is placed into the skin.

b. Itching around the site of injection is not considered significant.

c. Erythema or redness without induration is considered to be of no significance.

10. **Correct answer is c.** Ghon's tubercles, or calcified primaries, are primary tubercles that have healed over a period of several months through the formation of fibrous scars. These lesions contain living bacilli that can reactivate and reinfect the patient, even several years later.

a, b, and **d.** These are other stages in the infectious process of tuberculosis but do not involve formation of a calcifiednodule.

11. **Correct answer is a.** Active tuberculosis is usually treated with medication for at least 9 months.

b and **c.** Once drug therapy is begun, the patient will be instructed to have a sputum culture taken every 2–3 weeks until 2 successive cultures are free of the bacilli, verifying a noninfectious state.

d. The patient will not be immune to tuberculosis. The bacillus could become reactivated, even after treatment.

7

Cardiovascular Function

OVERVIEW

I. Structure and function of cardiovascular system
A. Structure of cardiovascular system
B. Function of cardiovascular system

II. General diagnostic tests
A. Laboratory tests
B. Radiographic and radioisotope studies
C. Echocardiography
D. Phonocardiography
E. Electrocardiography
F. Vectorcardiography
G. Exercise stress testing
H. Cardiac catheterization
I. Angiography
J. Arteriography
K. Hemodynamic monitoring

III. General nursing assessments
A. Patient history
B. Observation and physical examination
C. Diagnostic tests

IV. Nursing considerations with selected therapies and techniques
A. Cardiac surgery
B. Pacemaker insertion
C. Administration of heart medications
D. Prevention of heart disease

V. Selected disorders
A. Cardiac disorders
B. Vascular and peripheral disorders

NURSING HIGHLIGHTS

1. The nurse can play a critically important role in supporting the patient with cardiomyopathy by encouraging an attitude of realistic hope.
2. The nurse should provide detailed education about medications, diet, and weight control for the patient who has an acute episode of cardiac failure.
3. The cardiac surgery patient needs individualized, comprehensive nursing care directed toward meeting physical and psychosocial needs within the context of a family support system.
4. The nurse should be attentive to the needs of patient and family throughout the perioperative experience, setting realistic goals in collaboration with the patient; family members should be helped to support goals of self-care and eventual discharge.

GLOSSARY

aldosteronism—an electrolyte imbalance caused by excessive aldosterone secretion

angioplasty—procedure whereby narrow areas within blood vessels are eliminated

bradycardia—slow heartbeat, with a pulse rate of <60

cardioversion—elective procedure in which defibrillator and external electrodes are used to terminate rapid dysrhythmias

commissurotomy—separation of the thickened, adherent leaflets of a stenotic cardiac valve

cor pulmonale—right ventricular heart failure

Corrigan's pulse—jerky pulse with full expansion and sudden collapse

echocardiogram—a record of the position and motion of the walls and internal components of the heart made by the echo produced when beams of ultrasonic waves are directed through the chest wall

intermittent claudication—severe pain in calf muscles during walking due to inadequate blood supply

Marfan syndrome—hereditary condition affecting bones, connective tissue, ligaments, skeletal structures, and muscles

myxoma—tumor composed of mucous connective tissue

orthopnea—difficulty in breathing except in an upright position

pitting edema—abnormal fluid accumulation in the intercellular spaces in which the skin remains indented for several minutes after firm finger pressure has been removed

Valsalva's maneuver—forcible exhalation effort against the closed glottis; increases intrathoracic pressure

valvuloplasty—repair of a defective valve

ENHANCED OUTLINE

See text pages
_____

I. Structure and function of cardiovascular system

A. Structure of cardiovascular system
   1. Overall structure: fist-sized muscular pump with 4 chambers (the heart) connected to a system of tubes, including the aorta, pulmonary arteries, vena cava, and pulmonary veins
   2. Heart structure
      a) Layers
         (1) Endocardium: the endothelial membrane that lines the heart's cavities and the connective tissue bed on which the heart lies

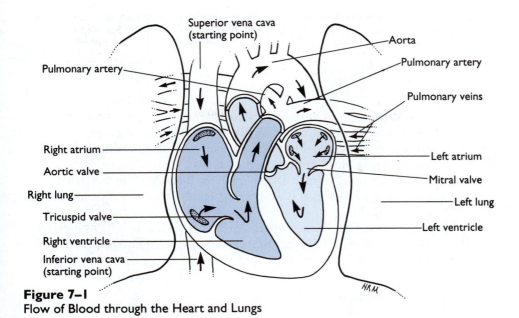

Figure 7–1
Flow of Blood through the Heart and Lungs

    (2) Myocardium: the thickest, middle layer of the heart wall, composed of cardiac muscle
    (3) Pericardium: the sac that surrounds the heart and the roots of the major blood vessels
    (4) Fibrous pericardium: the outermost covering of the heart
   b) Internal components
    (1) Chambers: right ventricle and left ventricle; right atrium and left atrium (plural: atria)
    (2) Valves: atrioventricular valves, including the tricuspid valve and the mitral (bicuspid) valve; semilunar valves, including the pulmonic valve and aortic valve
  3. Blood vessel structure: arterial system, consisting of arteries and arterioles; venous system, consisting of veins and venules; capillaries

B. Function of cardiovascular system
  1. Heart
   a) Heart chambers: The right and left ventricles send blood into arteries (right side into pulmonary circulation and left side into systemic circulation); the right and left atria receive incoming blood from veins and store blood until it is emptied into the ventricles.
   b) Heart valves
    (1) Atrioventricular valves: The tricuspid valve separates the right atrium from the right ventricle; the bicuspid (mitral) valve separates the left atrium from the left ventricle.
    (2) Semilunar valves: The pulmonic valve separates the right ventricle from the pulmonary artery; the aortic valve separates the left ventricle from the aorta.

2. Blood vessels
   a) Arterial system: Arteries carry blood from the heart; arterioles, which branch into capillaries, allow for exchange of gases (carbon dioxide and oxygen) and nutrients between blood and body cells and between blood and air in the lungs.
   b) Venous system: Veins transport venous blood back to the heart under low pressure; veins have valves that keep blood flowing toward the heart.
   c) Capillaries: Capillaries contact each organ's tissue cells and deliver oxygen and metabolic substances; once exchange takes place, venous blood is returned to the heart.

See text pages
_____

II. General diagnostic tests

A. Laboratory tests: may diagnose heart disease or determine patient's progress during and after treatment
   1. Blood chemistry: information on general physical status and/or part of diagnostic analysis
   2. Serum enzymes and isoenzymes: Elevated levels indicate cellular injury as a result of cardiac disease.

B. Radiographic and radioisotope studies: determine size and position of heart; damage to lungs due to heart disease; location of catheters, endotracheal tubes, and hemodynamic monitoring devices; and areas of myocardial damage

C. Echocardiography: uses ultrasound to assess cardiomyopathy, valvular disorders, cardiac tumors, pericardial effusion, and ventricular function

D. Phonocardiography: graphic recording of heart sounds during auscultation, used to diagnose heart valve and cardiac disorders

E. Electrocardiography (ECG): graphic recording of electrical current generated by heart

F. Vectorcardiography: type of ECG that shows a 3-dimensional view of the electrical current of the heart

G. Exercise stress testing: ECG taken during exercise (walking on treadmill, pedaling stationary bicycle) performed until target heart rate is reached; used to assess cardiac function

H. Cardiac catheterization: introduction of a flexible catheter into heart and coronary arteries to diagnose cardiac disease

I. Angiography: injection of contrast medium into arterial system to determine obstruction, narrowing, or aneurysm

J. Arteriography: injection of contrast medium to detect aneurysm or blockage of artery (e.g., aortogram) or arterial disease (e.g., peripheral arteriogram)

K. Hemodynamic monitoring: includes central venous pressure monitoring, systemic intra-arterial monitoring, and pulmonary artery monitoring; gives information on blood volume, vascular capacity, tissue perfusion, and pump effectiveness

III. General nursing assessments

See text pages

A. Patient history
1. Components: demographic information, personal and family history, socioeconomic data, diet, functional health pattern assessment
2. Emphasis: information pertaining to cardiovascular disease risk factors and symptoms

B. Observation and physical examination
1. General appearance: Look for evidence of anxiety, depression, pain, or irregular breathing pattern.
2. Temperature: If temperature is taken rectally, thermometer should be lubricated and inserted gently to prevent excessive vagal stimulation, which can produce bradycardia.
3. Pulse: Note rate, rhythm, and quality; check for pulse deficit and for pulse in other areas, including extremities and carotid artery; auscultate for heart sounds (first sound is S_1, opening of mitral and tricuspid valves; second is S_2, closing of aortic and pulmonic valves; third is S_3, ventricular gallop; fourth is S_4, atrial gallop). Procedure also reveals murmurs, clicks, and friction rubs.
4. Blood pressure: Measure while patient is standing, sitting, and lying down; assess for marked difference between left and right arms and for postural hypotension.
5. Respiration: Observe rate and character (easy or labored, deep or shallow, wet or dry, and wheezing or quiet) for 1 minute; auscultate for wheezes and crackles.
6. Skin color and temperature: Note cyanosis of mucous membranes, lips, ear lobes, skin, and nail beds; check for pallor, bearing in mind that white skin appears bloodless and black skin appears grayish.
7. Edema: Assess feet, ankles, fingers, hands, and sacral area; check for pitting edema.
8. Weight: Be alert for sudden weight gain of 2.2 lb or more, which may indicate the presence of edema.
9. Pain: Assess character, location, duration, radiation to other areas, changes, and relationship to events in daily life.
10. Diagnostic tests: Assist during diagnostic procedures.

C. Diagnostic tests: nursing responsibilities
1. Lab tests
   a) Blood chemistry: Ascertain that patient is appropriately prepared for collection of specimens.
   b) Serum cardiac enzymes and isoenzymes: Ascertain that patient is appropriately prepared for collection of specimens.

2. Radiographic and radioisotope studies
   a) Chest radiographs and fluoroscopy: Explain the purpose of the procedure and its components; prepare patient.
   b) Radioisotope studies: Explain purpose of procedure.
3. Electrocardiography (ECG): Explain procedure and its components.
   a) 12-lead ECG: Ask patient to lie as still as possible during test.
   b) Holter recorder: Instruct patient to keep a detailed diary; to avoid using heavy machinery, hair dryers, and electric shavers; and to refrain from bathing and showering.
   c) Stress test
      (1) Reduce anxiety by assuring patient that testing is done in a controlled environment, where nursing and medical assistance are available.
      (2) Advise patient to get adequate rest the night before the procedure and to dress in loose, comfortable clothing.
      (3) Instruct patient to fast for 2 hours before test and to refrain from smoking and drinking beverages containing alcohol or caffeine on day of test.
      (4) Caution patient to report cardiac symptoms experienced during test.
      (5) Caution patient to refrain from taking a hot shower for 2 hours after test.
   d) Vectorcardiography: Ask patient to lie as still as possible during test.
4. Cardiac catheterization
   a) Assess patient for allergies to contrast medium, iodine-containing substances, and local anesthetics.
   b) Shave and scrub area to be catheterized with antiseptic skin preparation.
   c) Inform patient that it is necessary to strap him/her to x-ray table during procedure.
   d) Check position of catheter.
   e) Assess insertion site for bloody drainage or hematoma formation.
   f) Assess vital signs at each dressing, pulse, and temperature check, and check pulses distal to catheterization site.
   g) Compare skin temperature of affected extremity with that of opposite extremity.
   h) Contact doctor or radiologist if bleeding or changes in vital signs occur.
5. Echocardiography: Assure patient that test is painless and will be over in 1 hour or less; instruct patient to lie quietly during procedure; and assist patient, if necessary, to lie on left side.

6. Hemodynamic monitoring: Explain purpose and components of procedure; reassure patient that medical and nursing assistance will be available at all times.
   a) Central venous pressure: Change dressing and IV tubing every 24 hours after procedure; inspect insertion site for signs of infection; take pressure reading, especially when patient is connected to bedside monitor (calibrate monitor, ensure that monitor functions properly, and follow institution's protocol).
   b) Systemic intra-arterial monitoring: Check for bleeding around intra-arterial catheter and for loose connections; monitor color and temperature at insertion site and pulse distal to insertion site for signs of systemic venous thrombosis or circulatory compromise; and take pressure reading, especially when patient is connected to bedside monitor.
   c) Pulmonary artery monitoring: Ensure that flush device functions properly after procedure; take periodic pressure readings.

IV. Nursing considerations with selected therapies and techniques

See text pages
_____

A. Cardiac surgery
   1. Preoperative
      a) Provide emotional support to patient and family members.
      b) Explain diagnostic tests, preoperative preparations, and postoperative care procedures.
      c) Insert indwelling Foley catheter, nasogastric tube, and IV line.
      d) Prepare skin over operative site by applying bacteriostatic soap scrub and shaving skin.
      e) Ensure that medications are discontinued 1–2 days before surgery and that antibiotics are ordered before surgery.
      f) Observe trauma patient for signs and symptoms of shock and cardiac compression (superficial neck veins, cyanosis, dyspnea, hypotension, and pulse rate or rhythm changes); take pulse frequently; and report fecal incontinence to physician immediately.
   2. Postoperative
      a) Provide reassurance and explain all procedures to patient.
      b) Monitor vital signs; measure central venous pressure, urine output, and nasogastric tube drainage.
      c) Inspect chest tubes hourly for compression, leakage, and free-flowing drainage.
      d) Assess endotracheal tube for patency; suction as needed; and encourage extubated patient to cough and deep breathe every 1–2 hours.
      e) Auscultate lungs hourly for normal, abnormal, or absent breath sounds; check for skin color, restlessness, or shallow respiration.
      f) Inspect dressings for signs of infection; monitor temperature every 4 hours.
      g) Monitor fluid intake and output; observe patient for signs of fluid imbalance.

       h) Administer prescribed analgesic; monitor blood pressure, pulse, and respiratory rates before and after giving narcotic.

       i) Palpate peripheral pulses; note color and temperature of extremities on an hourly basis; administer vasopressors if needed.

       j) Encourage patient to do leg exercises every 2 hours; assess for signs of peripheral thrombus or embolus formation.

       k) Document any behavior changes.

       l) Notify physician immediately in the event of condition change, renal shutdown, shock, thrombus formation, cardiac dysrhythmias, electrolyte imbalance, heavy drainage from chest tubes, chills, or sudden fever.

       m) Observe heart transplant patient for signs of organ rejection, including elevated WBC count, ECG changes, and fever.

       n) Develop patient teaching plan.

  B. Pacemaker insertion

    1. Provide patient and family members with emotional support.

    2. Inspect venous insertion site of external pacemaker daily for signs of irritation (especially several days postinsertion); report evidence of reddening near site or along pathway of vein.

    3. Change dressing over internal pacemaker insertion site daily; inspect site for infection.

    4. Educate patient with permanent internal pacemaker about its care (see Client Teaching Checklist, "Care of Permanent Internal Pacemaker").

  C. Administration of heart medications

    1. Nitroglycerin (Nitrostat)

       a) Instruct patient to keep tongue still and to avoid swallowing saliva until nitroglycerin tablet is dissolved; if pain is severe, tablet may be crushed with teeth to speed absorption.

       b) Advise patient to carry medication at all times.

       c) Explain to patient that fresh nitroglycerin causes a burning sensation under the tongue.

       d) Caution patient that because nitroglycerin is unstable and inactivated by heat, it should be kept in a dark-colored glass bottle.

       e) Instruct patient to renew supply of nitroglycerin every 6 months.

       f) Tell patient to take smallest amount of nitroglycerin that will relieve pain or prevent pain due to anticipated exertion.

       g) Advise patient to record frequency of doses and how long it takes for nitroglycerin to work.

       h) Caution patient to be alert for and report the following side effects of nitroglycerin: flushing, throbbing headache, hypotension, or tachycardia.

Care of Permanent Internal Pacemaker

Instruct the client with a pacemaker to do the following:

✔ Maintain follow-up care with physician.
✔ Check pulse rate daily, and contact physician immediately if rate is above or below target rate.
✔ Take prescribed drugs exactly as instructed.
✔ Notify physician if suture line becomes inflamed or sore.
✔ Avoid injuring insertion site, and wear loose-fitting clothes over that area.
✔ Check with physician about the dangers of proximity to outside electrical interference, including diathermy machines and microwave ovens.
✔ Follow physician's advice about lifting and exercise; resume activities at recommended pace.
✔ Carry ID information indicating physician's name, type of pacemaker, and pacemaker settings (rate and electrical output); pacemaker ID card provided by manufacturer should always be carried.
✔ Because pacemakers can trigger metal detector alarm systems, present pacemaker ID card and request hand scanning.
✔ Be aware that pacemaker replacement may be necessary in the future.

    i) Warn patient that failure of nitroglycerin to relieve pain may signal impending myocardial infarction.

    j) Explain to patient that nitroglycerin ointment is especially useful for nocturnal angina and during long periods of sustained activity; site of application should be rotated to prevent skin irritation.

2. Beta-adrenergic blockers

    a) The drug of choice is propranolol hydrochloride (Inderal), given at 6-hour intervals; it may also be given with sublingual isosorbide dinitrate (Isordil) for antiangina and anti-ischemia prophylaxis.

    b) Blood pressure and heart rate should be monitored 2 hours after administration, with patient in upright position.

    c) Side effects include precipitation of congestive heart failure and asthma, musculoskeletal weakness, hypotension, bradycardia, and mental depression.

    d) If blood pressure drops, a vasopressor may be needed; atropine sulfate (Atropisol) is the drug of choice for severe bradycardia.

    e) Abrupt discontinuation of propranolol hydrochloride (Inderal) may worsen angina and precipitate myocardial infarction.

3. Calcium ion antagonists and calcium channel blockers

    a) Drug should be administered every 4–6 hours in dose appropriate for individual patient.

    b) These drugs should be used with caution in patients with heart failure, since they block calcium, which supports contractility.

        c) Side effects include hypotension after IV administration, constipation, gastric distress, dizziness, and headache.

    4. Narcotic analgesics

        a) Nurse should always take blood pressure and respiratory and pulse rates before giving narcotic analgesics; if systolic blood pressure is <100 or respiratory rate is ≤10 breaths per minute, physician should be contacted before administration.

        b) Because serious adverse effects can follow analgesic administration, depression of respiration, nausea, dysrhythmias, and hypotension should be noted (especially with morphine).

        c) Nurse should take vital signs 30–45 minutes after drug is given and closely observe patient.

        d) Marked drop in blood pressure or respiratory rate should be reported to physician immediately, since narcotic antagonist or other therapy may be necessary.

  D. Prevention of heart disease

    1. Nurse should explain to patient that most forms of heart disease can be prevented by lifestyle modifications.

    2. Nurse should give patients the following suggestions for preventing heart disease: Stop smoking; lower blood pressure; decrease amount of fat in blood by dietary modification and exercise or, if necessary, by use of drugs; lower level of blood sugar; try to alter negative environmental factors and one's response to them (e.g., reduce stress and hostility).

V. Selected disorders

See text pages

A. Cardiac disorders

    1. Congestive heart failure

        a) Definition: inability of heart to meet demands of body tissues for oxygen and nutrients, followed by back-up and filling of many organs with blood and tissue fluid

        b) Pathophysiology and etiology

          (1) Pathophysiology

            (a) Left-sided failure: Left side fails to empty completely with each contraction; retained blood creates backpressure, causing lungs to become congested with blood, leading eventually to pulmonary edema.

            (b) Right-sided failure: Backpressure occurs in blood circulation from heart into venous system, causing distended neck veins; engorgement of gastrointestinal system, kidneys, and liver; and edema.

          (2) Etiology: Left-sided failure is caused by hypertension, aortic stenosis, anemia, hyperthyroidism, heart valve defect or

congenital heart defect, arrhythmias, myocardial infarction, or cardiomyopathy; right-sided failure is caused by pulmonary hypertension, valve defect, or congenital heart defect.

c) Symptoms
   (1) Left-sided failure: cough, dyspnea, orthopnea, tachycardia, heart gallop (S_3 or S_4), left displacement of apical pulse, moist crackles on lung auscultation, fatigue, insomnia, anxiety, restlessness, confusion
   (2) Right-sided failure: cough, dyspnea, swollen feet or ankles (pitting edema), nocturia, flatulence, anorexia, nausea

d) Diagnostic evaluation
   (1) Patient history, physical exam, chest radiography, ECG, arterial blood gas analysis, CBC, determination of serum electrolyte levels, hemodynamic monitoring
   (2) Right-sided failure: in addition to above, examination of extremities for edema, liver palpation for hepatomegaly

e) Medical treatment: rest; limitation of sodium intake and administration of diuretics to eliminate excess fluid; administration of digitalis (Digiglusin) to slow heart rate and strengthen ventricular contraction; administration of oxygen to improve ventilation

f) Complications: acute pulmonary edema

g) Essential nursing care for patients with congestive heart failure
   (1) Nursing assessment
      (a) Assess general physical appearance, vital signs, type and appearance of sputum, location and severity of edema, skin color, and mental status.
      (b) Examine jugular veins for distention.
      (c) Auscultate lungs for abnormal breath sounds.
   (2) Nursing diagnoses
      (a) Decreased cardiac output related to reduced stroke volume
      (b) Anxiety related to dyspnea
      (c) Activity intolerance related to fatigue
      (d) Sleep pattern disturbance related to nocturia
   (3) Nursing intervention
      (a) Provide complete bed rest, and answer call button promptly.
      (b) Record fluid intake and output, and monitor for signs of electrolyte imbalance.
      (c) Use appropriate bedding to prevent pressure ulcers.
      (d) Provide information about treatment necessary to prevent symptom recurrence and disease progression (see Client Teaching Checklist, "Heart Failure Prevention").
   (4) Nursing evaluation
      (a) Patient increases daily activities without respiratory distress.
      (b) Fluid volume excess is corrected.
      (c) Sleep pattern is normal.
      (d) Patient adheres to recommended treatment program.

2. Angina pectoris
   a) Definition: severe pain or a feeling of pressure in the anterior chest relieved by rest or antianginal drugs
   b) Pathophysiology and etiology
      (1) Pathophysiology: Attack is precipitated by increasing myocardial demand for oxygen due to physical exertion, exposure to cold, eating heavy meal, or emotional stress.
      (2) Etiology: lack of adequate blood supply to myocardium, usually caused by arteriospasms or atherosclerotic heart disease, and associated with significant obstruction of a major coronary artery
   c) Symptoms
      (1) Sudden chest pain or pressure, most severe over heart, under the sternum
      (2) Pain radiating to shoulders and arms, especially on left side, or to jaw, neck, or teeth

---

✔ CLIENT TEACHING CHECKLIST ✔

Heart Failure Prevention

Explain the following methods to patients for deterring the progression of heart disease:

✔ Rest to reduce fatigue and dyspnea.
✔ Increase activity level gradually; stop and rest if dyspnea occurs.
✔ Identify and avoid situations that produce stress.
✔ Elevate legs while sitting.
✔ Follow prescribed diet; avoid food products high in sodium and saturated fats.
✔ Avoid extreme heat, cold, and humidity.
✔ Take medications as prescribed; never omit a medication unless directed by your physician.
✔ Take diuretics early in the day to prevent frequent urination at night.
✔ Monitor pulse rate before taking digitalis; if pulse rate falls below 60, don't take the medication, and call physician immediately.
✔ Take blood pressure regularly, and know the signs of hypertension.
✔ Weigh yourself at the same time each day using the same scale.
✔ Report these symptoms immediately:
   — Weight gain of >2–3 lb over a few days
   — Appetite loss
   — Shortness of breath on activity or at rest
   — Swelling of ankles, feet, or abdomen
   — Persistent cough
   — Frequent urination at night

(3) Burning, squeezing, crushing tightness in upper chest or throat, with dyspnea, pallor, sweating, and faintness

(4) Attack usually lasting <5 minutes, usually in connection with physical or emotional stress

d) Diagnostic evaluation

(1) Patient history of symptoms and description of pain

(2) ECG and stress tests to identify coronary artery disease

(3) Coronary angiography to reveal collateral circulation and coronary artery condition

(4) Lab tests to determine serum cholesterol and triglyceride levels

e) Medical treatment

(1) Appropriate drug therapy should be administered, including antianginal drugs (e.g., nitroglycerin [Nitrostat] and isosorbide dinitrate [Isordil]); calcium channel blockers (e.g., diltiazem hydrochloride [Cardizem], nifedipine [Procardia]); or beta-adrenergic blocking agents (e.g., propranolol hydrochloride [Inderal], nadolol [Corgard]).

(2) Patient should be advised to modify lifestyle, including stopping smoking, exercising regularly, and losing weight.

(3) Vascularization may need to be improved with coronary artery bypass surgery and percutaneous transluminal coronary angioplasty.

f) Complications: dysrhythmia, myocardial infarction

g) Essential nursing care for patients with angina pectoris

(1) Nursing assessment

(a) Record patient's daily activities, and note those that cause angina.

(b) Ask patient to describe timing, onset, type, and duration of pain and how pain is relieved.

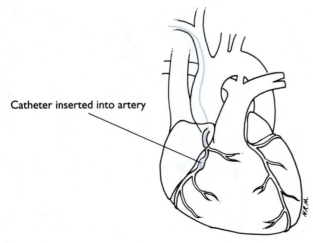

Catheter inserted into artery

Figure 7–2
Percutaneous Transluminal Angioplasty: Positioning of Catheter

(2) Nursing diagnoses
  (a) Anxiety related to fear of death
  (b) Pain related to myocardial ischemia
  (c) Knowledge deficit related to means of avoiding complications
  (d) Noncompliance with therapeutic regimen related to nonacceptance of prescribed lifestyle changes
(3) Nursing intervention
  (a) Instruct patient to be conservative about physical exertion.
  (b) Urge patient to try to minimize number of stressful situations.
  (c) Stay with hospitalized patient as much as possible to allay fears of death.
  (d) Inform patient about how to improve the quality of life with angina.
  (e) Teach patient about administration of nitroglycerin (Nitrostat; see section IV,C,1 of this chapter).
(4) Nursing evaluation
  (a) Patient's pain is controlled.
  (b) Patient avoids factors that precipitate angina attack.
  (c) Patient implements positive lifestyle changes.

3. Myocardial infarction
  a) Definition: destruction of myocardial tissue in areas of the heart that are deprived of sufficient blood supply due to reduced coronary blood flow; commonly called a "heart attack"

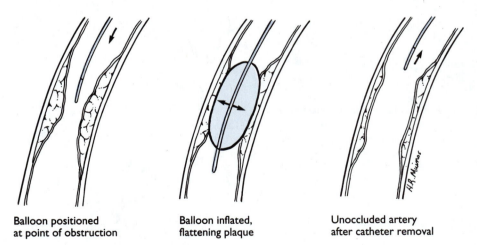

Balloon positioned at point of obstruction

Balloon inflated, flattening plaque

Unoccluded artery after catheter removal

Figure 7–3
Percutaneous Transluminal Angioplasty: Inflating the Balloon

b) Pathophysiology and etiology
  (1) Pathophysiology: ischemia and necrosis of myocardial cells, usually occurring in the left ventricle and involving part of the myocardium or subendocardial area
  (2) Etiology: narrowing of a coronary artery due to atherosclerosis; occlusion of artery by thrombus or embolus
c) Symptoms
  (1) Sudden, severe chest pain, more intense than that experienced in angina, that may or may not radiate to shoulder, arm, teeth, jaw, or throat
  (2) Pain that is not relieved by rest or antianginal drugs and that lasts for up to 2 days before changing to soreness and then disappearing
  (3) Pallor, sweating, faintness, severe drop in blood pressure, nausea, rapid weak pulse
  (4) Left-sided heart failure symptoms (dyspnea, cyanosis, and cough), which may appear if left ventricular pumping is impaired
d) Diagnostic evaluation
  (1) Perform ECG, noting that changes normally appear within 2–12 hours after infarction, but may take up to 3 days to appear.
  (2) Perform enzyme level tests, noting that creatine phosphokinase (CPK) levels rise within 2–6 hours and that isoenzyme CPK-MB is present in blood about 2 hours after infarction.
e) Medical treatment
  (1) Initiating appropriate drug therapy, including thrombolytic medications (within 6 hours of infarction), anticoagulants (to prevent thrombus formation), antiarrhythmics, analgesics, and tranquilizers (to promote rest and ease anxiety).
  (2) Maintaining complete bed rest immediately after infarction; increasing level of activity based on extent of infarction, presence of complications, and response to therapy.
f) Complications: heart failure; dysrhythmia; bleeding related to thrombolytic therapy, sometimes progressing to hypovolemic shock
g) Essential nursing care for patients with myocardial infarction
  (1) Nursing assessment
    (a) Obtain medical history, including nature and history of pain and any drugs taken.
    (b) Obtain vital signs; auscultate heart and lungs, noting cardiac rate and rhythm; and record peripheral pulse.
    (c) Examine extremities for edema.
    (d) Observe patient for pallor, diaphoresis, cyanosis, and signs of apprehension.
  (2) Nursing diagnoses
    (a) Activity intolerance related to impaired oxygen transport
    (b) Hyperthermia related to tissue necrosis
    (c) Anticipatory grieving related to perceived losses resulting from illness

  (3) Nursing intervention

   (a) Exhibit calm attitude, and provide emotional support to family and patient.

   (b) Check peripheral pulses and color and temperature of skin every 2–4 hours.

   (c) Auscultate lungs frequently for breath sounds; remind patient to breathe deeply every 2 hours while awake.

   (d) Auscultate for heart sounds; check cardiac monitor readings.

   (e) Measure fluid intake and output; notify physician if urine output falls below 500 ml in 24 hours.

   (f) Administer antianginal drug(s); notify physician if patient fails to respond.

   (g) Give analgesic every 3–4 hours for severe pain, but take blood pressure, pulse, and respiratory rates before administering narcotic analgesic.

   (h) Instruct patients to avoid Valsalva's maneuver by exhaling rather than holding breath when moving in bed.

   (i) Educate patient about follow-up treatment and rehabilitation.

  (4) Nursing evaluation

   (a) Patient maintains normal fluid balance.

   (b) Patient attains normal sleeping pattern.

   (c) Patient tolerates gradually increased activity.

   (d) Patient accepts necessary lifestyle changes.

4. Pericarditis

 a) Definition: inflammation of the pericardium

 b) Pathophysiology and etiology

  (1) Pathophysiology: Blood, excess fluid, pus effusion or exudates, or infections cause inflammation of the pericardium, producing partial or complete cardiac tamponade (compression), leading to decreased cardiac output.

  (2) Etiology: Condition occurs after infection, chest trauma, or myocardial infarction or in conjunction with malignant disorders, uremia, or connective tissue disorders.

 c) Symptoms: sharp pain aggravated by moving or breathing that radiates to neck and left arm; dyspnea; pericardial friction rub during heart auscultation

 d) Diagnostic evaluation: ECG to confirm clinical diagnosis made on presentation of signs and symptoms; radiography to show dilatation of heart with pericardial effusion; CT scan to confirm radiographic evidence, if necessary.

e) Medical treatment
   (1) Determining cause of pericarditis and administering therapy appropriate for that cause
   (2) Restricting patient to bed during acute phase; gradually increasing activity as condition permits
   (3) Administering appropriate drug therapy, including meperidine hydrochloride (Demerol) or morphine sulfate (Duramorph) for pain relief during acute phase; corticosteroids to control symptoms, resolve inflammation, and prevent further pericardial effusion; antibiotics to treat infections; salicylates to relieve pain and hasten fluid reabsorption in patient with rheumatic pericarditis
   (4) Performing pericardiocentesis in patient with chronic fluid accumulation to make a pericardial opening that allows fluid to drain into pleural space
   (5) Removing binding pericardium in patient with constrictive pericarditis to allow heart chambers to fill and contract more efficiently
f) Complications: pericardial effusion, cardiac tamponade
g) Essential nursing care for patients with pericarditis
   (1) Nursing assessment
       (a) Attempt to identify possible causes of condition by asking patient about recent dental work, infections, and recently prescribed drugs.
       (b) Determine nature of patient's pain by having him/her assume different positions.
   (2) Nursing diagnoses
       (a) Pain related to pericarditis
       (b) Activity intolerance related to decreased cardiac output
       (c) Hyperthermia related to inflammatory process
       (d) Altered nutrition related to anorexia
   (3) Nursing intervention
       (a) Administer analgesic; immediately report suddenly increasing pain to physician.
       (b) Monitor temperature every 4 hours and administer prescribed antipyretic; change perspiration-dampened bedding promptly.
       (c) Monitor patient's consumption of foods and fluids; notify physician if level of intake dramatically declines.
       (d) Explain importance of continued drug therapy and follow-up care to patient and family.
   (4) Nursing evaluation
       (a) Patient's inflammation is controlled.
       (b) Patient's activity tolerance is increased.
       (c) Patient's body temperature is normal.
5. Cardiomyopathy
   a) Definition: a group of diseases affecting myocardial structure and function

b) Pathophysiology and etiology
  (1) Pathophysiology
    (a) All types: impaired left ventricular pumping; lessened stroke volume, stimulating sympathetic nervous system and causing increased systemic vascular resistance; enlargement of left ventricle to accommodate demands, with eventual ventricular failure
    (b) Dilated or congestive cardiomyopathy: enlarged ventricular cavity with decreasing muscle wall thickness, left atrial enlargement, and stasis of blood in ventricle
    (c) Hypertrophic cardiomyopathy: increase in mass, weight, and size of heart
    (d) Restrictive cardiomyopathy: impaired ventricular stretch and volume
  (2) Etiology
    (a) All types: infection, metabolic disorders, immunologic disorders, pregnancy and postpartum disorders, congenital anomaly
    (b) Dilated or congestive cardiomyopathy: chronic alcoholism
    (c) Hypertrophic cardiomyopathy: associated with idiopathic hypertrophic subaortic stenosis (IHSS), possibly hereditary
    (d) Restrictive cardiomyopathy: amyloidosis, cancer, and other infiltrative diseases
c) Symptoms: exertional and paroxysmal nocturnal dyspnea, cough, fatigue, jugular vein distention, tachycardia, pitting edema, hepatic engorgement
d) Diagnostic evaluation
  (1) Patient history, noting predisposing factors, including alcoholism, family history of cardiomyopathy, and conditions associated with amyloidosis
  (2) Echocardiogram to visualize left ventricle
  (3) Cardiac catheterization and scans to rule out coronary artery disease
e) Medical treatment
  (1) Identifying and treating cause of heart failure
  (2) Performing heart transplant in severe cases, using ventricular assist devices until donor can be found, if necessary
f) Complications: heart failure, ventricular dysrhythmia
g) Essential nursing care for patients with cardiomyopathy
  (1) Nursing assessment
    (a) Obtain detailed history, including psychosocial history.
    (b) Determine extent of family support network.
    (c) Examine patient for signs of congestive heart failure.

(2) Nursing diagnoses
  (a) Ineffective breathing pattern related to myocardial failure
  (b) Anxiety related to diagnosis
  (c) Potential noncompliance related to self-care program
(3) Nursing intervention
  (a) Provide emotional support and allow patient to verbalize fears; initiate referral services.
  (b) Administer oxygen via nasal prongs.
  (c) Keep patient's environment clean and dust free.
  (d) Encourage patient to participate in brief activities.
  (e) Teach patient self-care program.
(4) Nursing evaluation
  (a) Patient demonstrates improved respiratory function.
  (b) Patient increases activity tolerance.
  (c) Patient complies with program of self-care.

6. Dysrhythmia
  a) Definition: disorder of heartbeat, originating in the sinus node, atria, atrioventricular node or junction, or ventricles, which may include a change in rate or rhythm, or both; can be minor or life-threatening in severity
  b) Pathophysiology and etiology
    (1) Sinus bradycardia
      (a) Pathophysiology: extremely low heart rate
      (b) Etiology: vagal stimulation, digitalis intoxication, increased intracranial pressure, myocardial infarction, extreme athletic conditioning, severe pain, some drug therapies, anorexia nervosa, hypoendocrine states
    (2) Sinus tachycardia
      (a) Pathophysiology: extremely high heart rate, up to 180 beats per minute
      (b) Etiology: anemia, acute blood loss, shock, pain, exercise, congestive heart failure, fever, hypermetabolic states, sympathomimetic or parasympatholytic drugs, anxiety
    (3) Premature atrial contractions
      (a) Pathophysiology: premature firing of a site in the atrium
      (b) Etiology: alcohol, caffeine, nicotine, stretched atrial myocardium, atrial ischemia, hypermetabolic states, hypokalemia, injury, myocardial infarction, anxiety, stress
    (4) Paroxysmal atrial tachycardia
      (a) Pathophysiology: extremely high heart rate, up to 250 beats per minute
      (b) Etiology: alcohol, caffeine, nicotine, fatigue, sympathomimetic drugs, stress
    (5) Atrial flutter
      (a) Pathophysiology: extremely high atrial heart rate accompanied by therapeutic block at the atrioventricular node, preventing some impulse transmission

      (b) Etiology: atrial ischemia, heart failure, mitral valve stenosis, fluid overload

(6) Atrial fibrillation

      (a) Pathophysiology: uncoordinated and disorganized twitching of atrial muscles

      (b) Etiology: valvular or atherosclerotic heart disease, congestive heart failure, congenital heart disease, cor pulmonale, thyrotoxicosis

(7) Premature ventricular contractions

      (a) Pathophysiology: increased automaticity of ventricular muscle cells

      (b) Etiology: digitalis or catecholamine toxicity, hypokalemia, hypoxia, fever, acidosis, exercise

(8) Ventricular bigeminy

      (a) Pathophysiology: alternation between normal and premature beats

      (b) Etiology: digitalis (Digiglusin) overdose, myocardial infarction, coronary artery disease, congestive heart failure

(9) Ventricular tachycardia

      (a) Pathophysiology: increased myocardial irritability

      (b) Etiology: coronary artery disease

(10) Ventricular fibrillation

      (a) Pathophysiology: rapid, ineffectual quivering of ventricles

      (b) Etiology: coronary artery disease

c) Symptoms: bradycardia, tachycardia, dyspnea, fatigue, dizziness, weakness, syncope, chest pain, pallor, sweating

d) Diagnostic evaluation: 12-lead ECG; Holter monitor

e) Medical treatment

(1) Sinus bradycardia: atropine sulfate (Atropisol) administration

(2) Sinus tachycardia: treatment of underlying cause, propranolol hydrochloride (Inderal) administration

(3) Premature atrial contractions: no treatment if infrequent; treatment of underlying cause if frequent

(4) Paroxysmal atrial tachycardia: treatment of underlying cause; administration of morphine, vasopressors, short-acting digitalis (Digiglusin), propranolol hydrochloride (Inderal), quinidine sulfate (Quinidex), or verapamil hydrochloride (Calan); carotid sinus pressure; cardioversion

(5) Atrial flutter: digitalis (Digiglusin), quinidine sulfate (Quinidex), calcium channel blocker, or beta-adrenergic blocker administration; cardioversion

(6) Atrial fibrillation: digitalis (Digiglusin), quinidine sulfate (Quinidex) administration

(7) Premature ventricular contractions: treatment of underlying cause; lidocaine hydrochloride (Xylocaine), procainamide hydrochloride (Procan), or quinidine sulfate (Quinidex) administration

(8) Ventricular bigeminy: lidocaine hydrochloride (Xylocaine), procainamide hydrochloride (Procan), or quinidine sulfate (Quinidex) administration; phenytoin (Dilantin) administration (if caused by digitalis [Digiglusin] overdose)

(9) Ventricular tachycardia: treatment of underlying cause, antidysrhythmic drugs, cardioversion

(10) Ventricular fibrillation: defibrillation

(11) Immediate treatment in life-threatening situation: cardiopulmonary resuscitation (CPR)

(12) Long-term treatment: implantation of temporary or permanent pacemaker

f) Complications: brain damage, sudden cardiac death

g) Essential nursing care for patient with dysrhythmia

  (1) Nursing assessment

    (a) Take complete medical history, including information on allergies, drug use history, and use of alcohol, caffeine, and tobacco.

    (b) Determine presence of symptoms that might indicate decreased cardiac output.

    (c) Assess pulse apically and peripherally; note presence of pulse deficit.

    (d) Auscultate heart for extra sounds.

    (e) Observe skin for signs of diminished cardiac output, including pallor and coolness.

  (2) Nursing diagnoses

    (a) High risk for activity intolerance related to dysrhythmia

    (b) Anxiety related to symptoms

    (c) Noncompliance with medical regimen related to fear of side effects

  (3) Nursing intervention

    (a) Monitor patient for potential recurrence of dysrhythmia.

    (b) Instruct patient about medication regimen, including possible adverse reactions and follow-up schedule.

    (c) Instruct patient with bradycardia to avoid Valsalva's maneuver.

    (d) Avoid vagal stimulation (caused by suctioning, enemas, or rectal thermometers or exams) in patient with bradycardia.

    (e) Instruct patients with premature beats and ectopic rhythms to avoid alcohol, caffeine, smoking, and stress.

  (4) Nursing evaluation

    (a) Patient tolerates increased activity.

    (b) Patient understands risks associated with alcohol and caffeine consumption.

    (c) Patient knows side effects of prescribed medication and knows what to do if they occur.

      7. Pulmonary edema
- a) Definition: abnormal collection of fluid in lungs, constituting acute emergency
- b) Pathophysiology and etiology
  - (1) Pathophysiology: Heart empties insufficient amount of blood with each contraction due to weakened left ventricle; right ventricle continues to pump blood toward lungs; pulmonary capillaries and alveoli become engorged; lungs fill with fluid, causing acute respiratory disease.
  - (2) Etiology: left ventricle weakened by heart failure, myocardial infarction, cardiac dysrhythmias, or arteriosclerosis; lung tissue injury (e.g., blast injury); condition that impairs pulmonary circulation (e.g., large embolus or emphysema); inhalation of irritants (e.g., ammonia); drug overdose; fluid overload
- c) Symptoms: sudden dyspnea, wheezing, moist or gurgling breath sounds, pink frothy sputum, orthopnea, cough, cyanosis, bounding pulse, elevated blood pressure, severe apprehension, restlessness
- d) Diagnostic evaluation: interpretation of patient's symptoms, chest radiograph, arterial blood gas analysis, and ECG
- e) Medical treatment
  - (1) Induce physical and emotional relaxation by administering morphine sulfate (Duramorph).
  - (2) Relieve hypoxia and improve ventilation by administering humidified oxygen.
  - (3) Delay venous return to heart with use of phlebotomy or rotating tourniquets, morphine sulfate (Duramorph) administration, and use of intermittent positive pressure or mechanical ventilator.
  - (4) Improve cardiovascular function when pulmonary edema is caused by heart failure by administering digitalis (Digiglusin) or related compound and a diuretic.
- f) Complications: respiratory failure, cardiac failure
- g) Essential nursing care for patients with pulmonary edema
  - (1) Nursing assessment
    - (a) Notify physician that pulmonary edema is suspected.
    - (b) Obtain patient's blood pressure, pulse, and respiratory rates; assess skin color and temperature.
    - (c) Auscultate lungs, and assess color and type of sputum.
    - (d) Determine patient's level of consciousness and degree of apprehension.
    - (e) Compare intake with output to detect fluid overload.
  - (2) Nursing diagnoses
    - (a) Ineffective airway clearance related to inability to remove airway secretions

   (b) Fluid volume excess related to low cardiac output

   (c) Knowledge deficit related to prevention of future episodes

  (3) Nursing intervention

   (a) Stay with patient, maintaining calm demeanor.

   (b) Administer morphine sulfate (Duramorph) and oxygen as prescribed.

   (c) Monitor vital signs regularly; watch for improvement in skin color.

   (d) Raise head of bed to upright position; use footboard to keep patient from sliding down; if possible, ask patient to dangle legs over side of bed to reduce venous return.

   (e) Administer diuretic, and record fluid intake and output hourly.

   (f) Run IV solutions at keep-vein-open rate to prevent fluid overload.

   (g) Provide teaching plan to help patient avoid future episodes.

  (4) Nursing evaluation

   (a) Patient's airway is clear, and pulmonary congestion is reduced.

   (b) Fluid volume excess is corrected, and urine output is normal.

   (c) Patient understands necessity of follow-up care.

8. Cardiac arrest

 a) Definition: sudden cessation of heartbeat and effective cardiac output

 b) Pathophysiology and etiology

  (1) Pathophysiology: ventricular asystole, consisting of complete absence of heart muscle activity; ventricular fibrillation, consisting of random contraction of individual heart muscle fibers

  (2) Etiology: myocardial infarction, respiratory arrest, electrical injury, hypothermia, blood loss, anaphylactic shock

 c) Symptoms: sudden collapse; loss of consciousness; absence of pulse, audible heart sounds, and respiratory movements; dilation of pupils after 45 seconds

 d) Diagnostic evaluation: absence of carotid pulsation

 e) Medical treatment

  (1) Performing cardiopulmonary resuscitation (CPR): maintaining open airway; providing artificial ventilation with rescue breathing; providing artificial circulation by external cardiac compression (see Nurse Alert, "How to Perform CPR")

  (2) Administration of appropriate oxygen and appropriate medication, including epinephrine hydrochloride (Adrenalin), isoproterenol (Vapo-Iso), dopamine hydrochloride (Dopastat), dobutamine hydrochloride (Dobutrex), sodium bicarbonate, and/or norepinephrine bitartrate (Levophed)

f) Complications: brain damage, pneumothorax, fat embolism, liver hematoma, fractured ribs or sternum

g) Essential nursing care for patient with cardiac failure

(1) Nursing assessment: Recognize that cardiac arrest is taking place.

(2) Nursing diagnoses

(a) Ineffective breathing pattern related to cardiac arrest

(b) Impaired gas exchange related to cardiac arrest

(c) Fluid volume excess related to cardiac arrest

(3) Nursing intervention

(a) Begin resuscitative measures immediately.

(b) Evaluate patient's response to CPR, observing pupils.

(c) Check peripheral pulses during cardiac compression.

(d) Observe patient closely after successful resuscitation, taking vital signs and measuring fluid output hourly.

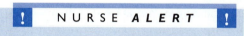

!   N U R S E   *A L E R T*   !

How to Perform CPR

Airway

- Create patent airway by removing material from the mouth; insert oropharyngeal airway.
- Attempt endotracheal intubation only if you have had sufficient training.

Breathing

- Begin mouth-to-mouth breathing (use bag-valve-mask device to eliminate danger of transmission of infectious diseases).
- Give 10–12 maximal insufflations before chest compression is started so that oxygenated blood will be circulated; with two rescuers, one inflation should be interposed after each five compressions without any halting of compression; with one rescuer, two breaths are interposed after each 15 compressions.
- Breather should see chest rise and fall, feel resistance of lungs as they expand, and hear noise of air escaping during exhalation.

Circulation: Cardiac compression

- Apply rhythmic pressure at the rate of 60–80 compressions per minute over lower half of sternum to compress heart.
- Use manual or automatic chest compressor (if available) to perform external cardiac compression.
- Assess effectiveness by palpating for carotid pulsation.

(4) Nursing evaluation
　　(a) Patient's color improves.
　　(b) Patient's breathing pattern returns to normal.
　　(c) Patient avoids dysrhythmias due to hypoxemia.

9. Valvular heart disease
　a) Definition: failure of the heart valves (aortic, tricuspid, or mitral) to open fully or close fully
　b) Pathophysiology and etiology
　　(1) Mitral stenosis
　　　(a) Pathophysiology: valve thickening caused by fibrosis and calcification, fusing together of leaflets, contraction and shortening of chordae tendineae, and narrowing of valvular orifice, leading to decreased cardiac output
　　　(b) Etiology: rheumatic fever, atrial myxoma, thrombus formation, calcium accumulation
　　(2) Mitral insufficiency (regurgitation)
　　　(a) Pathophysiology: valve thickening caused by fibrosis and calcification that causes mitral valve to fail to close completely, thus allowing backflow of blood and leading eventually to dilation and hypertrophy of left atrium and ventricle
　　　(b) Etiology: rheumatic heart disease, congenital anomaly, infective endocarditis, ischemic heart disease
　　(3) Mitral valve prolapse
　　　(a) Pathophysiology: enlargement and prolapse of valvular leaflets during systole, sometimes leading to marked mitral regurgitation
　　　(b) Etiology: endocarditis, myocarditis, rheumatic heart disease
　　(4) Aortic stenosis
　　　(a) Pathophysiology: narrowing of aortic valve orifice, which obstructs left ventricular outflow during systole, progressing to ventricular hypertrophy and right-sided heart failure
　　　(b) Etiology: congenital valvular disease or malformation, rheumatic heart disease, atherosclerosis, aortic valve calcification
　　(5) Aortic insufficiency (regurgitation)
　　　(a) Pathophysiology: failure of aortic valve leaflets to close properly during diastole, combined with dilated or loose annulus, leading to regurgitation of blood into left ventricle during diastole and eventual left ventricular hypertrophy
　　　(b) Etiology: infective endocarditis, congenital malformation, hypertension, Marfan syndrome, rheumatic heart disease (infrequent)

      (6) Tricuspid stenosis
         (a) Pathophysiology: narrowing of tricuspid valve orifice causing obstruction of blood flow from right atrium to right ventricle, proceeding to right atrial hypertrophy
         (b) Etiology: rheumatic heart disease

c) Symptoms
   (1) Mitral stenosis: fatigue, dyspnea, orthopnea, lowered systolic blood pressure, emaciation, anorexia, congestive heart failure, hemoptysis, hepatomegaly
   (2) Mitral insufficiency: fatigue, exertional dyspnea, orthopnea, pitting edema, palpitations, dysrhythmias, emboli, cough
   (3) Mitral valve prolapse: chest pain, palpitations, fatigue, heart failure, tachycardia; many patients asymptomatic
   (4) Aortic stenosis: dizziness, fainting, anginal pain, exertional dyspnea
   (5) Aortic insufficiency: exertional dyspnea, widened pulse pressure, angina, fatigue, Corrigan's pulse, palpitations, throbbing sensation in head
   (6) Tricuspid stenosis: diastolic murmur, noticeable pulse wave in neck veins, peripheral edema, ascites, hepatomegaly

d) Diagnostic evaluation
   (1) General: patient and family history, physical exam, heart auscultation
   (2) Mitral stenosis: ECG, phonocardiography, echocardiography, cardiac catheterization
   (3) Mitral insufficiency or valve prolapse: ECG, chest radiography, echocardiography, stress test, cardiac catheterization
   (4) Aortic stenosis: ECG, left-sided cardiac catheterization
   (5) Aortic insufficiency: cardiac angiography, echocardiography
   (6) Tricuspid stenosis: ECG, echocardiography

e) Medical treatment
   (1) Mitral stenosis: mitral commissurotomy, valvuloplasty, or valve replacement
   (2) Mitral insufficiency: mitral commissurotomy, prosthetic valve implantation, digitalis (Digiglusin), and anticoagulant therapy
   (3) Mitral valve prolapse: antiarrhythmic drugs or valve replacement; no treatment needed in many patients
   (4) Aortic stenosis: digitalis (Digiglusin), antiarrhythmic drugs, diuretics; antibiotics before and after dental procedures and invasive procedures; valve replacement
   (5) Aortic insufficiency: aortic valve replacement; digitalis (Digiglusin), antiarrhythmic drugs, and diuretics
   (6) Tricuspid stenosis: surgical repair or valve replacement

f) Complications: left atrial hypertrophy, left ventricular hypertrophy, right ventricular hypertrophy, right-sided cardiac failure

g) Essential nursing care for patients with valvular heart disease

    (1) Nursing assessment

        (a) Take thorough history, focusing on past infectious disorders, childhood diseases, familial history of heart disease, and activity tolerance.

        (b) Examine patient for signs and symptoms of valvular heart disease.

        (c) Assess patient's level of anxiety and coping skills of patient and family.

    (2) Nursing diagnoses

        (a) Activity intolerance related to dyspnea

        (b) High risk for infection related to invasive diagnostic procedures

        (c) Knowledge deficit related to benefits of surgery

    (3) Nursing intervention

        (a) Explain invasive diagnostic procedures according to patient's level of comprehension.

        (b) Report sudden fever, chills, or inflammation at site used for catheter insertion to physician.

        (c) Advise patients to contact physician for prophylactic antibiotic therapy before any dental or invasive procedure.

        (d) See section IV,A of this chapter for care after cardiac surgery.

    (4) Nursing evaluation

        (a) Patient maintains activity tolerance.

        (b) Patient exhibits no sign of infection.

        (c) Patient understands importance of antibiotic therapy before dental and invasive procedures.

B. Vascular and peripheral disorders

  1. Hypertension

    a) Definition: sustained elevation of arterial blood pressure >140/90

    b) Pathophysiology and etiology

      (1) Pathophysiology: increased heart workload and damage to arteries due to increased resistance of arterioles to blood flow

      (2) Etiology

        (a) Primary hypertension: cause unknown, but causative factors believed to include heredity, obesity, emotional stress, smoking, and increased serum cholesterol and sodium levels

        (b) Secondary hypertension: adrenal tumor, renal artery stenosis, oral contraceptive use, primary aldosteronism

    c) Symptoms: usually asymptomatic; if symptomatic, headache, dizziness, fatigue, insomnia, nervousness, nosebleeds, blurred vision, angina, shortness of breath

    d) Diagnostic evaluation
      (1) Primary hypertension
        (a) Physical exam: family history of hypertension or death of family member caused by stroke or heart disease
        (b) Blood pressure (taken in both arms while standing, sitting, and lying)
        (c) Lab tests, ECG, chest radiography, excretory urography
      (2) Secondary hypertension: procedures used to diagnose primary hypertension as well as studies to determine underlying cause, including renal arteriography, serum electrolyte levels, and funduscopic examination of eye
    e) Medical treatment
      (1) Primary hypertension
        (a) Sustained nutritional therapy, including weight reduction and consumption of low levels of sodium and saturated fats
        (b) Lifestyle modifications, including stopping smoking and reducing level of stress
        (c) Administration of antihypertensive drugs
      (2) Secondary hypertension: treatments used for primary hypertension as well as treatment of underlying cause
    f) Complications: congestive heart failure, myocardial infarction, cerebrovascular accident, renal failure, blindness
    g) Essential nursing care for patients with hypertension
      (1) Nursing assessment
        (a) Take complete medical, symptom, and family history.
        (b) Take blood pressure in both arms while patient is standing, sitting, and lying.
        (c) Take pulse in both wrists, noting rate, rhythm, and abnormal heart sounds.
        (d) Auscultate lungs, noting breath sounds.
        (e) Discuss treatment regimen, drugs prescribed, and side effects experienced in patient with recurrent hypertension.
      (2) Nursing diagnoses
        (a) Activity intolerance related to severity of hypertension
        (b) Fluid volume deficit related to diuretic effect of antihypertensive medication
        (c) Altered sexuality patterns related to adverse drug effects
      (3) Nursing intervention
        (a) Instruct patient to rise from a sitting position slowly and to sit down if feeling faint.
        (b) Check and record bowel movements daily; notify physician if constipation or diarrhea occurs.
        (c) Measure fluid intake and output.

(d) Examine skin and oral mucosa for changes.

(e) Report leg cramps and weakness to physician.

(f) Explain prescribed diet, exercise, medication (teach patient to monitor and report side effects as well as emphasizing the importance of not discontinuing medications even though he/she feels better), and weight reduction program.

(g) Teach and reinforce self-monitoring.

(4) Nursing evaluation

(a) Patient's bowel habits are normal.

(b) Patient maintains normal weight by eating well-balanced meals and exercising.

(c) Patient copes effectively with stressful situations.

(d) Patient demonstrates ability to monitor own blood pressure and pulse.

2. Arteriosclerosis and atherosclerosis

a) Definition: Arteriosclerosis is the hardening and loss of elasticity of arteries; atherosclerosis is the accumulation of fatty deposits (mostly cholesterol) on the walls of arteries.

b) Pathophysiology and etiology

(1) Pathophysiology: formation of fatty streak on surface of artery; development of fibrous plaque that partly or completely occludes arterial blood flow; calcification, hemorrhage, ulceration, or thrombosis of fibrous lesions

(2) Etiology: heredity, diet, smoking, hypertension, diabetes

c) Symptoms: intermittent claudication, coldness or numbness in extremities, skin and nail changes, ulcerations, gangrene, muscle atrophy, bruits

d) Diagnostic evaluation

(1) Lab studies, including measurements of low-density and high-density lipoproteins, triglycerides, serum creatinine, and blood urea nitrogen (BUN) concentrations

(2) Arteriography of lower extremities; Doppler ultrasonography and angiography; ECG

e) Medical treatment

(1) Risk factor modification, including stopping smoking and limitation of dietary fat and cholesterol intake

(2) Encouragement of routine exercise

(3) Administration of lipid-lowering agents, such as nicotinic acid and lovastatin (Mevacor)

(4) Laser angioplasty for severe cases

f) Complications: malnutrition, organ fibrosis, myocardial infarction, stroke

g) Essential nursing care for patients with arteriosclerosis and atherosclerosis

(1) Nursing assessment

(a) Obtain health history, focusing on patient's and family's history of cardiovascular problems and risk factors associated with lifestyle.

        (b) Examine patient for changes associated with reduced oxygen supply, including dry skin, loss of muscle size, thickened and clubbed nails, or rubor of the skin.

        (c) Check patient for early signs of ulcer formation, such as discoloration of extremities.

        (d) Auscultate heart and each large artery; be attentive for arterial bruit.

        (e) Palpate pulses at all major sites and note differences.

        (f) Check lower extremities for temperature differences and capillary filling.

    (2) Nursing diagnoses

        (a) Altered peripheral tissue perfusion related to obstructed arterial blood supply

        (b) Altered nutrition, greater than body requirements, related to high intake of saturated fats

        (c) Altered health maintenance related to difficulty in changing lifestyle

    (3) Nursing intervention

        (a) Encourage patient to stop smoking, to limit amount of dietary fat to 30% of day's calories, to limit cholesterol intake, and to exercise regularly.

        (b) Administer prescribed lipid-lowering agents.

    (4) Nursing evaluation

        (a) Patient's serum cholesterol level is <200 mg/dl.

        (b) Patient stops smoking.

        (c) Patient's episodes of dizziness and blurred vision are resolved.

  3. Peripheral vascular disease (PVD) (occlusive disorders of peripheral arteries and veins)

    a) Definition: diseases that obstruct or constrict the arteries that supply the extremities (include Raynaud's disease, thrombosis, thrombophlebitis, embolism)

    b) Pathophysiology and etiology

      (1) Pathophysiology: partial or total arterial occlusion, which disrupts the supply of oxygen and nutrients to body tissues

      (2) Etiology

        (a) Raynaud's disease: periodic constriction of arteries to extremities; underlying cause unknown; more prevalent in women

        (b) Thrombosis, phlebothrombosis, embolism: prolonged bed rest, pregnancy, shock, lower extremity paralysis, blood vessel trauma, endocarditis, dysrhythmias

        (c) Diabetes mellitus

c) Symptoms
  (1) Total occlusion: whiteness, cold, and extreme pain in affected extremity; absence of normal arterial pulse below area of obstruction; numbness, tingling, and cramping, followed by loss of sensation in affected area; loss of motion, shock, ischemia
  (2) Venous thrombosis: sudden edema, cyanosis, warmth, and tenderness over affected area; positive Homans' sign
  (3) Phlebothrombosis: symptoms often absent
  (4) Deep vein thrombosis: pain, swelling, and tenderness in affected extremity; mild fever; positive Homans' sign
d) Diagnostic evaluation
  (1) Examination of affected extremity, palpation of peripheral pulses, evaluation of symptoms
  (2) Phlebography to identify point of obstruction
  (3) Doppler ultrasonography to detect abnormalities in peripheral blood flow
e) Medical treatment
  (1) Arterial occlusive disease: Place extremity in dependent position; keep patient warm; wrap extremity to prevent radiation of heat; never apply direct heat; administer IV heparin (Lipo-Hepin), vasodilators, or narcotic drugs; thrombectomy, embolectomy, endarterectomy, or insertion of bypass graft may be required in severe cases.
  (2) Venous occlusive disease: Restrict patient to bed rest, with extremity elevated; administer analgesics and IV heparin (Lipo-Hepin); and apply continuous warm, moist heat to affected extremity; clot may be removed surgically, if necessary.
f) Complications: pulmonary embolism, gangrene, ulcerations
g) Essential nursing care for patients with peripheral vascular disease
  (1) Nursing assessment
    (a) Examine extremities for skin color, temperature, and abnormal changes.
    (b) Palpate peripheral pulses, noting absence or decreased intensity.
    (c) Assess patient's activity tolerance.
  (2) Nursing diagnoses
    (a) Activity intolerance related to pain
    (b) Impaired tissue integrity related to occlusive disorder of artery
    (c) Altered tissue perfusion related to occlusive disorder
  (3) Nursing intervention
    (a) Inspect patient's extremities for infection, color change, or skin breakdown; move patient carefully.
    (b) Encourage patient to move extremities and change position every hour; report severe pain to physician immediately.

              (c) Notify physician immediately if signs of pulmonary embolism are observed.

              (d) Offer suggestions to help reduce patient's discomfort, including wearing cotton gloves at night, lined latex gloves while washing dishes, and avoiding cold temperatures and sharp winds.

              (e) Advise patient to exercise moderately, avoid smoking, avoid factors that cause pain, refrain from sitting for long periods, and keep extremities warm.

          (4) Nursing evaluation

              (a) Patient tolerates moderate activity without discomfort.

              (b) Oxygen transport to tissues is improved.

              (c) Skin of extremities is intact, and there is no evidence of infection.

    4. Aortic aneurysm

      a) Definition: most common type of aneurysm (outpouching), located in aorta

      b) Pathophysiology and etiology

        (1) Pathophysiology: Arterial wall weakens, creating aneurysm that enlarges until it ruptures; massive tear in aorta causes death in a few minutes; occlusion of artery branching off aorta impairs dependent organs or structures.

        (2) Etiology: arterial disease, trauma, congenital defect

      c) Symptoms

        (1) Aneurysm detected prior to hemorrhage: pain, discomfort, and symptoms related to pressure on nearby structures

        (2) Aneurysm detected at time of hemorrhage: sudden acute illness, marked difference between left and right arm blood pressures, severe pain, shock

      d) Diagnostic evaluation: radiography, aortography

      e) Medical treatment: antihypertensive drugs until surgery can be performed; bypass or replacement grafting

      f) Complications: cardiac arrest, organ failure

      g) Essential nursing care for patients with aortic aneurysm

        (1) Nursing assessment

          (a) Preoperative: Monitor patient's general condition, blood pressure, pulse and respiratory rates, and skin color.

          (b) Postoperative: Observe patient for signs of blood loss and infection.

        (2) Nursing diagnoses

          (a) Pain related to pressure produced by aneurysm on adjacent structures

      (b) Fluid volume deficit related to abnormal fluid loss during surgery.

      (c) Ineffective airway clearance related to pain on coughing

(3) Nursing intervention

      (a) Preoperative: Notify physician if cramps begin or if a change in skin color or temperature is observed; instruct patient about coughing, deep breathing, and leg exercises.

      (b) Postoperative: Report sudden pain or pain in back, arm, or leg to physician; observe patient for signs of infection; monitor intake and output of fluids; encourage patient to cough, deep breathe, and exercise legs; instruct patient about follow-up care and preventive measures.

(4) Nursing evaluation

      (a) Patient does postoperative exercises.

      (b) Patient's skin color and color of extremities are normal.

      (c) Patient understands importance of follow-up anticoagulant therapy.

1. When teaching a patient with congestive heart failure, the nurse begins by explaining the normal functioning of the heart chambers. It would be important to tell the patient that the right atrium receives deoxygenated blood from the:

   a. Pulmonary veins.
   b. Lungs.
   c. Right ventricle.
   d. Upper and lower body.

2. Mr. Connor is being evaluated for paroxysmal atrial tachycardia, a dysrhythmia. He is to be placed on a Holter monitor. What instructions should the nurse give him to ensure that this test provides a comprehensive picture of his cardiac status?

   a. Remove the electrodes intermittently for hygiene measures.
   b. Exercise frequently while the monitor is in place.
   c. Keep a diary of all your activities while being monitored.
   d. Refrain from activities that precipitate symptoms.

3. Marian Barden, 68 years old, is scheduled for coronary arteriography during a cardiac catheterization. Which nursing intervention will be essential as she recovers from the diagnostic procedure on the hospital unit?

   a. Encouraging frequent ambulation to prevent deep vein thrombosis
   b. Limiting fluid intake to prevent fluid overload
   c. Evaluating cardiac status via continuous ECG monitoring
   d. Assessing arterial puncture site when taking vital signs

4. Nicholas Spagnola, 72 years old, is admitted to the Emergency Department with pulmonary edema. His symptoms include severe dyspnea, orthopnea, diaphoresis, bubbling respirations, and cyanosis. He states that he is afraid "something bad is about to happen." A recommended position for Mr. Spagnola would be:

   a. High Fowler's, with legs and feet in a dependent position.
   b. Trendelenburg, to drain the upper airways of congestion.
   c. Supine, to promote pooling of blood in the sacral area.
   d. Prone, to provide for maximal rest and decrease cardiac workload.

5. Upon further assessment of Mr. Spagnola, the nurse notes hepatomegaly, ascites, dependent edema, and jugular neck vein distention. The nurse understands that which of the following mechanisms accounts for these symptoms?

   a. End-stage cirrhosis of the liver
   b. Backward effects of right ventricular failure
   c. End-stage left ventricular failure
   d. Backward effects of lymphatic obstruction

6. Based upon the assessment data obtained on Mr. Spagnola when he was admitted to the Emergency Department, a priority nursing diagnosis is:

   a. Ineffective breathing pattern related to concern about hospitalization.
   b. Fluid volume excess related to decreased fluid intake.
   c. Decreased cardiac output related to insufficient cardiac muscle contractility.
   d. Anxiety related to ineffective breathing pattern.

7. Christopher O'Donnell has a high level of high-density lipoproteins (HDL) in proportion to low-density lipoprotein (LDL) level. How does this relate to his risk of developing coronary artery disease (CAD)?

   a. He is less likely to develop CAD.
   b. There is no direct correlation.
   c. His risk may be increased with exercise.
   d. His risk will increase with age.

8. Mr. Sheldon Levin, who is 82 years old and has been diagnosed with congestive heart failure, is hospitalized in a cardiac step-down unit. He is taking multiple cardiac medications, including digoxin and diuretics. What possible contributory factor must the nurse consider when he develops frequent premature ventricular contractions while attached to a cardiac monitor?

a. Hypocalcemia
b. Elevated creatine phosphokinase enzymes
c. Hypokalemia
d. Hyponatremia

9. Ms. Maria Vasquez, 30 years old, has a history of rheumatic fever. The nurse counsels her that a certain medical intervention should occur prior to many diagnostic tests and procedures. Which of the following interventions is indicated?

a. Anticoagulant therapy
b. Cardioversion
c. Antihypertensive therapy
d. Prophylactic antibiotic therapy

10. Sympathetic nervous system stimulation can result in essential hypertension by:

a. Causing a rebound parasympathetic nervous system response.
b. Causing the release of antidiuretic hormone (ADH), which induces vasoconstriction.
c. Causing aldosterone release and subsequent reabsorption of sodium and water.
d. Causing norepinephrine release, which constricts arterioles.

11. Bill Deutsch is a 72-year-old patient who had a total hip arthroplasty 8 days ago. He suddenly develops tenderness in his left calf, a slight temperature elevation, and a positive Homans' sign. Which of the following would be included in his initial nursing care?

a. Warm packs to the leg
b. Vigorous massage of the leg
c. Placing the leg in a dependent position
d. Applying an elastic stocking to the leg

12. Manny Esquerra, a 79-year-old patient, has congestive heart failure. When assessing Mr. Esquerra, nurse should be alert for which of the following?

a. Hepatomegaly, abdominal distention, and anascara
b. Exertional dyspnea, pulmonary rales, and cough
c. Anorexia, confusion, and jugular neck vein distention
d. Dependent edema, ascites, and cyanosis

ANSWERS

1. **Correct answer is d.** The right atrium of the heart receives deoxygenated blood from all peripheral tissues via the superior and inferior venae cavae. Additionally, the coronary sinus brings deoxygenated blood from the heart muscle itself into the right atrium. This deoxygenated blood is called venous return.

a. The pulmonary veins supply reoxygenated blood from the lungs to the left atrium.
b. Blood reoxygenated in the lungs returns to the left atrium.
c. The right ventricle receives venous blood from the right atrium during ventricular diastole.

2. **Correct answer is c.** The client should function according to his/her normal daily schedule unless directed to do otherwise by the physician. Keeping a diary or log of these daily activities is necessary so that it can be correlated with the continuous ECG monitor strip to determine whether the dysrhythmia occurs during a certain activity or at a particular time of day.

a. The Holter monitor is usually worn for only 24 hours, so it is not necessary to change the leads.
b. The client should function according to his/her normal routine unless otherwise instructed by the physician.

d. Activities that precipitate symptoms may be correlated with a dysrhythmia that can be treated, preventing further symptoms from occurring. Therefore, it would be helpful if the patient were symptomatic while attached to the Holter monitor.

3. **Correct answer is d.** Following a cardiac catheterization in which an arterial site is used for access, the puncture or cutdown site should be assessed at least as often as vital signs are monitored. The patient is at risk for development of bleeding, hemorrhage, hematoma formation, and arterial insufficiency of the affected extremity.

   a. When the arterial access site is used, the patient is on strict bed rest for at least several hours.
   b. Fluids are encouraged after catheterization to increase urinary output and flush out the dye used during the procedure.
   c. Patients are not routinely placed on a cardiac monitor after cardiac catheterization.

4. **Correct answer is a.** High Fowler's position decreases venous return to the heart by allowing blood to pool in the peripheral extremities. Decreasing venous return lowers the output of the right ventricle and decreases lung congestion. This position also allows the abdominal organs to fall away from the diaphragm.

   b. A Trendelenburg position would not promote venous pooling in the extremities but would actually increase pulmonary congestion.
   c. A supine position also would contribute to increased pulmonary congestion.
   d. A prone position, lying on the abdomen, would not allow blood to pool in the extremities.

5. **Correct answer is b.** When the right ventricle fails, congestion of the viscera and peripheral tissues results because the right side of the heart cannot adequately empty its blood volume. In addition, the heart cannot accommodate all the blood returning from the venous circulation.

a. End-stage cirrhosis is characterized by impaired gastrointestinal function, which causes esophageal varices, stomach hemorrhage, and chronic gastritis. Neurologic impairment is also evident.
c. Left ventricular failure results in symptoms that are pulmonary in nature, since the blood backs into the lungs when the left ventricle fails. Symptoms include dyspnea, cough, and fatigue.
d. Lymphatic obstruction causes symptoms that are mainly pulmonary.

6. **Correct answer is c.** Pulmonary edema usually results from heart disease that places an increased strain on the left ventricle. Although the symptoms are primarily pulmonary, intervention would focus on measures that increase cardiac output by increasing the efficiency of the heart muscle itself.

   a. Ineffective breathing patterns would be used as a nursing diagnosis in patients with pulmonary disorders, such as chronic obstructive pulmonary disease.
   b. Fluid volume excess is associated with increased fluid intake.
   d. Anxiety would not be a priority in a client who is not adequately oxygenated.

7. **Correct answer is a.** While elevated LDL levels in proportion to HDL levels are positively correlated with CAD, elevated HDL levels in proportion to LDL levels may decrease the risk of developing CAD.

   b. The relationship between HDL and LDL levels is correlated with the risk of developing CAD.
   c. HDL levels may increase with exercise, thereby decreasing a patient's risk.
   d. Age is not a predictor of HDL and LDL levels.

8. **Correct answer is c.** Serum potassium levels must be closely monitored in patients receiving digoxin and diuretics, since they are predisposed to dysrhythmias. Hypokalemia also increases sensitivity to digitalis, predisposing a patient to digitalis toxicity.

a. Hypocalcemia usually causes tetany.

b. Elevated CPK enzyme levels may indicate cardiac muscle damage.

d. Hyponatremia is not directly related to dysrhythmias.

9. **Correct answer is d.** Prophylactic antibiotic therapy is necessary to prevent complications such as rheumatic and infective endocarditis.

   a and c. Neither anticoagulant nor antihypertensive therapies would be indicated for a patient with a history of rheumatic fever prior to diagnostic tests or invasive procedures.

   b. Cardioversion is a procedure in which a pathologic cardiac rhythm is converted to a normal sinus rhythm.

10. **Correct answer is d.** Sympathetic nervous system stimulation eventually results in the release of norepinephrine, which causes blood vessels to constrict. Patients with hypertension are particularly sensitive to norepinephrine.

    a. A rebound parasympathetic response does not occur in essential hypertension.

b and c. Sympathetic nervous system stimulation does not cause ADH or aldosterone release.

11. **Correct answer is a.** Warm moist heat applied to the extremity reduces the discomfort associated with thrombophlebitis.

    b. Vigorous massage of the leg is contraindicated in any patient, since it may cause a thrombus to become dislodged.

    c. The leg should be elevated to prevent venous stasis.

    d. Elastic stockings are used for prophylaxis of deep venous thrombosis.

12. **Correct answer is b.** Signs of left-sided heart failure are pulmonary. The overworked left ventricle cannot accommodate the blood coming to it from the lungs. The increased pressure in the pulmonary circulation causes fluid to be forced into pulmonary tissues.

    a, c, and **d.** Abdominal distention, anascara, anorexia, ascites, confusion, cyanosis, dependent edema, hepatomegaly, and jugular vein distention are all signs and symptoms of right-sided heart failure.

8

Hematologic and Lymphatic Function

OVERVIEW

I. **Hematologic system**
   A. Structure and function
   B. General diagnostic tests
   C. General nursing assessments
   D. Nursing considerations with selected therapies and techniques
   E. Selected disorders

II. **Lymphatic system**
   A. Structure and function
   B. General diagnostic tests
   C. General nursing assessments
   D. Selected disorder

NURSING HIGHLIGHTS

1. Because the suffering involved in many hematologic diseases is intense, nurse should anticipate patient's concerns and crises and guide him/her toward optimal health.
2. The nurse must possess and employ excellent communication skills to determine which lifestyle and dietary modifications are beneficial for the patient with hematologic disease.
3. Since a diagnosis of leukemia may require major adjustments in the way in which patients view themselves, the nurse must help patient and family to understand the illness and treatment, redefine priorities, and maintain hope; nurse should make referrals to self-help groups such as "I Can Cope" and "Make Today Count."

GLOSSARY

cardiomegaly—hypertrophy of the heart
ecchymosis—a hemorrhagic spot on the skin that is larger than a petechia, commonly called a "bruise"
granulocyte—a cell that contains granules, especially a granular leukocyte
hemoglobinuria—the occurrence of free hemoglobin in the urine
hemolysis—the separation of free hemoglobin from erythrocytes

leukocyte—a white blood cell, whose primary function is protecting an organism against disease

lymphocyte—white blood cell

megakaryocyte—large bone marrow cell with multiple nuclei

myelogenous—producing or originating in bone marrow

petechia—a minute hemorrhagic lesion of the skin

purpura—a group of disorders in which purplish or red discoloration, caused by hemorrhage, is visible through the dermis

ENHANCED OUTLINE

I. Hematologic system

See text pages
_____

A. Structure and function
   1. Bone marrow produces blood cells, platelets, granulocytes, and some types of immune reactive cells, including lymphocytes and macrophages.
   2. Red blood cells (erythrocytes) transport hemoglobin, which carries oxygen from the lungs to tissues and carbon dioxide from tissues to the lungs for excretion.
   3. White blood cells (leukocytes), which are formed partly in bone marrow and partly in the lymphatic system, play an important role in the body's immune system.
   4. Platelets are an important part of the coagulation process; they adhere to injured blood vessel walls to form plugs, which stop the blood flow caused by injury.
   5. The spleen performs a number of functions that are critical to the hematopoietic system, including synthesizing antibodies, destroying imperfect red blood cells, and helping to metabolize iron.
   6. Kidneys produce erythropoietin, which stimulates production and differentiation of red blood cells.

B. General diagnostic tests
   1. Blood studies
      a) Purpose: to provide a range of information about hematopoietic function
      b) Representative tests: CBC, hemoglobin, prothrombin time, hematocrit, WBC count, differential, platelet count, total iron-binding capacity
   2. Bone marrow aspiration (to determine types and percentage of cells)

C. General nursing assessments
   1. Patient history: demographic and socioeconomic data; family history of hematologic problems; drugs taken, including aspirin, antibiotics, and cytotoxic agents; duration, severity, and consistency of symptoms
   2. Observation and physical examination: color of skin, mucous membranes, and nail beds; presence of skin lesions, petechiae, or ecchymoses; size of lymph nodes, spleen, and liver; signs of inflammation; exertional fatigue or shortness of breath; assistance during diagnostic test procedures

3. Diagnostic tests: nursing responsibilities
    a) Blood studies
        (1) Finger puncture procedure for obtaining blood for smears or counts: finger cleaned with alcohol and wiped dry to prevent alteration of test results due to alcohol; pulp of middle or index finger punctured
        (2) Procedure for drawing large amounts of blood: tourniquet placed around upper arm to make arm and hand veins prominent; straight vein identified and fixed in subcutaneous tissue; while stretching skin distal to vein with one hand, needle pushed through skin into vein with other hand
    b) Bone marrow aspiration
        (1) Procedure before aspiration: meperidine hydrochloride (Demerol) or minor tranquilizer administered to anxious patient; sensations that patient will feel during procedure described by nurse
        (2) Procedure during aspiration: each step in procedure explained by nurse
        (3) Procedure immediately after aspiration: pressure applied by nurse to site of entry for several minutes
        (4) Procedure for 24 hours after aspiration: aspiration site closely observed for signs of bleeding and infection; mild analgesic administered to control discomfort
D. Nursing considerations with selected therapies and techniques
    1. Blood transfusions
        a) Verify orders, explain procedure to patient, and check blood label with another nurse.
        b) Wear gloves during all procedures involving possible contact with blood.
        c) Record vital signs before transfusion; administer blood or packed red cells through 18-gauge or larger needle into large vein.
        d) Infuse blood products slowly (2 ml/min) for first 15 minutes; observe patient carefully for adverse effects; increase flow rate unless patient is at high risk for circulatory overload.
        e) Observe patient every 30 minutes during transfusion.
        f) Be aware of possible complications of blood transfusions.
            (1) Circulatory overload
                (a) Cause: pulmonary edema due to additional blood volume
                (b) Signs: dyspnea, orthopnea, cyanosis, sudden anxiety, coughing of pink frothy sputum, neck vein distention, rise in central venous pressure

(c) Medical management: patient placed in upright position with feet in dependent position; transfusion discontinued; physician notified

(d) Prevention: slow administration of packed cells rather than whole blood; careful monitoring

(2) Febrile reaction

(a) Cause: infection due to contaminated blood; sensitivity reaction to leukocyte or platelet antigens

(b) Signs

   i) Infection: fever, shaking chills within 30 minutes, shock; high mortality rate

   ii) Sensitivity reaction: fever during administration of blood or shortly thereafter, chills, malaise; good prognosis

(c) Medical management

   i) Infection: transfusion discontinued, temperature monitored for 30 minutes after chills, antipyretic administered

   ii) Sensitivity reaction: antipyretic administered

(d) Prevention

   i) Infection: scrupulous aseptic technique, blood products kept refrigerated, hospital protocol followed regarding hang times

   ii) Sensitivity reaction: avoidance of future transfusions in susceptible patients or premedication with antihistamines or antipyretics

(3) Allergic reaction

(a) Cause: sensitivity to plasma protein; passive transfer of donor antibodies that react with antigen to which recipient is exposed

(b) Signs: mild urticaria, generalized itching; wheezing or anaphylaxis (rare)

(c) Medical management: antihistamines administered; transfusion continued at slower rate if urticaria is only symptom; parenteral epinephrine administered if reaction severe

(d) Prevention: premedication of patient with antihistamines before future transfusions

(4) Septic reaction

(a) Cause: transfusion of blood or components contaminated with bacteria

(b) Symptoms: rapid onset of chills, high fever, vomiting, diarrhea, marked hypotension

(c) Medical management: transfusion discontinued immediately; blood cultures obtained; patient treated for septicemia, using antibiotics, IV fluids, vasopressors, and steroids

          (d) Prevention: blood administered within 4-hour period, before warm room temperature promotes bacterial growth; blood or components inspected before administration for gas bubbles, clotting, or abnormal color

     (5) Hemolytic reaction and delayed reaction

          (a) Cause: incompatibility of donor blood with that of recipient; hemolysis most rapid with ABO incompatibility, less severe with Rh factor incompatibility

          (b) Symptoms

               i) Immediate reaction (within 10 minutes): chills, low back pain, headache, nausea, chest tightness, fever, hypotension, vascular collapse, hemoglobinuria at next voiding

              ii) Delayed reaction (within 2–14 days): fever, mild jaundice, gradually falling hemoglobin level, possible acute hemolytic reaction caused by subsequent transfusions

          (c) Medical management: transfusion discontinued immediately, since severity of reaction proportional to volume of blood infused; IV colloid or mannitol (Osmitrol) given; urine output measured; fluids restricted and dialysis performed if evidence of acute tubular necrosis exists

          (d) Prevention: avoidance of future transfusions in susceptible patients

     (6) Nursing management for all transfusion reactions

          (a) Keep IV lines open with saline solution in case IV medication is needed.

          (b) Save blood container and tubing; send to blood bank for repeat typing and culture.

          (c) Draw patient's blood for plasma hemoglobin analysis, culture, and retyping.

          (d) Collect urine sample as soon as possible; send to lab for hemoglobin determination; and observe subsequent urinations.

          (e) Notify blood bank that suspected transfusion reaction has occurred.

  2. Bone marrow transplantation

    a) Wash hands often; follow all prescribed procedures when performing dressing changes or manipulating central venous catheter; follow hospital protocol for use of nurse and patient masks during manipulation of IV line.

    b) Remove any standing collections of water (e.g., glasses of water or denture cups) from patient's room.

c) Eliminate uncooked food from patient's diet.

d) Frequently assess patient for infection; inspect oral mucosa; auscultate lung sounds every 4 hours; inspect urine for odor or cloudiness; assess vital signs often; be aware that even a temperature elevation of 0.5°F above baseline is significant.

e) Turn patient every hour; lubricate skin; and perform pulmonary toilet every 2–4 hours, promoting coughing, deep breathing, and postural drainage.

f) Be alert for signs of graft-versus-host disease (GVHD), which is a common complication of bone marrow transplantation in which transplanted cells immunologically reject and attack the recipient's body.

   (1) Cause: attack on the immunocompromised recipient's cells, tissues, and organs by transplanted mature T lymphocytes; some degree of GVHD seen in 30%–70% of all allogeneic bone marrow transplant recipients, with a mortality rate >15%.

   (2) Signs: skin rash followed by gastrointestinal problems, including severe diarrhea and abdominal pain; fluid and electrolyte imbalances; liver disease; impaired immune function

   (3) Medical management: administration of immunosuppressive agents without overly suppressing immune system; support for tissue systems sustaining heaviest damage; no cure available

   (4) Prevention: histocompatibility testing; administration of immunosuppressant drugs combined with total body irradiation before transplantation to eliminate mature T lymphocytes, reduce risk of GVHD, and destroy malignant cells.

E. Selected disorders

  1. Anemia

    a) Definition: decrease in number of erythrocytes with abnormally low hemoglobin level, resulting in decreased oxygen to cells

    b) Pathophysiology and etiology

      (1) Anemia due to blood loss can be sudden, due to trauma, or slow, due to peptic ulcer or bleeding from intestines.

      (2) Anemia due to hemolysis can be caused by incompatible blood transfusion, infection, or exposure to toxic chemicals.

      (3) Anemia due to inadequate production of erythrocytes can be caused by bone marrow injury; lack of necessary nutrient building blocks, such as vitamin B_{12}, iron, or folic acid; or erythropoietin deficiency with renal disease.

    c) Symptoms: fatigue, anorexia, faintness, pallor

    d) Diagnostic evaluation

      (1) Blood loss: External blood loss is easily recognized; acute or chronic blood loss should be confirmed by lab tests, including CBC, hemoglobin, and hematocrit.

      (2) Severe blood loss: Total blood volume determination may be needed to guide replacement therapy.

(3) Iron deficiency: Blood smear and lab tests, including CBC, hemoglobin, hematocrit, red cell indices, and serum iron level, should be undertaken.

e) Medical treatment
   (1) Sudden blood loss: blood transfusion
   (2) Other causes: treatment of underlying condition, blood transfusion and/or iron supplementation

f) Complications: musculoskeletal injury due to falls; vascular collapse in the elderly; exacerbations of underlying cardiac disease, manifesting as angina or symptoms of congestive heart failure

g) Essential nursing care for patients with anemia
   (1) Nursing assessment
      (a) Perform physical exam, evaluating skin and mucous membranes for pallor, dryness, and jaundice.
      (b) Perform cardiac assessment, including noting of vital signs, weight, and dyspnea on exertion.
   (2) Nursing diagnoses
      (a) Activity intolerance related to decreased erythrocyte count
      (b) Altered nutrition, less than body requirements, related to anorexia
      (c) Knowledge deficit related to methods of prevention
   (3) Nursing intervention
      (a) Record daily activity level and establish activity goals; prevent falls; provide frequent rest; space timing of activities.
      (b) Provide information about treatment and follow-up care.
      (c) Explain appropriate use of iron or vitamin B_{12} supplements.
   (4) Nursing evaluation
      (a) Patient tolerates increased activity.
      (b) Patient's appetite improves; patient eats well-balanced meals.
      (c) Patient demonstrates understanding of treatment.

2. Sickle cell anemia
  a) Definition: incurable hereditary blood disease found primarily in blacks in which deformed, sickle-shaped red blood cells cause a chronic form of anemia
  b) Pathophysiology and etiology: Deformed red blood cells block small blood vessels, reducing blood flow.
  c) Symptoms
    (1) Chronic symptoms: anemia, jaundice, tachycardia, dyspnea, cardiomegaly, cardiac dysrhythmias, chronic leg ulcers, priapism

(2) Symptoms of sickle cell crisis: sudden fever, pain, and joint swelling
  d) Diagnostic evaluation
    (1) Sickle cell screening tests to determine presence of abnormal hemoglobin
    (2) Hemoglobin electrophoresis to determine whether patient is an asymptomatic carrier or has the disease
  e) Medical treatment
    (1) Chronic disorder: Treat infections promptly.
    (2) Sickle cell crisis: Provide patient with supplemental oxygen, bed rest, blood transfusions, analgesics, and increased fluids.
  f) Complications: tissue ischemia or infarction, necrosis of head of femur, or gallstones; renal failure, shock, pulmonary infarction, and cerebrovascular accident as a result of sickle cell crisis
  g) Essential nursing care for patients with sickle cell anemia
    (1) Nursing assessment
      (a) Examine patient for jaundice.
      (b) Check patient for early signs of chronic dermal ulcers on legs.
      (c) Assess patient for presence of dyspnea, cardiac dysrhythmias, tachycardia, and cardiomegaly.
    (2) Nursing diagnoses
      (a) Pain related to accumulation of deformed blood cells in peripheral vessels
      (b) Body image disturbance related to chronic leg ulcers
      (c) Personal identity disturbance related to unpredictable recurrence of sickle cell crisis
    (3) Nursing intervention
      (a) Administer analgesics (patients in crisis often require large amounts of narcotics), give whirlpool bath, position patient properly, and notify physician if pain suddenly becomes more intense.
      (b) Instruct patient to attempt to avoid situations and places that may lead to hypoxia and dehydration, including general anesthesia, extreme heat, and high altitudes.
    (4) Nursing evaluation
      (a) Patient and family members understand hereditary aspects of sickle cell disease and agree to undergo genetic counseling and testing.
      (b) Patient prevents permanent tissue damage by recognizing and responding to early signs of sickle cell crisis.
      (c) Patient avoids factors that may trigger sickle cell crisis, including excessive alcohol consumption, dehydration, fatigue, and emotional stress.
3. Aplastic anemia (bone marrow failure)
  a) Definition: depressed bone marrow activity with low production of erythrocytes, leukocytes, and platelets

b) Pathophysiology and etiology
    (1) Side effect of certain drugs (e.g., streptomycin sulfate, chloramphenicol [Chloroptic], or mechlorethamine [Mustargen]) and of exposure to toxic chemicals and radiation
    (2) May be intentionally caused in patients undergoing bone marrow transplants
c) Symptoms: severe anemia, leukopenia, thrombocytopenia, fatigue, weakness, exertional dyspnea, lowered resistance to infection, tendency toward bleeding
d) Diagnostic evaluation: patient history, general hematologic lab tests, bone marrow biopsy
e) Medical treatment: withdrawal of any causative agent(s); bone marrow transplantation; administration of immunosuppressive therapy with antithymocyte globulin (ATG); blood transfusions; antibiotics for treatment of infection; high doses of corticosteroids
f) Complications: extensive hemorrhage, severe infection
g) Essential nursing care for patients with aplastic anemia
    (1) Nursing assessment
        (a) Assess patient for signs of severe anemia and bleeding.
        (b) Check patient continually for early symptoms of infection, and report them immediately.
    (2) Nursing diagnoses
        (a) Knowledge deficit related to immunosuppressive therapy with ATG
        (b) Potential for infection related to poor nutrition
        (c) High risk for impaired skin integrity related to tissue hypoxia
    (3) Nursing intervention
        (a) Assist patient in taking steps to minimize exertion associated with daily activities.
        (b) Explain to patient the importance of maintaining normal bowel function, and help with meal planning.
        (c) Advise patient to avoid tasks that may injure skin and to practice good skin care.
    (4) Nursing evaluation
        (a) Patient understands that response to ATG therapy may be delayed for 6 months.
        (b) Patient avoids situations and behaviors that can cause infection.
        (c) Oral mucous membrane is intact, with no evidence of bleeding or ulceration.

4. Leukemia
   a) Definition: any of several types of cancer in which there is a disorganized proliferation of white blood cells in the bone marrow
   b) Pathophysiology and etiology
      (1) Red blood cells, platelets, and normal white blood cells are crowded out of the marrow by leukemic cells.
      (2) Other organs, including the liver and spleen, may stop functioning properly as they become infiltrated by leukemic cells.
      (3) The excessive number of abnormal white blood cells interferes with the body's ability to fight infection.
      (4) Knowledge of causes is incomplete, although exposure to toxic chemicals and radiation are recognized causes.
   c) Symptoms
      (1) Acute myelogenous leukemia (AML) or chronic myelogenous leukemia (CML): anemia, infection, bleeding, lymphadenopathy, splenomegaly, hepatomegaly, joint and bone pain, thrombocytopenia, leukopenia
      (2) Acute lymphocytic leukemia (ALL): fever, bleeding, enlarged lymph nodes, fatigue, weakness, symptoms of "blast crisis"
      (3) Chronic lymphocytic leukemia (CLL): no symptoms or mild symptoms, including anemia, weakness, fatigue, fever; blast crisis
   d) Diagnostic evaluation: examination of peripheral blood, bone marrow, computed tomography (CT), magnetic resonance imaging (MRI), lymphangiogram, and biopsy of lymph nodes
   e) Medical treatment
      (1) AML: chemotherapy with agents such as mercaptopurine (Purinethol) and daunorubicin hydrochloride (Cerubidine), red cell and platelet transfusions, bone marrow transplantation
      (2) CML: chemotherapy with agents such as busulfan (Myleran) and hydroxyurea (Hydrea)
      (3) ALL: chemotherapy with combinations of asparaginase (Elspar), daunorubicin hydrochloride (Cerubidine), prednisone (Deltasone), and vincristine (Vincrex), followed by maintenance therapy with mercaptopurine (Purinethol), methotrexate (Folex), prednisone (Deltasone), and vincristine (Vincrex); craniospinal irradiation
      (4) CLL: chemotherapy with steroids and chlorambucil (Leukeran)
   f) Complications: hemorrhage, severe infections that may not respond to antibiotic therapy
   g) Essential nursing care for patients with leukemia
      (1) Nursing assessment
         (a) Inquire about current symptoms and those experienced in the recent past.
         (b) Review results of laboratory tests.
         (c) Examine patient for evidence of bruising and bleeding.

      (2) Nursing diagnoses

        (a) Body image disturbance related to alopecia

        (b) Fear related to economic cost of treatment and need for assistance with activities of daily life

        (c) Pain related to accumulation of leukocytes in tissues

      (3) Nursing intervention

        (a) Provide emotional support, encouraging patient to talk about personal and financial concerns.

        (b) Monitor patient's vital signs every 4 hours and report any increase in temperature; administer acetaminophen (Tylenol) rather than aspirin (Easprin) for fever control.

        (c) Administer analgesic, if needed, and place pillows at patient's back and knees to increase comfort; practice symptom control for side effects of chemotherapy.

        (d) Provide information regarding continuing treatment at home to patient and family members (see Client Teaching Checklist, "Home Care for Leukemia Patients").

      (4) Nursing evaluation

        (a) Patient is able to carry out activities of daily living.

        (b) Patient assumes positions that cause the least amount of discomfort.

        (c) Patient understands the importance of continued follow-up care and monitoring after discharge from the hospital.

5. Multiple myeloma

    a) Definition: a malignant disorder in which immature plasma cells proliferate in bone marrow, forming single or multiple osteolytic tumors

    b) Pathophysiology and etiology

      (1) Proliferating plasma cells produce excessive amounts of a single type of immunoglobulin.

      (2) Production of other cell types is impaired, making patient prone to infection.

      (3) Neoplastic plasma cells eventually infiltrate liver, spleen, soft tissues, and kidneys.

    c) Symptoms: vague pain in pelvis, spine, or ribs, eventually becoming more severe and localized; pathologic fractures, with decreased resistance to infection; anemia

    d) Diagnostic evaluation: skeletal radiographic studies revealing punched-out bone lesions; aspiration or biopsy of bone marrow

    e) Medical treatment: chemotherapy including melphalan (Alkeran), cyclophosphamide (Cytoxan), and steroids to relieve bone pain and decrease tumor size; radiation; blood transfusions

    f) Complications: severe infection, renal failure

Home Care for Leukemia Patients

Instruct client with leukemia to follow these guidelines:

✔ Avoid physical injury and exposure to colds and infections.
✔ Maintain balanced diet.
✔ Obtain adequate rest.
✔ Continue normal activities unless otherwise directed.
✔ Contact physician or nurse if mouth sores occur rather than attempting self-treatment.
✔ Follow physician's directions concerning monitoring of temperature and weight; report for frequent monitoring of blood and bone marrow.
✔ Contact physician immediately if you experience:
— Severe nausea with prolonged vomiting
— Severe diarrhea
— Fever
— Chills
— Excessive bleeding or bruising
— Cough
— Chest pain
— Cloudy urine
— Rash
— Bloody stool or urine
— Severe headache
— Extreme fatigue
— Breathing problems

g) Essential nursing care for patients with multiple myeloma
   (1) Nursing assessment
       (a) Assess patient for signs of renal insufficiency.
       (b) Dispense with fasting requirement for diagnostic tests because of acute renal failure due to dehydration.
       (c) Determine patient's level of pain and efficacy of prescribed analgesics.
   (2) Nursing diagnoses
       (a) Pain related to osteolytic bone lesions
       (b) Anxiety related to diagnosis
       (c) Impaired physical mobility related to pathologic fractures
       (d) Fluid volume excess or deficit related to renal failure
   (3) Nursing intervention
       (a) Increase patient's comfort by administering analgesics and using back brace or bivalve cast.
       (b) Provide emotional support, and encourage patient to discuss feelings.

            (c) Encourage patient to continue to walk, but to do so with care.

            (d) Stress the necessity of adequate hydration; measure fluid intake and output.

      (4) Nursing evaluation

            (a) Patient undertakes activities at times of day when analgesic efficacy is greatest.

            (b) Patient verbalizes feelings and reports reduced anxiety.

            (c) Patient states understanding of the dangers associated with immobility.

            (d) Patient understands importance of avoiding infections and even minor injuries.

            (e) Patient attains and maintains normal fluid intake.

  6. Hemophilia

    a) Definition: hereditary clotting factor disorder characterized by prolonged coagulation time, which can result in persistent and severe bleeding

    b) Pathophysiology and etiology

      (1) Hemophilia A caused by deficiency of factor VIII clotting activity; hemophilia B by deficiency of factor IX clotting activity

      (2) Both forms of disorder transmitted from mother to son as an X-linked recessive characteristic

    c) Symptoms: persistent bleeding into soft tissues, muscles, and joints after even minor injuries; joint pain; spontaneous gastrointestinal bleeding and hematuria

    d) Diagnostic evaluation: symptom history, family history, and coagulant factor assay

    e) Medical treatment

      (1) Administration of factor VIII or IX (Konyne-HT) or cryoprecipitate to treat acute bleeding or as preventive measure before surgery or dental extraction

      (2) Administration of aminocaproic acid (Amicar) to slow dissolution of blood clots

    f) Complications: severe joint damage or destruction due to recurrent bleeding; AIDS and other infectious diseases from use of contaminated blood and blood products

    g) Essential nursing care for patients with hemophilia

      (1) Nursing assessment

          (a) Check patient's vital signs and hemodynamic levels for evidence of hypovolemia.

          (b) Assess patient for signs of internal bleeding.

          (c) Inspect joints for swelling, limited movement, and pain.

          (d) Examine torso and limbs for hematomas.

(2) Nursing diagnoses
    (a) Anxiety related to fear of uncontrolled hemorrhage
    (b) Pain related to disease process
    (c) Impaired tissue integrity related to bleeding episodes
    (d) Knowledge deficit related to methods of preventing future bleeding episodes
(3) Nursing intervention
    (a) Suggest ways in which patient can perform activities of daily living without incurring further joint damage.
    (b) Explain that crutches, braces, and other assistive devices are only beneficial if they are properly adjusted for patient.
    (c) After ruling out internal bleeding as a cause of pain, administer nonaspirin-based analgesics when ordered.
    (d) Inspect skin for presence of new ecchymotic lesions, and examine old lesions for evidence of new bleeding; check for bright red clumps of blood in stool and vomitus.
    (e) Avoid intramuscular injections whenever possible, and provide prolonged pressure on the injection site if IM administration is necessary and on venipuncture sites after needle is removed; avoid taking temperature or administering drugs rectally.
(4) Nursing evaluation
    (a) Patient has an increased ability to perform activities of daily living.
    (b) Patient's bleeding episodes are controlled or eliminated.
    (c) Joint pain is reduced or eliminated.
    (d) Patient is able to plan activities that are unlikely to result in bleeding and injury.

7. Autoimmune thrombocytopenic purpura
  a) Definition: deficient number of platelets circulating in the blood
  b) Pathophysiology and etiology
    (1) Antibodies are directed to and coat the surface of the body's own platelets, making them more susceptible to destruction by phagocytic leukocytes.
    (2) Antibody-coated platelets are destroyed, primarily in the spleen.
    (3) When platelet destruction rate exceeds platelet production rate, the number of circulating platelets decreases and blood clotting slows.
    (4) Etiology appears to be autoimmune, but it may be related to an immune system defect caused by viral infection.
  c) Symptoms: purpura; extensive bruising on arms, legs, upper chest, and neck; spontaneous bleeding from nose, oral mucous membrane, and gastrointestinal tract; excessive menstrual bleeding; hemorrhage after dental extraction or surgery

    d) Diagnostic evaluation
      (1) Blood tests to screen for decreased platelet count, bleeding, and clotting times; low hematocrit and hemoglobin levels; antiplatelet antibodies in peripheral blood
      (2) Bone marrow aspiration to screen for large numbers of megakaryocytes
    e) Medical treatment
      (1) Transfusion of whole blood or platelets in hemorrhagic emergency
      (2) Administration of corticosteroids for symptomatic relief when platelet count is depressed
      (3) Splenectomy if patient fails to respond to more conservative treatment
      (4) Administration of an immunosuppressive agent, such as cyclophosphamide (Cytoxan) or azathioprine (Imuran), if patient remains symptomatic after splenectomy
    f) Complications: spontaneous fatal gastrointestinal or central nervous system hemorrhage
    g) Essential nursing care for patients with autoimmune thrombocytopenic purpura
      (1) Nursing assessment
        (a) Examine patient for extensive bruising.
        (b) Assess patient for evidence of internal bleeding.
        (c) Inquire about frequent nosebleeds, bleeding from gums, and, in younger female patients, excessive menstrual bleeding.
      (2) Nursing diagnoses
        (a) Impaired tissue integrity related to bleeding episodes
        (b) Body image disturbance related to extensive bruising
        (c) Anxiety related to frequent nosebleeds
      (3) Nursing intervention
        (a) Advise patient to avoid agents that may increase bleeding, such as aspirin-based products and alcohol.
        (b) Teach patient to recognize and report immediately signs of internal bleeding.
      (4) Nursing evaluation
        (a) Patient understands that uncontrolled bleeding can result from routine procedures, such as dental extractions, and advises all health care professionals of his/her condition.
        (b) Patient wears medical alert identification.
        (c) Patient is aware of and is attentive to potentially dangerous side effects of steroid therapy.

II. Lymphatic system

A. Structure and function
   1. Central lymphoid tissues (thymus, bone marrow, spleen, and liver): stimulate lymphocyte development and differentiation
   2. Lymph nodes: bean-shaped bodies in the axilla, groin, and neck and along the large vessels of the thorax and abdomen that remove foreign bodies from lymph fluid
   3. Lymph fluid: substance that passes through lymph ducts and contains antibodies, lymphocytes, granulocytes, and enzymes

B. General diagnostic tests
   1. Blood studies: provide a range of information about hematopoietic function; typically include CBC, WBC count, differential
   2. Lymph node biopsy: primarily useful if malignant process is suspected
   3. Lymphangiography
      a) Determines lymph fluid flow and involvement of lymph nodes and lymphatic tissues in metastatic carcinoma, lymphomas, and infections
      b) Radiographs taken after radiopaque substance is injected into lymphatic vessels of hands or feet

C. General nursing assessments
   1. Patient history: If an infectious process exists, inquire about the onset of symptoms and the possible cause(s).
   2. Observation and physical examination: size, location, and texture of lymph nodes; condition of adjacent skin

D. Selected disorder: Hodgkin's disease (Hodgkin's lymphoma)
   1. Definition: a malignant disorder of the lymphoid tissue marked by proliferation of constituent cells and resulting in lymph node enlargement
   2. Pathophysiology and etiology: of unknown cause; characterized by enlarged, painless lymph nodes; occurring more often in men than women, usually in young adulthood
   3. Symptoms
      a) Generalized pruritus
      b) Presence of several enlarged but painless lymph nodes
      c) Fullness in stomach, epigastric pain
      d) Marked weight loss, fatigue, anorexia, weakness, chills and fever, anemia, thrombocytopenia
      e) Poor resistance to infection, with frequent staphylococcal skin infections and respiratory tract infections
   4. Diagnostic evaluation
      a) Biopsy of affected lymph nodes
      b) Chest radiography, bone scan, lymphangiography
      c) After diagnosis, exploratory laparotomy performed to determine extent of disease; disease staged as I through IV on the basis of number of affected lymph nodes and involvement of other organs and structures

5. Medical treatment
   a) Radiation therapy
   b) Drug therapy, including corticosteroids, antineoplastics (nitrogen mustard, vincristine [Vincrex], prednisone [Deltasone], procarbazine [Matulane]), and antibiotics
   c) Transfusions, if necessary
6. Complications: severe edema and life-threatening infections; sterility due to radiation treatments (males may bank sperm before treatments begin)
7. Essential nursing care for patients with Hodgkin's disease
   a) Nursing assessment: Check for involvement of additional lymph nodes.
   b) Nursing diagnoses
      (1) Ineffective individual coping related to diagnosis
      (2) Potential for infection related to decreased immune system activity
      (3) Altered nutrition, less than body requirements, related to abdominal and gastrointestinal involvement
      (4) Impaired skin integrity related to radiation therapy
   c) Nursing intervention
      (1) Help patient to identify sources of anxiety and to vocalize concerns; counsel patient regarding possible sterility due to radiation therapy.
      (2) Monitor vital signs every 4 hours, and assess for early signs of infection, especially in patient with leukopenia.
      (3) Serve soft, bland diet in small portions, 4–6 times per day.
      (4) Relieve pruritus with cool sponge baths, and, when prescribed for severe cases, administer antipruritic medication.
      (5) Explain all procedures and treatments to patient (see Client Teaching Checklist, "Home Care for Hodgkin's Disease Patients").
   d) Nursing evaluation
      (1) Patient and family identify and address problems related to diagnosis.
      (2) Signs of infection are absent, and vital signs are normal.
      (3) Patient eats a balanced diet, drinks extra fluids, and maintains weight.

Home Care for Hodgkin's Disease Patients

Instruct client with Hodgkin's disease to observe these guidelines:

✔ Resume normal activities as soon as possible.
✔ Avoid exposure to infection.
✔ Eat a well-balanced diet.
✔ Drink plenty of fluids.
✔ Immediately report the following symptoms to physician:
— Fever
— Cough
— Severe malaise
— Recurrence of enlarged lymph nodes

1. Which of the following actions would the nurse expect to perform after a patient has a bone marrow biopsy taken from the iliac crest?

   a. Apply pressure to the site for 1 minute.
   b. Administer a narcotic analgesic.
   c. Apply an adhesive bandage to the site.
   d. Place the patient in a recumbent position.

2. A patient with anemia is to receive 1 unit of packed red blood cells. The nurse will plan to administer the unit over which period of time?

   a. 30 minutes–1 hour
   b. 2–3 hours
   c. 4–5 hours
   d. 1–2 hours

3. Miriam Rothko, a patient with acute myelogenous leukemia (AML), had an allogeneic bone marrow transplant 3 days ago. To monitor Ms. Rothko for development of graft-versus-host disease (GVHD), the nurse will watch for:

   a. A temperature >101°F.
   b. Development of a skin rash.
   c. Bleeding from the gums.
   d. Crackles in the lungs.

4. The assessment data for a female patient with anorexia nervosa include: hemoglobin 6.0 g/dl; weight 70 lb; height 5´9´´; dyspnea on ambulation; and pale skin and mucous membranes. Based on this information, which of the following nursing diagnoses would have the highest priority in the nurse's care plan?

   a. High risk for impaired skin integrity related to decreased tissue perfusion
   b. Knowledge deficit related to dietary iron deficiency
   c. Activity intolerance related to dyspnea and weakness
   d. Altered nutrition, less than body requirements, related to anorexia

5. The nurse writes "Knowledge deficit regarding prevention of crisis" on the nursing care plan of Anthony Laker, 18-year-old male with sickle cell anemia. After Mr. Laker has been taught to avoid situations that can precipitate a crisis, which of the following actions would indicate a need for follow-up education?

   a. Applying for a driver's permit
   b. Planning a vacation at a beach resort
   c. Staying up until 3:00 A.M. to study for a test
   d. Applying antiseptic to a cut on his finger

6. In a patient suspected of having aplastic anemia, the nurse should plan to:

   a. Take a thorough history of medication and chemical exposures.
   b. Assess for renal disease, and administer prescribed folic acid.
   c. Teach the patient which foods have a high iron content, and administer prescribed iron.
   d. Assess the patient for signs of infection, and administer ordered prophylactic antibiotics.

7. Which of the following observations reported by a patient with acute myelogenous leukemia (AML) would the nurse first assess?

   a. Weakness and fatigue
   b. Bruising on the arm
   c. Drainage from a small finger cut
   d. Mild abdominal pain

8. The nurse has reviewed a discharge teaching checklist for Victor Sheets, a 65-year-old male with chronic lymphocytic leukemia (CLL). Which of the following statements by Mr. Sheets would indicate to the nurse that further review is necessary?

   a. "I'm retired, so I can sleep whenever I want."
   b. "I've got season tickets for all the basketball games."
   c. "I'll call the doctor if I have a fever over 99°F."

d. "I'm going to teach my grandson how to fish."

9. Maureen Jenkins, a patient with multiple myeloma, is admitted to the hospital with a pathologic fracture of the tibia and is ordered to be on bed rest. Which of the following nursing actions would be appropriate?

   a. Raising the head of the bed to a 10° angle
   b. Turning the patient on her side once a shift
   c. Having the patient fast before a scheduled x-ray
   d. Accurate recording of fluid intake and output

10. During the past 3 months, Rick Cassidy, a 13-year-old with hemophilia A, has suddenly had an increased number of admissions for bleeding episodes. In planning for his discharge, the nurse should:

    a. Advise the patient to stop going to school.
    b. Encourage him to depend on his parents to provide his care.
    c. Question him and his parents about possible exposure to trauma.
    d. Instruct his parents to give him aspirin for joint discomfort.

11. The nurse would give immediate consideration to which of the following assessment findings in a female patient with autoimmune thrombocytopenic purpura?

    a. Petechiae on the chest
    b. Cold moist skin
    c. Bruising on the arms
    d. Heavy menstrual flow

12. A patient newly diagnosed with Hodgkin's disease will most often report which of the following symptoms to the nurse when providing a history?

    a. Generalized pruritus
    b. Petechiae across the back
    c. Nausea and vomiting
    d. Weight gain

ANSWERS

1. **Correct answer is d.** The patient should lie in bed in a recumbent position on top of a pressure dressing that has been applied to the site. Hemorrhage poses a slight risk after this procedure.

   a and c. Pressure should be applied to the site for several minutes. A pressure dressing should then be applied for 1 hour to reduce the chances of bleeding or hemorrhage. **b.** An analgesic may be ordered and administered prior to the procedure. Use of deep breathing and relaxation techniques may also be helpful. There is seldom pain after the biopsy, although the site may ache for a few days.

2. **Correct answer is b.** The unit of packed cells should be infused over a period of 2–3 hours. If it is infused over a shorter period, there is a greater chance of circulatory overload.

   a and d. Periods of 30 minutes to an hour and 1–2 hours are too short. Such a time frame does not allow enough time to monitor the patient for an adverse reaction to the blood. The blood should run very slowly at 2 ml per minute during the first 15 minutes. **c.** The duration of administration of a blood transfusion should not exceed 4 hours.

3. **Correct answer is b.** A skin rash is usually the first sign of GVHD. Most tissues can be attacked by the disease, but the most common sites of symptoms are the skin, GI tract, and liver.

   a and d. A patient who has received a bone marrow transplant is at risk for developing an infection until the donor marrow has been accepted (usually within about 10 days). Taking the temperature and listening to the lungs would be done to monitor the patient for infection. Fever and crackles would not indicate GVHD. **c.** Monitoring the patient for bleeding from the gums would be done to detect a clotting abnormality. It would not indicate GVHD.

4. Correct answer is d. Anorexia nervosa is a severe eating disorder in which very limited amounts of food and nutrients are consumed. Among many other complications, anorexia results in anemia, as indicated in the assessment data. Inadequate intake of iron, vitamin B_{12}, and folic acid leads to anemia. If adequate nutrients are taken in and absorbed by the body through diet or supplementation, the anemia and its symptoms should improve. Thus, altered nutrition is the highest priority diagnosis.

a and **c.** High risk for impaired skin integrity and activity intolerance are other appropriate diagnoses related to anemia. Decreased hemoglobin levels lead to decreased oxygenation of the body tissues.

b. The patient does not necessarily have a knowledge deficit. Anorexia nervosa is an indirect self-destructive behavior.

5. Correct answer is c. Fatigue can precipitate a crisis. The patient needs to identify and change lifestyle patterns that can precipitate crises.

a and **b.** Becoming a licensed driver and taking a vacation are both appropriate activities. Patients with sickle cell anemia should be encouraged to lead as normal a life as possible.

d. Taking preventive action to avoid infection indicates that the patient is attempting to maintain his well-being.

6. Correct answer is a. The underlying cause of aplastic anemia is unknown, but exposure to certain drugs, chemicals, radiation, and infections has been linked to the disorder. It is believed that these agents cause depressed bone marrow activity and lead to the replacement of marrow by fat cells.

b. Administering folic acid is appropriate for patients in whom anemia is associated with renal disease. If the patient receives dialysis, folic acid should be given to replace what passes into the dialysate.

c. Recommending iron-rich foods and administering supplemental iron are appropriate for patients with iron deficiency anemia.

d. The patient with aplastic anemia is at risk for development of infection as a result of the development of granulocytopenia. However, administration of prophylactic antibiotics is not recommended for patients with neutropenia because resistant bacteria and fungi may emerge.

7. Correct answer is c. Because of the granulocytopenia associated with AML, these patients are at high risk for development of infection. Infection is the major cause of death in patients with leukemia, and therefore the slightest indications of infection must be assessed and treated at once.

a. Weakness and fatigue occur in patients with AML as a result of anemia caused by defective erythropoiesis.

b. Bruising occurs in patients with AML as a result of thrombocytopenia. Bleeding tendencies are usually associated with fever or infection.

d. Abdominal pain is often reported in patients with AML due to enlargement of the liver and spleen. Since the pain in this case is mild, it does not have priority over a possible infection.

8. Correct answer is b. Patients with leukemia must avoid exposure to respiratory colds and infections. Attending basketball games exposes Mr. Sheets to crowds and therefore to the risk (especially during basketball season) of acquiring a respiratory infection with life-threatening complications.

a. The patient needs to get adequate rest.

c. The patient is correct to contact the physician when his temperature is elevated.

d. Normal and pleasurable activities like fishing that are not associated with risk of infection or trauma should be continued and encouraged.

9. **Correct answer is d.** Patients with multiple myeloma must be well hydrated to prevent precipitation of Bence-Jones protein in the renal tubules, which could cause renal damage. Recording fluid intake and output allows the nurse to determine whether adequate amounts of fluids are being taken in.

a and **b.** Because patients with multiple myeloma are at risk for developing bacterial infections, especially pneumonia, preventive measures must be taken. Raising the head of the bed by 10° is not sufficient to allow for lung expansion; a 45° angle would be more appropriate. Turning the patient to prevent skin breakdown and improve lung expansion should be done every 2–3 hours.

c. Fasting for diagnostic tests should not be done, since the patient must be well hydrated to prevent renal damage and acute renal failure.

10. **Correct answer is c.** The patient and his parents should be questioned about the possible reasons for the increased number of bleeding episodes. They may need further education or counseling to prevent trauma exposure and thus reduce the number of bleeding episodes.

a and **b.** Patients with hemophilia should be encouraged to accept themselves and their disease. They should also be encouraged to be self-sufficient and to maintain their independence rather than becoming dependent. The nurse should not discourage school attendance but may need to discuss ways to avoid injury at school.

d. Aspirin should not be given to patients with hemophilia, since it may cause bleeding. Other analgesics and pain reduction methods should be used.

11. **Correct answer is b.** Cold moist skin is one of the signs of shock. This finding indicates possible internal bleeding, which is a complication of autoimmune thrombocytopenic purpura.

a, c, and **d.** Petechiae, bruising, and heavy menstrual flow are all symptoms of this disease. Antiplatelet antibodies are produced in the body; these attack the platelets, causing a decreased platelet count and increased risk of bleeding.

12. **Correct answer is a.** Generalized pruritus may be the first and only symptom of Hodgkin's disease to appear for months. Along with lymph node enlargement, it is a common symptom of Hodgkin's disease.

b. Thrombocytopenia is a possible complication of Hodgkin's disease, but development of petechiae is not the most frequently reported symptom.

c. Nausea and vomiting are not the most common symptoms, although fullness in the stomach and epigastric pain are frequently reported.

d. Weight loss is usually reported.

9

Nervous System Function

OVERVIEW

I. Structure and function of nervous system
  A. Central nervous system
  B. Peripheral nervous system

II. General diagnostic tests
  A. Electroencephalography
  B. Lumbar puncture
  C. Contrast studies
  D. Imaging

III. General nursing assessments
  A. Patient history
  B. Observation and physical examination
  C. Diagnostic tests

IV. Nursing considerations associated with selected therapies and techniques
  A. Nursing assessment
  B. Nursing diagnoses
  C. Nursing intervention
  D. Nursing evaluation

V. Selected disorders
  A. Head injury
  B. Migraine
  C. Seizure disorders
  D. Myasthenia gravis
  E. Guillain-Barré syndrome
  F. Brain tumor
  G. Spinal cord injury
  H. Alzheimer's disease
  I. Stroke
  J. Parkinson's disease
  K. Multiple sclerosis

NURSING HIGHLIGHTS

1. Nurse should emphasize caring and quiet concern as patients deal with the intense psychologic trauma associated with neurologic deficits.
2. Nurse must constantly encourage and praise each patient during rehabilitation for a neurologic deficit; showing interest in each accomplishment may help patients accept what they cannot do.
3. Management of a patient with a neurologic disorder requires the cooperation of all health care team members.
4. Most neurologic disorders do not affect cognition or intellect but do affect their expression or performance. Nurse should treat each individual as a mature adult.

acetylcholine—a neurotransmitter at cholinergic synapses in the central and peripheral nervous systems

automatism—unconscious performance of a nonreflex action

dementia—loss of intellectual function due to organic or inorganic causes

dopamine—an intermediate product of norepinephrine synthesis that acts as a neurotransmitter in the central nervous system

graphesthesia—recognition of a number or letter when it is traced onto a body surface, usually the palm of the hand

myelin—the fatty substance that surrounds the axon of many types of nerve fibers

oculogyration—movement of the eye about the anteroposterior axis

pill-rolling tremor—a characteristic sign of Parkinson's disease in which the thumb moves along the distal second and third digits of the hand

plasmapheresis—removal of plasma from blood withdrawn from the body, followed by retransfusion

stereognosis—recognition of an object placed in the hand by its feel

ENHANCED OUTLINE

I. Structure and function of nervous system

See text pages
_____

A. Central nervous system (CNS)
   1. Brain
      a) Major anatomic divisions: anterior fossa (frontal and cerebral hemispheres); middle fossa (parietal, temporal, and occipital lobes); posterior fossa (brain stem and medulla)
      b) Coverings of brain
         (1) Skull
         (2) Meninges (membranes)
            (a) Dura mater: the outermost membrane that covers the brain and spinal cord, consisting of the falx cerebri, which longitudinally separates the 2 brain hemispheres, and the tentorium, a shelf that supports the hemispheres and keeps them separate from the posterior fossa
            (b) Arachnoid: the middle membrane, which resembles a delicate spider's web, in which cerebrospinal fluid (CSF) is produced and partially absorbed
            (c) Pia mater: the inner membrane, which covers every part of the brain
      c) Functional units of brain
         (1) Cerebrum: the largest part of the brain, comprising a frontal and cerebral hemisphere and the following 4 lobes:
            (a) Frontal lobe: located in the anterior fossa, controlling personality, judgment, affect, and inhibitions

           (b) Parietal lobe: located in the middle fossa, controlling the interpretation of sensations and affecting all senses except smell

           (c) Temporal lobe: located in the middle fossa, controlling taste, smell, hearing, and short-term memory

           (d) Occipital lobe: located in the middle fossa, controlling visual interpretation

        (2) Additional structures within middle fossa

           (a) Thalamus: memory and pain impulse control; coordination of all senses except smell

           (b) Hypothalamus: autonomic nervous system, emotion, and weight control; water, temperature, sleep, and blood pressure regulation

           (c) Pituitary gland: kidney, pancreas, and reproductive organ control

        (3) Structures of posterior fossa

           (a) Brain stem

              i) Midbrain, which connects the pons and cerebellum to the cerebral hemispheres

              ii) Pons, which connects the 2 halves of the cerebellum and the medulla oblongata and cerebrum

           (b) Medulla oblongata, which transmits motor fibers from the brain to the spinal cord and sensory fibers from the spinal cord to the brain; controls heart, respiration, and blood pressure; contains the origin of the fifth through eighth cranial nerves

  2. Spinal cord

    a) A continuous structure, protected by the vertebral column, extending from the foramen magnum at the base of the skull to the second lumbar vertebra

    b) Functions as a passageway for ascending sensory and descending motor neurons and as a center for reflex action

B. Peripheral nervous system (PNS)

  1. Cranial nerves: 12 pairs of nerves identified by roman numerals

  2. Spinal nerves: 31 pairs, each pair consisting of a dorsal root (motor fibers) and a ventral root (sensory fibers)

  3. Autonomic nervous system

    a) Sympathetic nervous system, which regulates energy expenditure and the body's response to stress, and which has 2 associated neurohormones, epinephrine and norepinephrine

    b) Parasympathetic nervous system, which conserves energy by controlling food digestion and waste elimination and by slowing heart rate

II. General diagnostic tests

See text pages
_____

A. Electroencephalography
  1. Definition: the mapping of electrical activity generated by the brain via electrodes on the scalp or microelectrodes within the brain
  2. Purpose: to diagnose seizure disorders; to screen for organic brain syndrome, tumor, abscess, scarring, or clots; to determine brain death

B. Lumbar puncture (spinal tap)
  1. Definition: insertion of a spinal needle into the subarachnoid space between the third and fourth lumbar vertebrae, or sometimes between the fourth and fifth vertebrae
  2. Purpose: to take pressure readings, obtain CSF for analysis, inject contrast medium or air for diagnostic purposes, check for spinal blockage, inject spinal anesthetic or other drugs, or reduce minor intracranial pressure (ICP)

C. Contrast studies
  1. Myelography
     a) Definition: injection, after lumbar puncture, of radiopaque substance into spinal canal, followed by removal of dye through spinal needle
     b) Purpose: to highlight abnormal spinal canal due to tumors or ruptured disks
  2. Cerebral angiography
     a) Definition: radiologic study of cerebral circulation, which is highlighted by contrast dye injected into artery
     b) Purpose: to diagnose vascular disease, aneurysms, or arteriovenous malformations; to help visualize cerebral arteries and veins before craniotomy; to explore cerebral circulation

D. Imaging
  1. Computed tomography (CT) scan
     a) Definition: use of narrow x-ray beam to scan head in layers, providing noninvasive cross-sectional view of brain in which lesions are recorded as variations in tissue density
     b) Purpose: to detect tumor, brain infarction, displaced ventricles, or cortical atrophy
  2. Positron emission tomography (PET)
     a) Definition: use of computer-based nuclear imaging to provide views of brain function
     b) Purpose: to help diagnose Alzheimer's disease and tumor; to identify blood flow and oxygen metabolism in patients with stroke; to reveal biochemical abnormalities in mental illness
  3. Single photon emission computerized tomography (SPECT)
     a) Definition: 3-dimensional imaging technique that uses radionuclides and devices emitting and detecting single photons, allowing viewing behind overlying structures or background
     b) Purpose: to detect, localize, and size stroke before it can be seen with CT; to localize seizure foci in epilepsy; to evaluate perfusion before and after surgery

4. Magnetic resonance imaging (MRI)
   a) Definition: use of powerful magnetic field to obtain images of brain
   b) Purpose: to identify cerebral abnormalities, including chemical changes within cells, at an earlier stage than is possible with other tests

See text pages
_____

III. General nursing assessments

A. Patient history
   1. Ask especially about disorders that may affect the nervous system, including diabetes, lung diseases, and hypertension.
   2. Inquire about previous neurologic problems, such as headaches, eye problems, trauma, or seizures.
   3. Ask about use of chemical agents that affect the nervous system, such as alcohol and prescription, nonprescription, and illicit drugs.
   4. Determine level of daily activity and recreational activities.
   5. Inquire about sleep, bowel, and bladder habits and any recent changes experienced in them.

B. Observation and physical examination
   1. Assess mental status, including level of consciousness, memory, attention span, language, copying ability, and cognition.
   2. Assess function or nonfunction of cranial nerves.
   3. Assess sensory function, including response to pain, temperature, and light touch; touch discrimination; position sense; vibration sense; graphesthesia; stereognosis; and abnormal sensory findings.
   4. Assess motor function, including tremors, involuntary movements, range of motion, hand strength, cerebral or brain stem integrity, and peripheral motor problems.

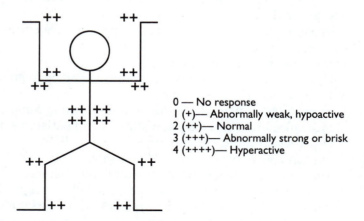

0 — No response
1 (+)— Abnormally weak, hypoactive
2 (++)— Normal
3 (+++)— Abnormally strong or brisk
4 (++++)— Hyperactive

Figure 9–1
Diagram for Recording Reflex Activity

5. Assess cerebellar function, including fine motor coordination, gait, and equilibrium.
6. Assess reflex activity, including deep tendon, cutaneous, plantar, and abdominal reflexes, paying particular attention to instances of asymmetry.

C. Diagnostic tests: nursing responsibilities
   1. Electroencephalography
      a) Refrain from administering CNS depressants and stimulants for 24 hours before test.
      b) If patient is to be "sleep deprived" for test, he/she should be awake from 2–3 A.M. on.
      c) If normally prescribed anticonvulsants are withheld, monitor patient for seizure activity.
      d) Withhold coffee and other stimulants, but urge patient to eat normally.
      e) Ensure that hair is clean and free of hairpins.
      f) Remove jelly and glue from patient's scalp after test.
      g) Reinstitute withheld medications per physician's orders, and encourage sleep-deprived patient to take nap.
   2. Lumbar puncture (spinal tap)
      a) Ask patient to empty bladder.
      b) Position patient on most comfortable side, with back close to edge of table or bed.
      c) Assist patient to assume and maintain fetal position.
      d) Restrict patient to bed for 4–12 hours after procedure.
      e) Encourage patient to increase fluid consumption to 3000 ml for 1–2 days to encourage CSF production.
      f) Be alert for development of complications, such as headache, infection, hematoma formation, and CSF leakage.
   3. Contrast studies
      a) Myelography
         (1) Avoid use of phenothiazines and CNS depressants for 48 hours before test.
         (2) Increase amounts of oral or IV fluids on evening and morning before study to promote hydration.
         (3) Ascertain whether patient has history of seizures, allergies to iodine or seafood, or liver or renal dysfunction.
         (4) Caution patient not to move and to maintain neck hyperextension during procedure.
         (5) Depending on type of contrast medium used, keep patient in appropriate position for required period of time after procedure.
         (6) Monitor neurologic signs carefully for 24 hours after procedure.
         (7) Inspect injection site regularly, and report any leakage immediately.
         (8) Allow patient to stand at bedside or to use bedside commode for voiding during period of bed rest if physician permits.

b) Cerebral angiography
  (1) Ascertain that patient has no known allergies to iodine or contrast agents.
  (2) Explain that patient cannot move during procedure and will feel a warm sensation as contrast medium is injected.
  (3) Allow nothing by mouth for 6–8 hours before test.
  (4) Ask patient to remove jewelry, hairpins, dentures, and hearing aids.
  (5) Administer a prescribed hypnotic, sedative, or analgesic before test.
  (6) Restrict patient to bed rest for 6–24 hours after test, with extremity kept straight and motionless.
  (7) Check extremity for adequate circulation and evidence of bleeding.
  (8) Check neurologic and vital signs frequently.
  (9) Increase fluid intake to facilitate excretion of contrast material.
4. Imaging
  a) Computed tomography (CT) scan
    (1) Ascertain whether patient is allergic to iodine.
    (2) Ask patient to remove wigs, hairpieces, and hairpins.
    (3) Withhold stimulants for 4–6 hours, but do not withhold food.
    (4) Suggest sedation if patient seems unusually apprehensive.
    (5) Advise patient to remain completely still during test.
    (6) Check for allergic response to contrast medium after test.
  b) Positron emission tomography (PET)
    (1) Withhold tobacco, caffeine, and alcohol for 24 hours before test.
    (2) Serve meal 3–4 hours before test; diabetic patients should have final pretest insulin at that time.
    (3) Withhold drugs that alter glucose metabolism.
    (4) Advise patient that he/she will need to be still for up to 90 minutes.
  c) Single photon emission computerized tomography (SPECT): same as for PET

IV. Nursing considerations associated with selected therapies and techniques: intracranial surgery

See text pages
_____

A. Nursing assessment
  1. Preoperative: Assist in neurologic exam; review diagnostic test results.
  2. Postoperative: Assess vital signs, level of consciousness, motor and sensory responses, pupils, speech, posture, reflexes, and evidence of complications (e.g., cerebral edema or intracranial bleeding).

B. Nursing diagnoses
   1. Impaired verbal communication related to level of consciousness
   2. Ineffective airway clearance related to level of consciousness
   3. Sensory alterations related to cerebral edema

C. Nursing intervention
   1. Reinforce patient's dressing if necessary, and report blood or straw-colored fluid discharge (CSF leakage) on dressing or from nose immediately.
   2. Monitor temperature every 2–4 hours; order cooling blanket if fever does not respond to antipyretic drugs.
   3. Touch and talk to patient, since increased stimulation may help reduce disorientation.
   4. Prepare family members for appearance of patient after surgery, and encourage them to ask questions.
   5. Provide teaching program, including information about medication, home care management, agency referrals, and rehabilitation program.

D. Nursing evaluation
   1. Patient and family state ability to cope with diagnosis.
   2. Patient demonstrates improved ability to communicate verbally.
   3. Patient's cerebral edema is successfully treated.
   4. Patient and family state realistic goals about recovery.

V. Selected disorders

See text pages
_____

A. Head injury
   1. Definition: trauma to the brain caused by an external force
   2. Pathophysiology and etiology
      a) Concussion: temporary loss of neurologic function after violent jarring of brain due to blow to head, from which there is complete recovery; generally involves brief loss of consciousness
      b) Contusion: more severe cerebral injury with bruising or hemorrhage of superficial cerebral tissue; may be unconscious for some time
      c) Epidural hematoma: collection of blood on top of the dura usually caused by rapid arterial bleeding after injury
      d) Subdural hematoma: collection of blood in the space between the dura and underlying brain caused by head injury, rupture of cerebral aneurysm, or various bleeding disorders
      e) Skull fracture: caused by impact against another object; simple fracture seldom serious; fracture at base of skull or depressed skull fracture, causing bone fragments to penetrate contents of skull, potentially life threatening
   3. Symptoms
      a) Concussion or contusion: loss of consciousness, headache, irritability, dizzy spells, confusion, unsteady gait; low blood pressure, rapid or weak pulse, pale or cool skin (with contusion)

b) Epidural hematoma: unconsciousness followed by period of lucidity, proceeding to deteriorating consciousness, dilation or fixation of pupils, or paralysis of extremity; followed in untreated patients by death

c) Subdural hematoma: coma in acute and subacute cases; in chronic cases, severe intermittent headache, alternating focal neurologic signs, personality changes, mental deterioration, and focal seizures

d) Skull fracture: pain, swelling, and hemorrhage from nose, pharynx, or ears in depressed fracture; drainage of CSF in basal skull fracture

4. Diagnostic evaluation: patient history; radiograph for suspected concussion or contusion; CT scan and MRI for suspected contusion, hematoma, or skull fracture; neurologic exam for suspected hematoma or skull fracture

5. Medical treatment

a) Concussion or contusion: patient observed closely; mild analgesic administered for headache

b) Epidural or subdural hematoma: holes burred in skull to relieve pressure, remove clot, and stop bleeding; craniotomy performed if bleeding cannot be located

c) Skull fracture: patient confined to bed and observed closely for simple fracture; craniotomy performed to remove bone fragments, control bleeding, and repair damaged tissue for depressed fracture

6. Complications: cardiac arrhythmias, hypotension, infection, respiratory failure, renal failure, post-traumatic seizures

7. Essential nursing care for patients with head injury

a) Nursing assessment

(1) Obtain patient history (including time and cause of accident) and summary of patient's condition from time of accident to present.

(2) Examine patient's external head surface for bleeding, cuts, and abrasions.

(3) Monitor vital signs and motor and eye function; assess level of consciousness; look for signs of increased ICP.

(4) Assess for complications (e.g., systemic infections, neurosurgical infections, or focal nerve palsies).

b) Nursing diagnoses

(1) Fluid volume deficit related to disturbances of consciousness

(2) Ineffective airway clearance related to decreased level of consciousness

(3) Altered thought processes related to head injury

c) Nursing intervention

(1) Monitor patient's temperature every 4 hours; notify physician of fever; administer antipyretics if necessary.

(2) Monitor fluid intake and output, serum electrolytes, and glucose values; test urine for acetone; administer IV fluids if ICP increases and fluids are restricted.

(3) Elevate head of bed to about 30° to decrease intracranial pressure; instruct patient to breathe deeply every hour, but to avoid coughing; guard against aspiration and respiratory insufficiency.

(4) Use mechanical ventilation if breathing is shallow and irregular; monitor arterial blood gases to assess adequacy of ventilation.

(5) Provide all care for patient, and do not interrupt patient's sleep-wake cycle.

(6) Avoid restraints whenever possible; pad side rails and wrap hands in mitts; avoid stimulation; provide adequate light to avoid hallucinations.

(7) Provide home care information to family when patient is discharged.

d) Nursing evaluation

(1) Patient's fluid and electrolyte values are within normal limits.

(2) Patient is oriented to place, time, and person.

(3) Patient's family states understanding of treatment and exhibits adaptive coping mechanisms.

B. Migraine

1. Definition: a symptom complex characterized by recurrent headache

2. Pathophysiology and etiology: believed to be the result of constriction and dilation of cerebral arteries caused by emotional stress, foods or food additives, fatigue, and hereditary factors

3. Symptoms

a) Aura: lasts up to 30 minutes and includes visual disturbances, fatigue, malaise, pallor, puffy face, facial numbness, confusion, irritability, dizziness

b) Headache: severe, incapacitating headache starting on one side but sometimes spreading to entire head with photophobia, nausea, and vomiting, and lasting several hours to a day or more

c) Recovery: muscle ache in neck, localized tenderness, exhaustion

4. Diagnostic evaluation: symptom description; CT or MRI to rule out tumor and aneurysm

5. Medical treatment: daily prophylactic use of beta blockers, which inhibit the activities of heart and brain cells controlling blood vessel dilation; administration of ergotamines or black coffee when attack is imminent; antiemetics to control acute nausea and vomiting

6. Complications: ergotamine intoxication; toxicity or side effects associated with other drugs being taken

7. Essential nursing care for patients with migraine

a) Nursing assessment: Obtain patient history, including record of occurrences, nature of pain, and precipitating circumstances; assess vital signs; assist in neurologic examination.

        b) Nursing diagnoses

          (1) Pain related to vascular changes

          (2) Anxiety related to unpredictability of headaches

          (3) Knowledge deficit related to precipitating factors

        c) Nursing intervention

          (1) Administer medications as prescribed, and explain drug regimen and dosage.

          (2) Eliminate light and noise; elevate head of bed 30°.

          (3) Instruct patient to keep record of occurrences, activities that often precede occurrences, and other possible causes.

          (4) Encourage patient to modify lifestyle to decrease frequency and severity of headaches (see Client Teaching Checklist, "Handling Migraine Headaches").

        d) Nursing evaluation

          (1) Patient is aware of foods that may trigger attacks.

          (2) Patient states stressful situations to avoid.

          (3) Patient states methods to prevent or abort headaches.

    C. Seizure disorders

      1. Definition

        a) Seizure: abnormal electrical disturbance in one or more specific areas of the brain

---

✔ CLIENT TEACHING CHECKLIST ✔

Handling Migraine Headaches

Explain the following suggestions to clients with migraine headaches:

✔ Get enough rest, and awaken at the same time each day.

✔ Eat a balanced diet, and avoid foods that contain tyramine, monosodium glutamate, milk products, and nitrite, including chocolate, many processed foods, and aged cheese.

✔ Avoid long intervals between meals.

✔ Relax and exercise regularly.

✔ Avoid stressful situations whenever possible; deal with unavoidable stress through meditation, counseling, or biofeedback.

✔ Avoid birth control pills, since they may increase the severity and frequency of attacks.

✔ Identify and avoid factors that precede attacks.

✔ Contact the National Headache Foundation for the location of a nearby headache clinic.

    b) Epilepsy: symptom complex consisting of several disorders of brain function characterized by recurrent seizures

2. Pathophysiology and etiology
   a) Pathophysiology: electrical disturbance of nerve cells in one area of the brain, causing abnormal discharge and sometimes leading to disturbances in other areas of the brain
   b) Etiology: genetic or developmental defect (idiopathic seizures); high fever, electrolyte imbalance, uremia, hypoglycemia, hypoxia, brain tumor, drug withdrawal, head injury, allergies (acquired seizures); perinatal brain or head injury, inborn metabolic errors (epilepsy)

3. Symptoms
   a) Partial seizure, elementary symptoms: jerking movements, hallucinations, mumbling, nonsense words; consciousness maintained
   b) Partial seizure, complex symptoms: wide variety of sensory and motor symptoms lasting <1 minute, inappropriate automatisms, emotional reactions, distorted visual or auditory sensations, memory impairment
   c) Absence (petit mal) seizures: brief loss of consciousness, blank stare, fluttering eyelids, moving lips; rarely accompanied by falling
   d) Myoclonic seizures: sudden excessive jerking of torso and extremities, sometimes accompanied by falling
   e) Tonic-clonic (grand mal) seizures
      (1) Prodromal phase: depression, anxiety, nervousness (lasting minutes or hours); aura (auditory or olfactory hallucination or sensation); epileptic cry (spasm of respiratory muscle) preceding loss of consciousness
      (2) Ictal phase: muscular contractions, jerking or thrashing of extremities; cyanosis and spasmodic respiration; frothing and clenched jaws; incontinence
      (3) Postictal phase: headache, fatigue, deep sleep, confusion, nausea, muscle soreness

4. Diagnostic evaluation: thorough patient and family history, careful observation, neurologic exam, serology, measurement of serum electrolytes, EEG, CT scan

5. Medical treatment: administration of anticonvulsive agents (e.g., phenytoin, carbamazepine); surgical intervention for seizure disorder or epilepsy caused by brain tumor, abscess, or other organic problem

6. Complications: trauma, aspiration pneumonia, depression

7. Essential nursing care for patients with seizure disorders
   a) Nursing assessment: Obtain patient and family history; assist with neurologic exam; carefully time and record events of seizure to assist in medical diagnosis.
   b) Nursing diagnoses
      (1) High risk for injury related to violent movements during seizure
      (2) Social isolation related to stigma accompanying epilepsy
   c) Nursing intervention
      (1) Provide safe, nonthreatening environment.
      (2) Remove pillows and elevate padded side rails if patient is in bed.

(3) Protect head with pad and loosen tight clothes.

(4) Refrain from prying open clenched jaws during a seizure to insert anything; do not restrain patient.

(5) Place patient on one side with head flexed forward; clear secretions.

(6) Keep patient turned on one side after seizure to prevent aspiration; make sure airway is patent.

(7) Check oral cavity and teeth for injury after seizure; notify physician in event of profuse bleeding, cuts on tongue surface, or loose or broken teeth.

(8) Expect short period of confusion or apnea to occur immediately after seizure.

(9) Reorient patient upon awakening and provide gentle restraint, since patient may experience severe excitement after seizure.

(10) Provide emotional support, and refer patient and family for counseling related to lifestyle factors affected by diagnosis of epilepsy.

    d) Nursing evaluation

      (1) Patient's seizures are controlled.

      (2) Patient states knowledge of measures that minimize possible side effects of anticonvulsant medication.

      (3) Patient keeps appointment for counseling, and talks openly about epilepsy.

D. Myasthenia gravis

  1. Definition: a neuromuscular disorder characterized by severe skeletal muscle fatigue

  2. Pathophysiology and etiology

    a) Pathophysiology: autoimmune disease in which antibodies attack acetylcholine (ACh) receptors, decreasing acetylcholine activity and leading to impaired transmission of impulses from nerve to muscle cells

    b) Etiology: uncertain

  3. Symptoms: fatigue after minimal exertion, extreme muscular weakness, ptosis, chewing or swallowing problems, double vision, weak voice, masklike facial expression

  4. Diagnostic evaluation: patient history and physical examination, administration of IV anticholinesterase drug, electromyography

  5. Medical treatment: administration of anticholinesterase drugs; immunosuppressive therapy, including corticosteroids, plasmapheresis, and thymectomy; plasma exchange to produce temporary reduction in number of circulating antibodies

  6. Complications: respiratory distress, myasthenic crisis, aspiration pneumonia

7. Essential nursing care for patients with myasthenia gravis
    a) Nursing assessment: Obtain patient history, including information about symptoms, allergies, and drugs taken; evaluate airway, breathing, circulation, consciousness, and vital signs.
    b) Nursing diagnoses
        (1) Ineffective breathing pattern related to weak respiratory muscles
        (2) Impaired physical mobility related to muscle weakness
        (3) High risk for aspiration related to weak bulbar muscles
    c) Nursing intervention
        (1) Monitor respiratory rate and depth and breath sounds if myasthenic crisis occurs due to undermedication with anticholinesterase drugs; maintain patent airway; institute artificial respiration.
        (2) Encourage rest before meals, and administer anticholinesterase agent at least 1 hour before mealtime to ensure maximum muscle strength; place patient in upright position with neck slightly flexed to ease swallowing; mix food in blender if choking occurs too often.
        (3) Tape eyes open for short intervals; instill artificial tears to prevent corneal damage if eyelids fail to close completely; place patch on eye(s) if patient experiences double vision.
        (4) Advise patient to consult with physician regarding pharmacotherapeutics.
        (5) Provide teaching plan for home care.
    d) Nursing evaluation
        (1) Patient and family demonstrate positive attitude toward disability.
        (2) Patient does not aspirate food.
        (3) Patient avoids myasthenic crises.

E. Guillain-Barré syndrome
    1. Definition: clinical syndrome that affects the peripheral nerves and spinal nerve roots
    2. Pathophysiology and etiology
        a) Pathophysiology: inflammatory edema and demyelination with some lymphocytic infiltration (especially in spinal nerve roots); patient normal after 1 year, sometimes with residual disability
        b) Etiology: unknown, although recent respiratory or gastrointestinal infection was experienced by most patients
    3. Symptoms: progressive ascending motor weakness, which may move to upper body and affect respiratory muscles, sometimes proceeding to complete paralysis; sensory disturbances, including numbness and tingling; problems with chewing, talking, and swallowing
    4. Diagnostic evaluation: patient history, physical examination, lumbar puncture to detect increase in CSF protein level, electrophysiologic testing to reveal nerve conduction velocity slowing

5. Medical treatment: tracheostomy and mechanical ventilation if respiratory muscles involved; enteral tube feedings or IV fluids if eating difficulties arise; plasmapheresis; continuous ECG monitoring; administration of propranolol to prevent tachycardia and hypertension as well as atropine to prevent bradycardia during physical therapy

6. Complications: deep vein thrombosis, pulmonary embolism, aspiration pneumonia

7. Essential nursing care for patients with Guillain-Barré syndrome
   a) Nursing assessment
      (1) Monitor patient's vital capacity continually, assessing for breathlessness while talking, shallow or irregular breathing, rising pulse rate, and other changes in respiratory pattern.
      (2) Monitor strength of diaphragm.
      (3) Observe patient for signs of deep vein thrombosis and pulmonary embolism.
   b) Nursing diagnoses
      (1) Ineffective breathing pattern related to progressive weakness
      (2) Altered nutrition related to inability to swallow
      (3) Impaired verbal communication related to intubation or cranial nerve dysfunction
   c) Nursing intervention
      (1) Administer IV or nasogastric feedings if prescribed; gradually resume oral feeding when swallowing reflex returns.
      (2) Provide mechanical ventilation if respiratory function deteriorates.
      (3) Provide patient with alternate forms of communication, such as flash cards, pad and pencil, or an eye blink code; refer to speech pathologist if ventilation continues for long periods.
      (4) Administer range-of-motion exercises at least twice daily; support extremities in functional positions.
      (5) Reduce patient isolation by involving family and friends with care; try to maximize patient's sense of control.
      (6) Caution patient about overexertion after discharge from hospital.
   d) Nursing evaluation
      (1) Patient regains normal breathing pattern.
      (2) Patient recovers mobility.
      (3) Patient can swallow and speak.

F. Brain tumor
   1. Definition: abnormal growth in or on the brain; may or may not be malignant

2. Pathophysiology and etiology
   a) Pathophysiology: abnormal growth or proliferation of cells normally found within CNS (primary tumor); metastasis of malignant cells from outside CNS (secondary tumor)
   b) Etiology: unknown in most instances; radiation; genetic factors
3. Symptoms: depending on area and extent of tumor, increased ICP with early morning headache, vomiting, papilledema, convulsions; speech difficulty, paralysis, double vision; deep, labored, noisy, slow respirations; hyperthermia; deepening coma
4. Diagnostic evaluation: symptom history, neurologic exam, CT scan, MRI, brain scan, cerebral angiography
5. Medical treatment: surgery, radiation, and chemotherapy, depending on location, size, and type of tumor and patient's age and general condition
6. Complications: vasogenic edema, herniation of brain tissue, hydrocephalus
7. Essential nursing care for patients with brain tumor
   a) Nursing assessment: Obtain patient history; assist with neurologic exam.
   b) Nursing diagnoses
      (1) Ineffective individual coping related to diagnosis
      (2) Self-care deficit related to tumor's effect on motor and sensory areas
      (3) Altered nutrition related to decreased level of consciousness
   c) Nursing intervention
      (1) Provide emotional support and reassurance about quality of care; listen to concerns of patient and family and offer to refer them to counselors and support groups.
      (2) Administer analgesics as required, including IV morphine for intractable pain.
      (3) Offer food when patient is rested and pain free; measure intake and output; inform physician if patient's intake is insufficient and administer IV fluids or parenteral nutrition if necessary.
      (4) Encourage patient to participate in personal care as condition allows.
   d) Nursing evaluation
      (1) Patient states strategies for coping.
      (2) Patient maintains normal food and fluid intake.
      (3) Patient and family make plans for home care.

G. Spinal cord injury
   1. Definition: injury to vertebrae, most commonly the fifth, sixth, and seventh cervical vertebrae, the 12th thoracic vertebra, and/or the first lumbar vertebra
   2. Pathophysiology and etiology
      a) Pathophysiology: transient concussion; fracture or collapse of 1 or more vertebrae; pressing of fragmented bone into spinal cord, interrupting transmission of nerve impulses; contusion, laceration, and compression of cord, causing bleeding and swelling; complete cord transection, causing paralysis below level of injury
      b) Etiology: trauma to the back

3. Symptoms: acute pain in back or neck, breathing problems, numbness, or paralysis, dependent upon location and degree of injury
4. Diagnostic evaluation: history of trauma; neurologic exam, radiographic studies, and continuous ECG monitoring
5. Medical treatment
   a) All injuries: head and back immobilized at scene of injury; IV line inserted; vital signs assessed; corticosteroids given to reduce swelling; hyperbaric oxygenation provided
   b) Cervical spine injury: head immobilized with cervical collar or traction; surgical removal of bone fragments to stabilize spine
   c) Lumbar spine or thoracolumbar injury: patient placed in special bed, such as Stryker frame; surgery performed to correct spinal cord compression; vertebrae fused at later time using bone from iliac crest
6. Complications: venous thrombosis, chronic dermal ulcers, infections, hemorrhage, contractures, autonomic dysreflexia
7. Essential nursing care for patients with spinal cord injury
   a) Nursing assessment
      (1) Monitor vital signs, and assess patient for presence of spinal shock (see Nurse Alert, "Dealing with Spinal Shock").
      (2) Assess patient's breathing pattern and cough reflex; auscultate lungs.
      (3) Monitor patient for changes in motor and sensory function and symptoms of progressive neurologic damage.
   b) Nursing diagnoses
      (1) Ineffective breathing patterns related to paralysis
      (2) Impaired physical mobility related to spinal cord injury
      (3) Incontinence, total, related to spinal cord injury
   c) Nursing intervention
      (1) Measure vital capacity and arterial blood gas values.
      (2) Administer analgesics as ordered, giving injection above level of paralysis.

! NURSE *ALERT* !

Dealing with Spinal Shock

- Support patient's respiratory and cardiac systems.
- Decompress gastrointestinal tract.
- Insert indwelling urethral catheter.
- Suction patient.
- Be prepared to administer mechanical ventilation.

     (3) Assess patient's skull for signs of infection when tongs, calipers, or pins are in place.

     (4) Observe pins for signs of loosening; in case of detachment, stabilize head and notify neurosurgeon immediately.

     (5) Insert indwelling urethral catheter, and measure fluid intake and output.

     (6) Auscultate abdomen for bowel sounds; administer stool softener or rectal suppository to encourage daily bowel elimination.

     (7) Perform chest physical therapy; encourage early clearing of secretions if patient is conscious.

     (8) Maintain proper body alignment; perform full range-of-motion exercises 4 or 5 times daily.

  d) Nursing evaluation

     (1) Normal breath sounds are audible.

     (2) Patient can move within the limits of injury.

     (3) Patient maintains continence or controls incontinence within the limits of injury.

H. Alzheimer's disease

  1. Definition: a progressive, degenerative, irreversible neurologic disease that causes dementia

  2. Pathophysiology and etiology

    a) Pathophysiology: reduced level of enzyme that produces acetylcholine; deposits of amyloid proteins; formation of neurofibrillary tangles and neuritic plaques, resulting in decreased cerebral cortex size

    b) Etiology: unknown, although heredity plays role in some cases

  3. Symptoms: progressively severe disturbances in short-term memory, cognition, self-care, awareness, language, learning skills, behavior, personality, and problem-solving ability

  4. Diagnostic evaluation: definitive diagnosis only at autopsy; probable diagnosis established by symptoms, MRI, PET, CT scan, and EEG

  5. Medical treatment: supportive care; administration of tranquilizers, antidepressants, and anticonvulsants

  6. Complications: traumatic injury, aspiration pneumonia

  7. Essential nursing care for patients with Alzheimer's disease

    a) Nursing assessment: Obtain medical history from patient or family member; evaluate patient's behavior, emotion, cognitive and motor skills, self-care ability, and level of orientation.

    b) Nursing diagnoses

     (1) Altered thought processes related to decreased mental function

     (2) Impaired physical mobility related to ataxia

     (3) High risk for injury related to progressive dementia

    c) Nursing intervention

     (1) Maintain structured routine; encourage patient to participate as much as possible in activities of daily living.

     (2) Help patient to ambulate; raise side rails while patient is in bed.

                (3) Listen attentively to patient; provide concise, easy-to-understand directions.

                (4) Encourage family to contact community agencies.

          d) Nursing evaluation

                (1) Patient ambulates safely.

                (2) Family states understanding of probable course of disease.

I. Stroke (cerebrovascular accident [CVA])

    1. Definition: sudden loss of brain function caused by a disrupted blood supply

    2. Pathophysiology and etiology

        a) Pathophysiology: brain ischemia, leading to hypoxia or anoxia, and hypoglycemia, which cause neuronal death

        b) Etiology: cerebral embolus or thrombus, hemorrhage, hypertension, or ischemia; main risk factors identified as diabetes and hypertension

    3. Symptoms: highly variable, including weakness, nausea, vomiting, headache, numbness, motor loss, communication loss, perceptual disturbances, impaired mental activity, psychologic disturbances, bladder dysfunction, coma, and breathing problems

    4. Diagnostic evaluation: patient history, neurologic exam, CT scan, MRI, brain scan, cerebral angiography, transcranial Doppler ultrasonography, lumbar puncture

    5. Medical treatment: maintenance of patent airway and circulation to brain; administration of anticoagulants for thrombosis or embolus, steroids to reduce inflammation, and diuretics to reduce cerebral edema; supportive treatment

    6. Complications: contractures, chronic dermal ulcers, deep venous thrombosis, aspiration pneumonia

    7. Essential nursing care for patients with stroke

        a) Nursing assessment: Obtain history from patient or family member; assist with neurologic assessment; assess bladder function.

        b) Nursing diagnoses

            (1) Incontinence related to flaccid bladder

            (2) Impaired verbal communication related to aphasia

            (3) Ineffective individual coping related to permanent neurologic deficit

        c) Nursing intervention

            (1) Change patient's position every 2 hours; use prone position several times daily; perform range-of-motion exercises on both sides.

            (2) Keep airway patent by suctioning (if necessary); encourage conscious patient to cough, deep breathe, and swallow.

(3) Measure fluid intake and output; offer bedpan or urinal regularly once catheter is removed; notify physician in event of urinary retention.

(4) Ask patient to speak slowly or to communicate by pointing, writing, nodding, or blinking; work with speech therapist by using words practiced during therapy.

(5) Provide emotional support; maintain consistent routines; surround patient with familiar people and objects.

d) Nursing evaluation

(1) Patient achieves mobility.

(2) Patient attains continence.

(3) Patient participates in cognitive improvement program.

J. Parkinson's disease

1. Definition: brain disorder that causes muscle tremor, stiffness, and weakness

2. Pathophysiology and etiology

a) Pathophysiology: degeneration of substantia nigra causing decreased dopamine levels, leading to an imbalance between dopamine and acetylcholine levels

b) Etiology: drugs, head injuries, encephalitis; dopamine deficiency in basal ganglia (idiopathic parkinsonism)

3. Symptoms

a) Idiopathic parkinsonism: stiffness, pill-rolling tremor, movement problems (early stage); head tremors, masklike expression, stooped posture, speaking in monotone, shuffling gait, weight loss (mid stage); slurred speech, chewing and swallowing problems, contractures, increased salivation and drooling, oculogyric crises (late stage)

b) Drug-induced parkinsonism: symptoms of idiopathic parkinsonism and rhythmic involuntary movements of jaw, tongue, and neck; facial grimaces

4. Diagnostic evaluation: symptoms, patient history, neurologic exam

5. Medical treatment: drug therapy, including dopaminergics, anticholinergics, and antihistamines; rehabilitation, including physical and occupational therapy; stereotaxic thalamotomy in some cases

6. Complications: musculoskeletal trauma, pneumonia

7. Essential nursing care for patients with Parkinson's disease

a) Nursing assessment: Obtain patient history; assist with neurologic exam; evaluate patient's ability to perform activities of daily life.

b) Nursing diagnoses

(1) Activity intolerance related to fatigue

(2) Impaired physical mobility related to muscle rigidity

(3) Impaired verbal communication related to inability to articulate words

(4) Self-esteem disturbance related to impaired physical mobility

c) Nursing intervention

(1) Administer antiparkinsonian drugs as ordered.

(2) Work with therapists to plan exercise regimen; perform passive exercises of extremities.

(3) Encourage patient to perform personal duties by allowing ample time for them and adapting clothing, eating, and grooming utensils for easy use.

(4) Provide emotional support, and encourage patient to interact with others.

(5) Advise patient to speak slowly; if necessary, provide pen and paper.

(6) Offer frequent, small meals of high-protein food that is easy to swallow; follow each meal with good oral care.

  d) Nursing evaluation

(1) Patient exhibits decrease in muscle rigidity.

(2) Patient sustains no contractures, muscle atrophy, or deformities.

(3) Patient demonstrates improvements in communication.

K. Multiple sclerosis

  1. Definition: chronic progressive disease of the nervous system, eventually causing muscle paralysis

  2. Pathophysiology and etiology

    a) Pathophysiology: Destruction of myelin nerve sheath interrupts impulse transmission, causing weakness and paralysis.

    b) Etiology: unknown

  3. Symptoms: blurred or double vision, nystagmus, weakness, clumsiness, numbness and tingling in extremities, paralysis of lower extremities, bowel and bladder dysfunction, tremor, mood swings, slurred speech

  4. Diagnostic evaluation: patient history, CT scan, MRI, myelography; lumbar puncture to identify presence of oligoclonal (IgG) bands

  5. Medical treatment: administration of adrenocorticotropic hormone and corticosteroids to reduce edema and inflammatory response, and carbamazepine or acetaminophen to treat pain and paresthesias; immunosuppressive therapy

  6. Complications: musculoskeletal injury, respiratory arrest, chronic dermal ulcers

  7. Essential nursing care for patients with multiple sclerosis

    a) Nursing assessment: Obtain patient history and assist in neurologic assessment; evaluate airway, breathing, circulation, and vital signs; auscultate abdomen for bowel sounds and bladder for distention; note evidence of incontinence.

    b) Nursing diagnoses

(1) Activity intolerance related to muscle weakness

(2) Self-care deficit related to paralysis

(3) Dysfunctional grieving related to body function loss

c) Nursing intervention
   (1) Change position of patient every 2 hours; encourage him/her to get out of bed and ambulate, if possible.
   (2) Plan activities to avoid extreme fatigue, but urge patients to perform activities of daily living.
   (3) Listen for subtle references to sexual dysfunction, and discuss them with physician.
   (4) Encourage patient and family to set goals and solve problems, perhaps with the help of a community agency.
d) Nursing evaluation
   (1) Patient's skin and mucous membranes remain intact.
   (2) Patient shows improvement in physical mobility and begins to use trapeze and wheelchair.
   (3) Patient identifies financial and home management problems.

1. 24 hours after a diagnostic lumbar puncture, Carol Mack is complaining of a severe, throbbing headache. Which of the following may have contributed to the headache?

   a. Fluid intake totaled 1000 ml in 24 hours.
   b. The patient remained on bed rest for 6 hours.
   c. An analgesic was taken immediately after the test.
   d. The patient did not remain in the fetal position.

2. The nurse is providing postoperative care to a patient who has had a craniotomy. Which of the following observations would require immediate attention?

   a. Continued unresponsiveness to verbal stimuli
   b. Negative glucose reading in nasal mucus
   c. Increased blood pressure and decreased pulse rate
   d. Pale, warm skin and a temperature of 99°F

3. Mark Drucker, who is being admitted with a concussion after a motor vehicle accident, tells the nurse that he cannot remember anything about the accident. The nurse explains that this:

   a. Is a cause for concern that should be reported to the doctor.
   b. Results from jarring of the brain and unconsciousness.
   c. May indicate that he has a skull fracture.
   d. Indicates that he may develop an epidural hematoma.

4. Sonya West, who is 25 years old, has a history of migraine headaches. Which of the following statements by Ms. West would indicate to the nurse that an immediate teaching review is necessary?

   a. "I'm starting to take birth control pills."
   b. "I'm going to a wine and cheese party."

   c. "I've been using biofeedback techniques."
   d. "The doctor told me to taper the propranolol (Inderal)."

5. Which of the following assessments would the nurse expect to find in a patient experiencing the postictal phase of a tonic-clonic seizure?

   a. Hallucinations and anxiety
   b. Clenched jaws and cyanosis
   c. Blank stare and fluttering eyelids
   d. Confusion and fatigue

6. The home health nurse visits 40-year-old Cathy Frye, who has myasthenia gravis. During the visit, Ms. Frye discusses her frustration with trying to accomplish basic activities of daily living. Which of the following is the most appropriate nursing diagnosis in this situation?

   a. Altered comfort level related to chronic pain
   b. Activity intolerance related to involuntary muscle movements
   c. Fatigue related to voluntary muscle weakness
   d. Self-care deficit related to the tumor's effect on motor areas

7. The nurse would expect to find which of the following assessments in a patient with a frontal lobe brain tumor?

   a. Disturbances in position and space of the body
   b. Personality changes and inappropriate judgment
   c. Inability to remember current events
   d. Visual hallucinations and partial blindness

8. While the community health nurse is visiting Ms. Tomko, Mr. Tomko falls off a high ladder and lies prone on the floor, calling for help. The nurse's first action is to:

   a. Immobilize Mr. Tomko, and assess him for injuries.

b. Turn him over, and assess for head injury.

c. Call for an ambulance to transport Mr. Tomko to the hospital.

d. Ask him to move his legs, and evaluate the strength of movement.

9. Dick Nelson, a 21-year-old patient with a complete fracture of the cervical spine at the seventh vertebra (C7), tells the nurse that he knows he will never walk again and asks why he should go to physical therapy. The nurse's best response is:

a. "You seem a little depressed today. Should I cancel your PT appointment?"

b. "If you keep strengthening all your muscles, you may be able to walk again."

c. "I know how you must feel, but lying around in bed isn't going to change anything."

d. "PT strengthens the upper body muscles and teaches you to become as mobile as possible without walking."

10. Monica Garland, the daughter of a 67-year-old female patient with Alzheimer's disease, expresses her frustration with caring for her mother. Ms. Garland explains that she never gets any rest because her mother is so forgetful and wanders around day and night. The nurse suggests which of the following?

a. Placing a restraining jacket on the mother at night

b. Calling the local Alzheimer's support group for help

c. Tiring the mother out during the day so that she sleeps at night

d. Locking the doors and allowing the mother to wander

11. Edward Roper, a 75-year-old patient with Parkinson's disease, was started on levodopa and carbidopa (Sinemet) therapy 1 month ago. On his follow-up clinic visit, he exhibits a dramatic improvement in his symptoms and declares to the nurse that he is cured of the disorders. Which of the following is the best response?

a. "There is no cure, and your symptoms will come back."

b. "These medications can cure the disease so long as you take them."

c. "There is no cure, but your symptoms are definitely decreased."

d. "You are cured, but now we need to plan an exercise regimen."

12. Rose Nawata, a 35-year-old patient, has multiple sclerosis (MS). Which of the following activities would help Ms. Nawata improve her physical mobility?

a. Exercising each extremity for 15 minutes

b. Gradually lengthening aerobic workouts

c. Performing passive range-of-motion exercises for all joints

d. Learning relaxation and coordination exercises

ANSWERS

1. **Correct answer is a.** 1000 ml is insufficient fluid to promote cerebrospinal fluid (CSF) production. A fluid intake of 3000 ml for 1–2 days post test is recommended. Decreased CSF level may cause a headache.

b. Bed rest is recommended for 4–12 hours after the test to prevent CSF leakage from the puncture site.
c. Taking an analgesic after the procedure should not cause a headache.
d. The fetal position is the recommended position during the test but need not be maintained thereafter.

2. **Correct answer is c.** Increased blood pressure and decreased pulse rate may indicate increased intracranial pressure (ICP). Further assessment and treatment must be undertaken promptly.

a. Any changes in responsiveness should receive consideration; decreased responsiveness may indicate increased ICP.
b. A negative glucose reading is a normal finding. A positive glucose reading would indicate the presence of CSF and a possible leak.

d. Pale, warm skin is a normal finding. If the skin were pale and cool or moist, it would indicate active bleeding and development of shock. The temperature may be normal in this patient. Although the nurse would monitor for an increase in temperature, it would not require immediate attention.

3. **Correct answer is b.** A concussion is a temporary loss of neurologic function after a blow to the head. In such a situation, it is common for patients to have no recollection of the accident that caused the injury.

   a, c, and **d.** These statements are inaccurate. The patient will be monitored for headache, dizziness, irritability, and anxiety, which would indicate more extensive head injury. Epidural hematomas may result from fractures of the skull; a subdural hematoma is usually caused by trauma.

4. **Correct answer is a.** Since birth control pills may increase the severity and frequency of migraine attacks, this statement would indicate the most immediate need for education.

   b. Ms. West may attend the party, but foods that contain nitrites, tyramine, milk products, and aged cheese should be avoided, since they may cause a migraine attack.
   c. Biofeedback and other measures to reduce stress are recommended, since stress may increase the risk of attacks.
   d. Migraine drug therapy may be gradually tapered, since natural remissions do occur.

5. **Correct answer is d.** Fatigue and a short period of confusion are expected after a seizure.

   a. These symptoms characterize the prodromal phase of tonic-clonic seizures. Hallucinations are part of the preseizure aura, and the accompanying anxiety occurs as a warning sign of the pending seizure.
   b. Clenched jaws and cyanosis are symptoms of the ictal phase of a tonic-clonic seizure.
   c. Blank stare and fluttering eyelids are symptoms of an absence seizure.

6. **Correct answer is c.** Myasthenia gravis is a neuromuscular disease characterized by severe muscle fatigue that has a strong impact on the patient's ability to accomplish any activities. These patients need frequent rest periods, since even chewing and talking can cause fatigue.

   a, b, and **d.** Patients with myasthenia gravis do not have chronic pain, involuntary muscle movements, or a tumor. Myasthenia gravis is an autoimmune disease in which antibodies attack acetylcholine receptors, impairing neuromuscular transmission.

7. **Correct answer is b.** The frontal lobe of the brain controls judgment, affect, and personality.

   a. The parietal lobe is a sensory lobe that controls the interpretation of sensations and the perception of body position and space.
   c. The temporal lobe controls taste, smell, hearing, and short-term memory.
   d. The occipital lobe controls visual interpretations.

8. **Correct answer is a.** It is essential to immobilize any victim of a fall, an auto accident, or trauma until head, neck, and spinal cord injuries are ruled out. Correct handling and immobilization prevent further damage and loss of neurologic function.

   b. The victim should not be turned or moved until trained personnel arrive.
   c. The victim should be immobilized and assessed before emergency medical assistance is summoned.
   d. The victim should not be asked to move, since that may exacerbate existing injuries.

9. **Correct answer is d.** A patient with a C7 fracture is likely to have partial arm and hand function and paralysis of the lower body and legs. Upper body strength is important so that the patient can transfer from wheelchair to bed to car and achieve vocational and recreational goals.

   a. Patients with paraplegia do grieve for the loss of their body function and experience a period of depression. Canceling PT is not therapeutic.

b. Offering false hope is inappropriate. The patient will not be able to walk again and needs encouragement and support as he adapts to major lifestyle changes.

c. The patient needs encouragement and opportunities to verbalize and work through his feelings, and judgmental comments are not helpful.

10. **Correct answer is b.** Families of patients with Alzheimer's disease often feel frightened, frustrated, angry, guilty, and helpless. Resources within the community can help Ms. Garland cope with the problems associated with her mother and her disease.

a. Restraints are inappropriate because they may cause increased agitation and accidental injury.

c. Suggesting that Ms. Garland tire her mother out is not specific enough. Daily activities and exercise should be balanced with short rest periods. If too much activity is attempted at one time, the mother may become tired, agitated, and uncooperative.

d. Unlocked doors are only 1 safety hazard for a patient with Alzheimer's disease. To reduce the risk of injury and to decrease the daughter's worrying, the nurse should help Ms. Garland create a hazard-free environment.

11. **Correct answer is c.** Parkinson's disease is a progressive neurologic disorder that is not curable, although drug therapy can be very effective in managing the disorder. This response corrects the patient while still confirming the improvement in his condition.

a. Although it is true that the patient's symptoms may come back, Mr. Roper also needs some encouragement and support. The beneficial effects of levodopa that occur during the first few years of therapy begin to decrease, while side effects may become severe.

b. Levodopa and carbidopa (Sinemet) do not cure Parkinson's disease. The patient may experience sudden immobility ("off effect") followed by a sudden return of mobility ("on effect") while on drug therapy. When this occurs, "drug holidays," during which the patient goes off the drugs, may be planned.

d. There is no cure for Parkinson's disease.

12. **Correct answer is d.** Relaxation and coordination exercises promote muscle efficiency, and diminishing muscle power is a major problem in patients with multiple sclerosis.

a and **b.** Aerobic workouts and long exercise sessions should be avoided, since vigorous exercise will increase body temperature and may aggravate symptoms. Prolonged exercise may cause paresis, numbness, and a lack of coordination. Fatigue may exacerbate symptoms.

c. Passive range-of-motion exercises should not be necessary. It would be more appropriate for the patient to do relaxation and coordination exercises, taking frequent rest periods.

10

Musculoskeletal Function

OVERVIEW

I. Structure and function of musculoskeletal system
A. Skeletal system
B. Muscular system

II. General diagnostic tests
A. Diagnostic tests
B. Laboratory tests

III. General nursing assessments
A. Patient history
B. Observation and physical examination
C. Diagnostic tests

IV. Nursing considerations associated with selected therapies and techniques
A. Casts
B. Traction
C. Orthopedic surgery
D. Joint replacement
E. Amputation

V. Selected disorders
A. Fractures
B. Osteoporosis
C. Osteomyelitis
D. Rheumatic disorders
E. Bone tumors

NURSING HIGHLIGHTS

1. Because musculoskeletal diseases vary in severity and symptoms, the nurse is challenged to identify the patient's problems, rather than the disease, in determining nursing diagnoses, in applying interventions, and in achieving realistic outcomes.
2. Nurse should help the patient adjust to the changes involved in musculoskeletal trauma.

GLOSSARY

arthrography—radiography of a joint
crepitation—grating sound heard when the ends of broken bones are moved
kyphosis—convex curvature of the dorsal spine; "dowager's hump"
myelography—radiography of the spinal canal after contrast medium has been injected
sequestrectomy—surgical removal of a fragment of necrosed bone
synovial fluid—lubricating fluid secreted by the synovial membrane of a joint

I. Structure and function of musculoskeletal system

See text pages
_____

A. Skeletal system
1. Bones: provide framework for body, support and protect tissues and vital organs, produce blood cells, and store minerals
2. Joints: allow range of motion between bones
3. Ligaments: bands of fibrous tissue that connect freely movable bones to one another
4. Bursae: sacs of synovial fluid that cushion joints at shoulder, elbow, knee, and elsewhere
5. Cartilage: fibrous connective tissue that is attached to articular surfaces of bone

B. Muscular system
1. Muscles: provide movement and produce heat
2. Tendons: cords of fibrous tissue that connect muscles to bones
3. Aponeuroses: flat sheets of connective tissue that connect muscles to bones, connective tissue, soft tissue, other muscles, or skin

II. General diagnostic tests

See text pages
_____

A. Diagnostic tests
1. Radiography and imaging
   a) Radiography: used to detect trauma or bone disorders (malignant bone lesions, joint deformities, calcification, degeneration, osteoporosis, or joint disease)
   b) Computed tomography scans (CT scans): used to detect musculoskeletal problems, especially in vertebral column
   c) Magnetic resonance imaging (MRI): used to diagnose problems with muscles, tendons, or ligaments
   d) Indium imaging: detects bone infection by labeling patient's leukocytes, reinjecting them, and scanning for their accumulation
2. Arthroscopy: visual inspection of joint with arthroscope; knee and shoulder most common sites
3. Arthrocentesis: aspiration of synovial fluid from joint to relieve discomfort or to inject drugs; may test fluid for culture or sensitivity studies
4. Bone scan: injection of radioactive material to visualize entire skeleton; used to detect tumors, arthritis, osteomyelitis, osteoporosis, vertebral compression fractures, or bone pain
5. Bone biopsy: extraction of bone specimen for microscopic examination; used to detect neoplasm or infection

B. Laboratory tests
1. Blood tests: detect infection, inflammation, or anemia
2. Synovial fluid tests: reveal disorders such as traumatic or septic arthritis, gout, rheumatic fever, or systemic lupus erythematosus

See text pages
_____

III. General nursing assessments

A. Patient history: Inquire about previous illnesses and accidents, family history of musculoskeletal disorders, nutritional history (including intake of calcium and protein and exposure to sunlight), obesity, and exercise regimen.

B. Observation and physical examination
   1. Assess posture, gait, and mobility.
   2. Assess major bones, joints, and muscles by inspection, palpation, and determination of function; check for muscle strength or wasting.
   3. Assess for pain, tenderness, swelling, redness, stiffness, abnormal size, and alignment.
   4. Assess vital signs.
   5. Look for external bleeding, wounds, debris, and injury beyond original area.

C. Diagnostic tests: nursing responsibilities
   1. Radiography: Caution patient to remain still during procedure.
   2. Arthroscopy
      a) Before surgery, explain procedure, post-test care, and exercises necessary after test.
      b) After surgery, monitor status of extremity every hour for first 4 hours, decreasing to every 4 hours for next 24 hours; administer analgesic as prescribed.
   3. Bone scan: Assure patient that radioactive material is not dangerous.
   4. Magnetic resonance imaging (MRI): See Nurse Alert, "Considerations for Patients Preparing for MRI."
   5. All diagnostic tests: Assist physician and other staff as needed.

See text pages
_____

IV. Nursing considerations associated with selected therapies and techniques

A. Casts
   1. Prepare patient for application of cast by describing the procedure.
   2. Handle damp cast with palms of hands, and prevent cast from resting on hard surfaces or edges to avoid denting, which can create pressure areas.
   3. Inspect cast every 2–4 hours during first few days for drainage, crackling, crumbling, alignment, and fit; circle, date, and monitor areas of drainage on cast. (If area increases, notify physician.)
   4. Report sudden increases in drainage or changes in cast integrity to physician immediately (see Nurse Alert, "Warning Signs for Patients with Casts").

N U R S E *A L E R T*

Considerations for Patients Preparing for MRI

Nurse should check prospective MRI candidate for:
- Pregnancy
- Excess weight (>260 lb)
- Presence of magnetic metal fragments or implants
- Presence of pacemaker or electronic implant
- IV catheter

Nurse should assess patient's ability to:
- Communicate clearly and understand verbal communication
- Survive without life-support equipment
- Lie still for 20–30 minutes
- Breathe without supplemental oxygen for 1 hour
- Withstand close, confining quarters

5. Check color and temperature of skin at the ends of the cast; notify physician immediately if skin is cold, white, or blue. Check sensation and ability to move distal to cast; report numbness, increase in pain, or decrease in movement.
6. Cover plaster cast completely with plastic while bathing patient and tuck plastic into ends of cast to prevent water seepage into cast. If cast becomes moist, use hand-held hair dryer on low setting for drying.
7. Relieve pain by elevating involved part and by applying cold to both sides of the cast.
8. Monitor patient's vital signs every 4 hours; report fever or chills.

! N U R S E *A L E R T* !

Warning Signs for Patients with Casts

- Never ignore pain complaints from a patient in a cast. (A pressure ulcer or compromised perfusion may exist.)
- Immediately report unrelieved pain to physician to avoid possible necrosis or paralysis.
- Pain associated with compartment syndrome is relentless; it is not controlled with elevation, cold, or analgesics. Irreversible damage can occur in 4–6 hours.
- Severe pain over a bony prominence warns of developing pressure ulcer; pain decreases when ulcer occurs.
- Infection warnings include the following: "hot spot," stain over one area of cast, musty odor, and fever; notify physician immediately if present.
- Thoroughly investigate pain above, below, or underneath cast before administering analgesic; compression of nerve or blood vessel can be crippling, causing tissue necrosis and possible necessity for amputation.

9. Clean soiled cast with mild detergent and damp cloth.
10. Monitor for complications of immobility such as skin breakdown, thromboembolism, or constipation.
11. Inspect edges of cast for any areas that might create skin integrity impairment.

B. Traction
1. Check traction equipment for alignment, fraying, loosening, and proper functioning; weights must hang freely at all times; lift, release, increase, or decrease weights only with a written order from the physician.
2. Encourage range-of-motion exercises in the unaffected limbs.
3. Inspect skin every 4–8 hours for signs of irritation or inflammation; pay particular attention to entry points of pins, wires, or screws; monitor pressure points with use of skin traction and ropes and pulleys.
4. Report severe pain due to muscle spasm to physician if body realignment fails to reduce pain.
5. Use a footboard to avoid footdrop.
6. Encourage participation in daily care.
7. Monitor for signs of complications of impaired mobility, including skin breakdown, pneumonia or respiratory problems, muscle atrophy, contractures, footdrop, and urinary tract infection.
8. Keep bottom sheet taut and wrinkle free; use sheepskin pads, foam rubber supports, or alternating pressure mattress for prevention of skin breakdown.
9. Check for signs of neurovascular and circulation problems: discoloration, coolness of extremity, absence of peripheral pulse, or decrease in movement or tactile sensation.

C. Orthopedic surgery
1. Preoperative care
    a) Elevate affected extremity, apply ice, and administer analgesics as prescribed.
    b) Monitor patient for color, temperature, pulse, pain, edema, paresthesia, and motion of extremity; notify physician immediately if compromised neurovascular activity is noted.
    c) Clean skin to reduce risk of infection.
    d) Assist patient in moving affected extremity while providing adequate support.
    e) Explain all preoperative preparations; demonstrate postoperative management (moving, deep breathing, and coughing).
2. Postoperative care
    a) Administer narcotic analgesics as prescribed.
    b) Monitor temperature every 4 hours, and inspect surgical site every 2–4 hours for infection; immediately report any signs of infection to physician (fever, increase in pain, or wound drainage with odor).

c) Demonstrate range-of-motion and isometric exercises.

d) Provide emotional support to anxious, stressed patients.

e) Prevent constipation by assuring fluid intake and adequate fiber; administer stool softener or laxative as needed.

f) Monitor patient for development of shock.

g) Monitor breath sounds, and encourage deep breathing and coughing exercises.

h) Provide information on home care.

D. Joint replacement
1. Preoperative care
   a) Assess patient for signs of infection (infection 2–4 weeks before surgery requires rescheduling).
   b) Clean and shave skin according to hospital protocol prior to surgery.
   c) Administer prophylactic antibiotics as prescribed.
   d) Explain all preoperative and postoperative procedures; demonstrate coughing and deep breathing exercises.
2. Postoperative care
   a) Administer analgesics as prescribed.
   b) Monitor vital signs; check dressing every 4 hours; report fever.
   c) Auscultate lungs each shift; encourage patient to deep breathe and cough every 2–4 hours.
   d) Inspect surgical site every 2–4 hours for color, temperature, and peripheral pulses; drain fluid with suction device.
   e) Teach patient protective positioning: Use pillow between legs when lying on back or side or when turning; do not sleep on operated side until given permission by surgeon; do not cross legs, stoop, or acutely flex hip.
   f) Review physician's instructions with patient.

E. Amputation
1. Preoperative care
   a) Provide emotional support and time to talk.
   b) Administer preoperative medications (e.g., narcotic analgesics or antibiotics) before surgery as prescribed.
   c) Assess site closely for gangrene or loss of circulation, as evidenced by pain, changes in color, or lack of peripheral pulse.
   d) Explain all preoperative preparations; review postoperative procedures with patient.
2. Postoperative care
   a) Explain phenomenon of phantom limb sensation or phantom pain.
   b) Report excess drainage or signs of infection immediately; monitor vital signs at regular intervals; continue to administer prophylactic antibiotics as prescribed.
   c) Inspect skin over pressure areas regularly.
   d) Encourage patient to exercise, to use the trapeze, and to deep breathe and cough every 2 hours while awake.
   e) Avoid placing residual limb on pillow in order to prevent contractures of proximal joints.

f) Auscultate lungs daily.

g) Watch closely for signs of bleeding.

h) To condition residual limb for prosthesis, have patient push limb into soft pillow, then into firm pillow, and finally against hard surface; teach patient to massage limb to ease tenderness and improve vascularity.

i) Provide discharge teaching plan, including information on care of prosthesis.

V. Selected disorders

See text pages

A. Fractures

   1. Definition: breaks or disruptions in the continuity of bone

   2. Pathophysiology and etiology

      a) Pathophysiology: Fractures occur when bone experiences stress it cannot absorb, caused by direct blow, crushing force, sudden twisting motion, or extreme muscle contraction.

      b) Etiology: Fractures are commonly caused by automobile accidents or falls; conditions such as osteoporosis, arthritis, and cancer increase the risk of fracture because of decreased bone strength; diseases such as Parkinson's disease and multiple sclerosis may be associated with an increase in the risk of fracture because of the increased risk of falls.

   3. Symptoms: pain, false motion, loss of function, deformity, shortening, crepitation, local swelling, discoloration

   4. Diagnostic evaluation: radiography, CT scan, or MRI

   5. Medical treatment

      a) Reduction

         (1) Closed: realignment of bone parts by external manipulation

         (2) Open: surgical exposure and realignment of bone

      b) Cast: rigid plaster or fiberglass device for immobilizing a reduced fracture

      c) Traction

         (1) Skin traction: uses weights connected to tapes, Velcro boot, or strips attached to skin with elastic bandages

         (2) Skeletal traction: uses weights connected to wire, screw, or pin inserted into bone when greater pull is needed

      d) External fixation: metal pins inserted into bone from outside skin and attached to compression device

      e) Internal fixation: metal pins, screws, or plates surgically inserted into bone

   6. Complications: compartment syndrome; shock; fat embolism; thromboembolism; infection; avascular necrosis; delayed union,

malunion, or nonunion; reflex sympathetic dystrophy; disseminated intravascular coagulation (DIC)
  7. Essential nursing care for patients with fractures
      a) Nursing assessment
          (1) Assess for changes in bone alignment, shape, and length.
          (2) Assess skin integrity.
          (3) Assess neurovascular status.
      b) Nursing diagnoses
          (1) Pain related to fracture
          (2) Impaired physical mobility related to injury
          (3) Self-care deficit related to restricted mobility
      c) Nursing intervention
          (1) Splint and support patient's fracture; perform position changes gently; apply ice; administer medications as prescribed.
          (2) Encourage patient to discuss problems associated with injury.
          (3) Encourage active participation in activities of daily living within the limits of treatment.
          (4) Encourage patient to exercise nonimmobilized joints and muscles and to perform isometric exercises on immobilized extremities.
      d) Nursing evaluation
          (1) Patient states that pain is reduced or eliminated.
          (2) Patient exhibits increased physical mobility.
          (3) Patient increases performance of activities of daily living.

B. Osteoporosis
   1. Definition: an age-related metabolic disorder in which bone density decreases
   2. Pathophysiology and etiology
      a) Pathophysiology: may be result of decreased osteoblast (bone-forming cell) activity or of increased osteoclast (bone-resorbing cell) activity
      b) Etiology: Exact cause is unknown; lack of calcium and vitamin D increases risk; estrogen may be protective (postmenopausal women at highest risk).
   3. Symptoms: kyphosis, back pain with tenderness and voluntary restriction of spinal movement, fatigue
   4. Diagnostic evaluation: radiography, laboratory studies, single-photon absorptiometry, dual-photon absorptiometry, CT scan
   5. Medical treatment: analgesics for bone pain; diet high in calcium, protein, and vitamin D; oral calcium supplements; regular weight-bearing and strengthening exercise; estrogen and progesterone replacement therapy
   6. Complication: fractures
   7. Essential nursing care for patients with osteoporosis
      a) Nursing assessment
          (1) Obtain full patient history, including age; family history of osteoporosis; alcohol, tobacco, and caffeine use; exposure to sunlight; amount of exercise; history of falls or sudden movements; previous fractures; body build; and weight.

        (2) Perform physical assessment, including musculoskeletal system; assess for kyphosis.

    b) Nursing diagnoses

        (1) Potential for injury related to loss of bone density

        (2) Pain related to fracture

        (3) Impaired physical mobility related to pain

    c) Nursing intervention

        (1) Provide ambulatory support as needed.

        (2) Eliminate hazards in patient's environment, and teach patient to maintain safety precautions at home; provide ample lighting.

        (3) Administer analgesics, anti-inflammatory drugs, and/or muscle relaxants as prescribed.

        (4) Work with physical therapist to ensure that orthotic devices fit the patient properly; inspect patient's skin for irritation.

        (5) Encourage patient to practice range-of-motion, isometric, resistive, weight-bearing, and breathing exercises.

    d) Nursing evaluation

        (1) Patient uses ambulatory aids as needed.

        (2) Patient identifies potential hazards in his/her environment and avoids injury.

        (3) Patient states that pain is reduced or eliminated.

        (4) Patient uses orthotic devices as prescribed.

        (5) Patient performs exercises on regular basis.

C. Osteomyelitis

    1. Definition: infection of bone

      a) Acute osteomyelitis: bone infection lasting <4 weeks

      b) Chronic osteomyelitis: bone infection lasting >4 weeks

    2. Pathophysiology and etiology

      a) Pathophysiology: After invasion by pathogen, the following occur: bone and soft tissue inflammation, edema formation, bone ischemia, bone necrosis (sequestrum formation), bone abscess, and superimposed infection.

      b) Etiology: may be caused by bacteremia, underlying disease, nonpenetrating trauma, urinary tract infection, long-term hemodialysis, long-term IV catheterization, *Salmonella* infection of GI tract, or penetrating trauma (e.g., puncture wound, gunshot wound, open fracture, animal bite, bone surgery)

    3. Symptoms: fever, swelling, sensation of heat, draining ulcers on hands or feet, bone pain

    4. Diagnostic evaluation: blood studies (elevated leukocyte level and sedimentation rate), radiography, bone scan, CT scan, MRI, bone biopsy

5. Medical treatment
  a) Prevention
    (1) Treatment of local infections to limit spread; management of soft tissue infections to prevent bone erosion
    (2) Administration of prophylactic antibiotics at surgery and up to 48 hours after
    (3) Performance of aseptic postoperative wound care to reduce incidence of infection
  b) Antibiotic therapy
  c) Surgical intervention
    (1) Sequestrectomy
    (2) Bone segment transfers
    (3) Bone grafts
    (4) Muscle flaps
    (5) Amputation
6. Essential nursing care for patients with osteomyelitis
  a) Nursing assessment
    (1) Assess patient for risk factors, injury, infection, or previous orthopedic surgery.
    (2) Perform physical exam, noting warm, inflamed, or swollen areas, purulent drainage, and elevation in temperature.
  b) Nursing diagnoses
    (1) Pain related to inflammation
    (2) Impaired physical mobility related to pain
    (3) Potential for injury related to bone infection
  c) Nursing intervention
    (1) Immobilize affected part with a splint to decrease pain and relieve muscle spasm; elevate affected extremity to relieve swelling; provide warm saline soaks for 20 minutes each hour for 48–72 hours.
    (2) Administer antibiotics as prescribed, and monitor patient's response to them.
    (3) Inform patient of rationale for activity restrictions; encourage participation in activities of daily living.
  d) Nursing evaluation
    (1) Patient states that pain is reduced or eliminated.
    (2) Patient demonstrates improved mobility.
    (3) Patient sustains no additional injuries.

D. Rheumatic disorders
  1. Definition
    a) A group of diseases varying in manifestation and severity involving the muscles, tendons, connective tissue, ligaments, and joints
    b) More than 100 types of rheumatic disorders, including rheumatoid arthritis, ankylosing spondylitis, lupus erythematosus, systemic sclerosis, and gout
  2. Pathophysiology and etiology
    a) Pathophysiology: disruption of protein components and collagen portion of connective tissue and widespread systemic inflammation

        b) Etiology: other than for disorders such as gout and infectious arthritis, etiology unknown (but possibly a combination of genetic, environmental, autoimmune, and viral factors)

   3. Symptoms: pain, enlargement, redness, deformity, or tenderness of joint; skin problems; alopecia; eye problems; altered bowel habits; abnormal reflexes

   4. Diagnostic evaluation: arthrocentesis; radiography; bone and joint scans; MRI; electromyelography; myelography; arthrography; muscle, arterial, or skin biopsy; serum lab studies for rheumatoid factor analysis

   5. Medical treatment
      a) Anti-inflammatory, antirheumatic medication
      b) Exercise for joint motion and muscle strength improvement
      c) Thermal treatments
      d) Plasmapheresis
      e) Joint protection, splints, and adaptive devices

   6. Essential nursing care for patients with rheumatic disorders
      a) Nursing assessment
         (1) Obtain patient history, inquiring about occupation, participation in sports, trauma, and family history of rheumatic disorders.
         (2) Perform physical exam, noting any joint pain, crepitation, joint enlargement, or fluid accumulation.
      b) Nursing diagnoses
         (1) Chronic pain related to inflammation
         (2) Impaired physical mobility related to joint deformity or pain
      c) Nursing intervention
         (1) Apply heat or cold (as tolerated) to relieve pain, stiffness, and muscle spasm; teach relaxation and imagery techniques to reduce pain.
         (2) Encourage patient to move and to be as self-sufficient as possible.
         (3) Introduce available assistive devices.
      d) Nursing evaluation
         (1) Patient states that pain is reduced or eliminated.
         (2) Patient exhibits an increased level of mobility.

E. Bone tumors
   1. Definition: neoplasms of the skeletal system that include a variety of types, either benign or malignant
   2. Pathophysiology and etiology
      a) Malignant tumors may originate in the bone (primary tumor) or may originate elsewhere and metastasize to the bone (secondary tumor).

b) Primary malignant tumors are called sarcomas; they generally metastasize to other body parts.
3. Symptoms: persistent pain, swelling, tender palpable mass, disability, weight loss, malaise, fever
4. Diagnostic evaluation: radiography (including bone scans, tomography, and arteriography), biochemical assays of blood and urine (serum alkaline phosphatase may be elevated), surgical biopsy
5. Medical treatment
    a) Primary malignant tumors: surgical removal of tumor by amputating extremity or by wide local resection, chemotherapy, or radiation therapy
    b) Benign tumors: curettage or local excision
6. Essential nursing care for patients with bone tumors
    a) Nursing assessment
        (1) Obtain patient history, noting previous radiation therapy for cancer, as well as patient's understanding of disease and his/her coping mechanisms.
        (2) Perform physical exam, which should include palpating mass; noting size, swelling, pain, or tenderness; and assessing range of motion of extremity and patient's ability to perform activities of daily living.
    b) Nursing diagnoses
        (1) Pain related to tumor
        (2) High risk for injury related to tumor
        (3) Ineffective individual coping related to prognosis
        (4) Self-esteem disturbance related to loss of body part
    c) Nursing intervention
        (1) Prepare patient and provide emotional support during painful procedures; work with patient to combine use of prescribed medication with psychologic and environmental pain management techniques.
        (2) Handle affected bones gently; provide external supports, and follow weight-bearing restrictions.
        (3) Teach patient how to use ambulatory aids safely.
        (4) Encourage patient and family to express their feelings; provide emotional support; refer them for counseling, if needed.
        (5) Encourage self-care and socialization; involve patient and family in treatment process.
    d) Nursing evaluation
        (1) Patient states that pain is reduced or eliminated.
        (2) Patient experiences no additional injuries.
        (3) Patient demonstrates effective coping patterns and positive self-concept.
        (4) Patient exhibits no complications.

1. Juan Husepa had an open reduction of a fractured right femur completed 8 hours ago. He was placed in balanced skeletal traction after surgery. Which sign would indicate that Juan is experiencing a complication of his injury?

   a. Continuous dry, hacking cough
   b. Urticaria on the chest and neck
   c. Tachypnea and tachycardia
   d. Bounding pulse in the right foot

2. Which nursing action should be implemented to promote optimal healing and health while Juan is in traction?

   a. Assess pin sites for infection each shift.
   b. Encourage fluid intake up to 2500 ml per day.
   c. Administer 30 ml of milk of magnesia at bedtime each day.
   d. Keep head of bed elevated at a 30° angle.

3. At which area of the body would Juan be most likely to experience skin breakdown while in traction?

   a. Left lateral malleolus
   b. Right ischium
   c. Scapula
   d. Sacrum

4. 24 hours ago, Vang Woo had a fiberglass cast applied to immobilize a fracture of the right ankle. He now reports a tight feeling in the toes of his right foot. The nurse's first action is to:

   a. Notify the orthopedist.
   b. Elevate the foot on 2 pillows.
   c. Bivalve the cast.
   d. Assess capillary refill time.

5. Bill Finley is to be discharged to his home with crutches. Which exercise does the nurse teach him in order to strengthen the triceps muscles for crutch-walking?

   a. Pushing the buttocks up off the mattress
   b. Pulling the body up, using an overhead trapeze

   c. Raising the legs straight up and down
   d. Squeezing a ball in each hand

6. Health promotion teaching for a 75-year-old patient who has osteoporosis would include information about:

   a. Increasing calcium intake to 1500 mg per day.
   b. Planning a 2-hour activity-free rest period each day.
   c. Applying ice to inflamed joints for 20 minutes t.i.d.
   d. Taking 2 tablets of acetaminophen every 4 hours p.r.n. for pain.

7. Heloise Hanson sustained a Colles' fracture of her left wrist and is awaiting surgical repair. During assessment of Ms. Hanson, the nurse observes edema, pallor, and numbness in the fingers of the left hand. Which analysis and follow-up action most accurately reflect these data?

   a. The data reflect expected inflammatory changes related to the injury; no action is needed.
   b. The data indicate possible compartment syndrome; the physician should be notified.
   c. The data indicate impaired tissue perfusion; the extremity should be elevated.
   d. The data indicate high risk for crush syndrome; the patient should be monitored for shock.

8. Faith Lightfeather, 16, experienced a traumatic above-knee amputation of her right leg during a motor vehicle accident. Which nursing diagnosis would be included in her care plan?

   a. High risk for infection related to traumatic injury
   b. Ineffective individual coping related to change in appearance
   c. Impaired physical mobility with high risk for falls related to imbalance
   d. Self-care deficit related to loss of body part

9. Which nursing action would be most helpful in preventing possible complications associated with Faith's injury?

   a. Reminding Faith to cough and deep breathe every 2 hours
   b. Elevating the stump on 2 pillows while the patient is in bed
   c. Helping the patient to lie prone for 20 minutes each shift
   d. Providing an overhead frame and trapeze

10. Joel Hirshbaum, 15, is admitted to the hospital for diagnostic testing for possible bone cancer. Which lab results are most indicative of bone cancer?

    a. Elevated alkaline phosphatase and lactate dehydrogenase levels
    b. Decreased serum calcium and phosphorus levels
    c. Elevated potassium level and erythrocyte sedimentation rate (ESR)
    d. Decreased hemoglobin and lymphocyte levels

11. Joel is scheduled for a bone biopsy and a bone scan. He asks the nurse, "Why do I need these tests?" The best response is:

    a. "The tests will help the doctor determine the prognosis for your illness."
    b. "Have your parents talked with you about your illness?"
    c. "Your blood tests indicated a need for these tests."
    d. "What has your doctor told you about the tests to be done?"

12. Kelly Linn has newly diagnosed rheumatoid arthritis. What information would the nurse share with Kelly when t eaching her about the management of this condition?

    a. Prevent gastric ulcers by avoiding the use of salicylates.
    b. Reduce swelling by elevating inflamed joints.
    c. Eat foods that are good sources of iron and vitamin C at each meal.
    d. Schedule lab visits twice a year to monitor IgG levels.

ANSWERS

1. **Correct answer is c.** Fracture of the femur is associated with a high risk of development of fat emboli. The major manifestations of fat emboli are dyspnea, chest pain, tachypnea, tachycardia, hypertension, fever, and petechiae over neck, upper arms, chest, and abdomen.

   a. Any cough would be expected to be moist. Such a cough would be secondary to pulmonary edema, which forms as a result of the presence of the emboli.
   b. The petechial rash is characteristic of fat emboli, whereas urticaria is characteristic of hypersensitivity reactions.
   d. A weak, easily obliterated pulse or an absent pulse would indicate impaired circulation to the distal portion of the extremity.

2. **Correct answer is b.** Common complications of immobility include stasis pneumonia, anorexia, constipation, urinary tract infection (UTI), depression, and skin breakdown. Increasing the patient's fluid intake to 2500–3000 ml per day during periods of immobility is recommended to support physiologic processes of healing and to prevent constipation and UTI.

   a. While assessing pin sites is an essential nursing function, it will not prevent infection from occurring.
   c. The first-line nursing intervention to promote bowel elimination during periods of immobility is to increase fluids and fiber in the diet. Milk of magnesia is typically given on a p.r.n. basis on the evening of the third day without a bowel movement.
   d. Keeping the head of the bed elevated 30° at all times increases the pressure and shearing forces on the buttocks and sacrum as the patient is pulled to the foot of the bed by traction weights. Besides preventing this problem, lying flat for periods of time promotes drainage of secretions from the lower lobes of the lungs.

3. **Correct answer is d.** When a patient is in traction, the 2 most common sites of skin breakdown are the heel of the noninvolved leg and the sacrum.

   a, b, and **c.** The left lateral malleolus, right ischium, and scapula are incorrect sites, for the reason just given.

4. **Correct answer is d.** The nurse must first assess the situation before taking appropriate action. The patient's report of tightness 24 hours after cast application indicates the possibility of impaired circulation. Prompt intervention to prevent possible circulatory collapse in the foot is necessary. A circulation, movement, sensation (CMS) check, which includes assessing capillary refill time, is indicated.

   a, b, and **c.** Assessment should precede the interventions suggested in these answers.

5. **Correct answer is a.** Pushing one's buttocks up off the mattress is a resistive exercise that improves the strength and tone of the triceps muscles.

   b. Pull-ups strengthen the biceps muscles.
   c. Straight leg raises strengthen the hip flexor and quadriceps.
   d. Squeezing a ball strengthens finger flexors.

6. **Correct answer is a.** Osteoporosis is weakening of the matrix of bone caused by loss of calcium. Current recommendations for improving health and preventing complications in persons with osteoporosis are increasing daily calcium and vitamin D intake and initiating estrogen replacement therapy. Recommended supplementation is to take calcium, 1500 mg/day, and vitamin D, 400 IU/day.

   b. Persons with osteoporosis need to remain active to move calcium into bones.
   c. Joints are inflamed and swollen in arthritic conditions, not in osteoporosis.
   d. Acetaminophen is a direct intervention for pain, not a health-promoting activity.

7. **Correct answer is b.** Compartment syndrome is a serious complication of fractures of the wrist that requires emergency medical intervention. Manifestations of compartment syndrome include edema, pain, pallor or cyanosis, numbness, tingling, paresthesia, and weak thready pulse or pulselessness.

   a. Although it is true that inflammation occurs with fractures, the additional signs of pallor and numbness indicate the possibility of a more serious complication that the nurse needs to assess.
   c. Compartment syndrome is a serious form of impaired circulation that requires prompt medical intervention.
   d. Crush syndrome occurs with massive tissue injury.

8. **Correct answer is b.** The primary developmental task of adolescence is defining personal identity. During this time, body image becomes a focus of interest and concern. Traumatic loss of a body part typically results in identity and body-image threats that require adaptation.

   a. Potential for infection does exist, but the etiologic factor is impaired skin integrity, rather than the initial accident.
   c. Impaired mobility is a concern, although the risk of falls is not necessarily an associated factor.
   d. Self-care deficits are associated with arm and hand amputations.

9. **Correct answer is c.** The primary complication of an above-knee amputation is flexion contracture of the hip muscles. Lying prone results in hip extension.

   a. It is expected that this patient will soon be out of bed and active. Coughing and deep breathing prevent the complications of immobility, not those of the amputation injury.
   b. Controversy exists regarding the advisability of elevating the stump. Positioning in this manner causes the hip muscles to flex and may contribute to the formation of flexion contractures. Stumps are typically

elevated for 24 hours after surgery to decrease edema formation.

d. An overhead trapeze provides for mobility in bed but does not prevent complications associated with the amputation.

10. **Correct answer is a.** Alkaline phosphatase is an enzyme that originates in the bone. It is used as a tumor marker and an index of bone disease. Lactate dehydrogenase level also increases in bone cancer.

    b. Calcium and phosphorus levels are elevated in bone cancer.

    c. Potassium levels are not associated with bone cancer. ESR is elevated in infections and inflammation of bones, but it is not specific to cancer.

    d. Anemia may be present, but it is not specific to bone cancer. White blood cell (WBC) counts are not associated with bone cancer.

11. **Correct answer is d.** The nurse applies the principles of therapeutic communication to ascertain the patient's understanding of his or her condition before appropriate responses to his or her questions can be made.

In this situation, the nurse needs to determine how much information this adolescent has been given about his illness and needs to use feedback techniques to validate the message being sent.

a and **c.** Simply indicating that the tests are necessary does not invite the patient to discuss his concerns.

b. Asking the patient about his parents is an evasive response.

12. **Correct answer is c.** Anemia commonly coexists with rheumatoid arthritis (RA), and teaching patients to choose foods that are high in iron, vitamin C, and folic acid will improve their health.

    a. Salicylates are the drugs of choice in the treatment of RA.

    b. Moist heat or ice may be applied to inflamed joints in RA.

    d. IgG is measured during the initial diagnostic work-up for RA. ESR values are monitored on a regular basis to determine the effectiveness of anti-inflammatory drug therapy.

11

Senses (Eyes, Ears)

OVERVIEW

I. Eyes
    A. Structure and function of
       visual system
    B. General diagnostic tests
    C. General nursing
       assessment
    D. Nursing considerations
       with selected therapies and
       techniques
    E. Selected disorders

II. Ears
    A. Structure and function of
       auditory system
    B. General diagnostic tests
    C. General nursing
       assessments
    D. Nursing considerations
       associated with ear
       surgery
    E. Selected disorders

NURSING HIGHLIGHTS

1. Eye disorders with the potential to cause vision impairment or blindness produce profound anxiety in patients; nurse should listen supportively and suggest ways in which patient can control anxieties, such as complying fully with treatment regimens and establishing a support system.
2. Loss of hearing and total deafness can be devastating consequences of ear problems; nurse should help patient learn to cope with loss and to use friends, family, and support groups to maintain functional ability.

GLOSSARY

aqueous humor—the fluid produced in the eye that fills the spaces in front of the lens
diplacusis—perception of a single auditory stimulus as two separate sounds
gonioscope—an instrument used to examine the anterior chamber of the eye
Hallpike maneuver—a test for benign paroxysmal positional vertigo or induced dizziness in which the head of a supine patient is rotated to the side for 1 minute
labyrinthectomy—total removal of the labyrinth to treat severe vertigo
miotic—an agent that causes the pupil to constrict
mydriatic—an agent that dilates the pupil
myringectomy—removal of the tympanic membrane

nystagmus—involuntary rapid horizontal, vertical, or rotatory movement of eyeball

recruitment—an abnormally rapid increase in the loudness of a sound caused by a slight increase in its intensity

tympanoplasty—surgical reconstruction of the tympanic membrane

ENHANCED OUTLINE

I. Eyes

See text pages

_____

A. Structure and function of visual system
  1. Structure
     a) The eyeball sits in the skull's bony cavity, protected by eyelids and tears on its anterior surface.
     b) The eyeball consists of 3 layers: the external layer, called the *fibrous coat,* including the sclera and cornea; the middle layer, called the *uvea,* including the choroid, ciliary body, and iris; and the inner layer, called the *retina,* which is bordered by the vitreous body.
  2. Function: Light rays enter the cornea and pass through the pupil, lens, and vitreous body to the retina, stimulating sensory receptors to send impulses to the brain, where they are registered.

B. General diagnostic tests
  1. Fluorescein angiography: detects retinal circulation and disorders, including diabetic retinopathy and eye tumors, by injection of sodium fluorescein into arm vein, followed by taking of photographs that record the appearance of dye in the retinal vessels
  2. Corneal staining: diagnoses conditions caused by trauma, abrasions, and ulcers by application of dye into conjunctival sac to detect irregularities
  3. Tonometry: diagnoses glaucoma
     a) Applanation (most common): measures force required to flatten a small standard area of cornea
     b) Indentation: measures deformation of globe in response to standard weight placed on cornea

C. General nursing assessment
  1. Patient history
     a) Obtain information about overall health, lifestyle, family history, and independence level.
     b) Assess symptoms, including visual impairment, headaches, vertigo, ocular pain, and eye discharge.
  2. Observation and physical examination
     a) Inspect external eye structures, cornea, anterior chamber, and extraocular muscles.
     b) Assess ocular tension and visual field.

3. Diagnostic tests: nursing responsibilities
    a) Fluorescein angiography: Explain that test is intended to provide a permanent record of ocular circulation that is especially valuable in showing damage to arterioles; obtain informed consent; ask about allergies to dyes; instill mydriatic 1 hour before test; advise patient to drink fluids, avoid bright light, and rest after procedure.
    b) Corneal staining: Explain that coloration is used to determine irregularities of the corneal surface, thus indicating trauma to the eye; ask patient to remove contact lenses, if worn; explain that test is painless; apply dye and ask patient to blink; after test, remove dye from cheeks and advise patient not to rub eyes.
    c) Tonometry
        (1) Noncontact tonometry: Explain that this is a screening procedure to measure intraocular pressure (IOP); caution patient that he/she will feel a puff of air on the eye; direct air against cornea using tonometer; record pressure reading (reading >24 mm Hg suggests glaucoma).
        (2) Applanation tonometry: Explain that this procedure is a more accurate way to measure IOP; anesthetize eyes by instilling anesthetic into conjunctival sacs; urge patient not to rub eyes; touch flattened cone to cornea; record amount of pressure that causes flattening.

D. Nursing considerations with selected therapies and techniques
    1. Ocular irrigations
        a) Place pH paper in cul-de-sac of eye, and instill proparacaine hydrochloride as ordered.
        b) Ask patient to lie down, with head turned slightly toward affected side.
        c) Position eyelid speculum or irrigating contact lens.
        d) Direct solution across globe toward lateral canthus and into receptacle.
        e) Irrigate eyes simultaneously if both are affected, using separate equipment and personnel.
    2. Eyedrops (see Nurse Alert, "Instilling Eyedrops for Glaucoma Patients")
        a) Instruct patient to tilt head, open eyes, and look up.
        b) Pull lid down and forward; holding bottle like pencil, rest wrist on patient's cheek, and squeeze bottle gently.
        c) Release eyelid, and instruct patient to close eyes.
        d) Instruct patient not to squeeze eyes, since that will force medication into nasolacrimal system, reducing absorption.
        e) To achieve maximal absorption, wait 5 minutes before instilling another drop.

3. Eye surgery
   a) Preoperative: Administer eyedrops, enema or laxative, tranquilizer, antiemetic, and analgesics; scrub around eyes or shampoo hair, if needed.
   b) Postoperative
      (1) Remind patient not to touch dressing.
      (2) Orient patient to physical surroundings and to location of call button, telephone, and other important objects; maintain quiet, restful atmosphere.
      (3) Caution patient to maintain position appropriate for particular type of surgery performed.
      (4) Check condition of dressing, and report bleeding or other drainage immediately.
      (5) Report any signs of infection immediately.
      (6) Report sharp eye pain or pain associated with nausea immediately, since it may be a sign of altered intraocular pressure (IOP).
      (7) Remind patient to avoid activities that can increase IOP, such as coughing, sneezing, vomiting, straining to defecate, bending at waist, lifting objects heavier than 15 lb, and lying on affected side; if necessary, obtain order to administer drugs to prevent coughing, sneezing, vomiting, or constipation.
   c) Post-discharge
      (1) Instruct patient in aseptic technique of eye medication instillation.
      (2) Caution patient to wear eye shield at night for one month after surgery and when around young children and pets.
      (3) Discuss with patient ways to avoid eye injury or other injury associated with limited vision in the home setting.

E. Selected disorders
   1. Glaucoma
      a) Definition: a group of diseases caused by increased intraocular pressure

    b) Pathophysiology and etiology
      (1) Pathophysiology: imbalance in production and drainage of aqueous humor in anterior chamber
      (2) Etiology: heredity, age, diabetes, hypertension
    c) Symptoms: discomfort, aching, temporary blurring of vision, halos around lights, reduced peripheral vision, frequent need to change glasses
    d) Diagnostic evaluation: ocular, medication, and health history; tonometry; gonioscopy; ophthalmoscopy
    e) Medical treatment
      (1) Drug therapy
        (a) Agents that enhance pupillary constriction, allowing better circulation of aqueous humor to absorption site: miotics, such as pilocarpine hydrochloride and carbachol
        (b) Agents that inhibit aqueous humor formation: beta-adrenergic blocking agents, such as timolol (Timoptic); and carbonic anhydrase inhibitors, such as acetazolamide (Diamox)
      (2) Surgery, including iridectomy, trabeculectomy, seton procedures, laser surgery
    f) Complication: blindness
    g) Essential nursing care for patients with glaucoma
      (1) Nursing assessment: Obtain symptom, medical, and allergy history; determine amount of vision.
      (2) Nursing diagnoses
        (a) Knowledge deficit related to need for lifelong treatment
        (b) Sensory/perceptual alterations (visual) related to destruction of nerve fibers by increased IOP
        (c) Pain related to increased IOP
        (d) Potential for injury related to reduced peripheral vision
      (3) Nursing intervention
        (a) Explain that drug therapy for glaucoma must continue throughout patient's life; be alert for signs of noncompliance.
        (b) Administer medications to reduce IOP and stabilize vision.
        (c) Administer analgesic if prescribed; evaluate often for pain relief.
        (d) Remove obstacles that may be hazardous to ambulatory patients.
        (e) Follow standard nursing procedures for postoperative care of patient who has undergone eye surgery, as outlined in section I,D,3 of this chapter.

(4) Nursing evaluation
 (a) Patient maintains existing vision.
 (b) Patient states that pain is reduced or eliminated.
 (c) Patient's self-care needs are met.

2. Cataracts
 a) Definition: lens opacities that reduce the amount of light reaching the retina, distorting images
 b) Pathophysiology and etiology
  (1) Pathophysiology: slow deterioration of vision as lens becomes opaque
  (2) Etiology: aging, congenital defect, eye injury, eye diseases, medications, radiation exposure
 c) Symptoms: halo around lights, reading problems, changes in color vision or acuity, glare, object distortion, blurry or double vision
 d) Diagnostic evaluation: tests of visual acuity (Snellen's chart, brightness acuity tests); A-scan ultrasound; ophthalmoscopic slit-lamp exam
 e) Medical treatment: surgical removal of lens, followed by use of corrective lenses; implants
 f) Complications: impaired vision, blindness
 g) Essential nursing care for patients with cataracts
  (1) Nursing assessment: Obtain symptom, medical, drug, and family history; perform ophthalmoscopic exam.
  (2) Nursing diagnoses
   (a) Sensory/perceptual alterations (visual) related to disease
   (b) Potential for injury related to cataract surgery
   (c) Self-care deficit related to vision problems

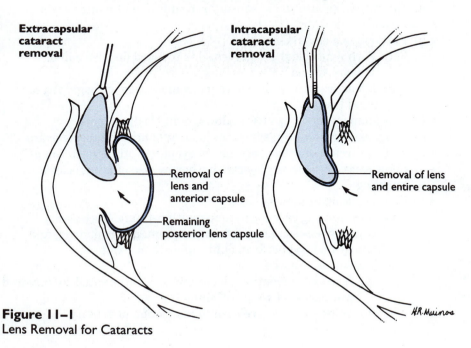

Extracapsular cataract removal

Intracapsular cataract removal

Removal of lens and anterior capsule

Remaining posterior lens capsule

Removal of lens and entire capsule

H.R. Muinos

Figure 11–1
Lens Removal for Cataracts

        (3) Nursing intervention

           (a) Follow standard nursing procedures for postoperative care of patient who has undergone eye surgery, as outlined in section I,D,3 of this chapter.

           (b) Position patient in semi-Fowler's position or on unaffected side.

           (c) Instill steroid antibiotic eyedrops if ordered by ophthalmologist.

           (d) Apply cool compresses to reduce itching, and administer mild analgesic, such as acetaminophen, for pain.

           (e) Tell patient to advise ophthalmologist immediately of any symptoms of retinal detachment, including seeing dark spots, bright flashes, or an increased number of floaters or experiencing decreased visual field.

        (4) Nursing evaluation

           (a) Patient demonstrates improved ability to process visual stimuli.

           (b) Patient avoids infection and other complications of cataract surgery.

           (c) Patient is able to participate in some aspects of daily care.

3. Retinal detachment

    a) Definition: separation of sensory retina from pigmented layer of retina

    b) Pathophysiology and etiology

        (1) Pathophysiology: vision loss due to blood deprivation of sensory retina

        (2) Etiology: trauma, eye surgery, tumors, hemorrhage, vitreous fluid loss

    c) Symptoms: vision gaps or shadows, light flashes, spots

    d) Diagnostic evaluation: symptom history, ophthalmoscopic exam

    e) Medical treatment: bed rest, use of eyepatch, administration of mydriatics, cryosurgery, electrodiathermy, use of laser, scleral buckling

    f) Complication: blindness

    g) Essential nursing care for patients with retinal detachment

        (1) Nursing assessment: Obtain symptom, medical, drug, and family history; perform ophthalmoscopic exam.

        (2) Nursing diagnoses

           (a) Sensory/perceptual alterations (visual) related to impaired processing of visual stimuli

           (b) Self-care deficit related to restriction of activity

      (3) Nursing intervention
         (a) Follow standard nursing procedures for postoperative care of patient who has undergone eye surgery, as outlined in section I,D,3 of this chapter.
         (b) If gas or silicone oil was used to promote retinal reattachment, position patient on abdomen, with head turned to operative eye; patient can also sit on side of bed, with head on bedside stand.
         (c) Be aware that nausea is common after surgery for retinal detachment; to prevent vomiting, which can raise IOP, administer antiemetic as soon as patient complains of nausea.
         (d) Administer meperidine or acetaminophen and codeine to control pain.
         (e) Caution patient not to engage in activities that involve rapid eye movements, such as reading, writing, and doing fine needlework, for 1 week.
      (4) Nursing evaluation
         (a) Patient demonstrates improved ability to process visual stimuli.
         (b) Patient is able to participate in some aspects of daily care.

4. Infectious and inflammatory eye disorders
   a) Definition: infection or inflammation of the conjunctiva, uveal tract, cornea, or eyelid
   b) Pathophysiology and etiology
      (1) Conjunctivitis: inflammation of conjunctiva caused by infection
      (2) Uveitis: inflammation of uveal tract of unknown cause
      (3) Keratitis/corneal ulcer: inflammation of cornea caused by trauma or infection
      (4) Blepharitis: inflammation of eyelids caused by dry eyes
      (5) Stye and chalazion: inflammation, infection, and formation of cyst of eyelid oil gland caused by excess oil
   c) Symptoms: redness, tearing, swelling, pain, drainage, itching, congestion, reduced vision, photophobia
   d) Diagnostic evaluation: visual exam, noting of symptoms, slit-lamp exam, cultures, use of fluorescein drops
   e) Medical treatment: drugs, irrigation, drainage
   f) Complications: astigmatism, decreased vision, blindness
   g) Essential nursing care for patients with infectious and inflammatory eye disorders
      (1) Nursing assessment: Obtain medical, symptom, and allergy history; examine eye and surrounding structures.
      (2) Nursing diagnoses
         (a) Anxiety related to pain
         (b) Potential for infection related to pathogen transfer
      (3) Nursing intervention
         (a) Teach patient aseptic technique for self-administration of eye medications.
         (b) Caution patient to avoid rubbing eyes.

(4) Nursing evaluation
    (a) Patient states that pain is reduced.
    (b) Patient experiences no spread of infection.

See text pages
_____

II. Ears

A. Structure and function of auditory system
  1. Structure: external ear, middle ear (tympanic membrane, malleus, incus, stapes, window membranes), inner ear (semicircular canals, cochlea, distal end of vestibulocochlear nerve)
  2. Function: to permit hearing and maintenance of balance
    a) Mechanism of hearing: transfer of sound by eardrum to malleus, incus, and stapes, through cochlea; transduction of vibrations by receptors into action potentials sent to brain as neural impulses
    b) Mechanism of balance: Vestibular structures filled with fluid and hair cells are connected to nerves in the brain; fluid bends hair cells as head position changes, providing information about body's position.

B. General diagnostic tests
  1. Otoscopic examination: examination of ear canal and eardrum to detect cerumen buildup and presence of infection, inflammation, or foreign body
  2. Air/bone conduction test: evaluation of hearing by placing vibrating fork on mastoid process and then in front of pinna
  3. Miscellaneous tests of vestibular function: test for falling (sense of balance), past pointing (sense of position), gaze nystagmus assay (involuntary eye movements), Hallpike maneuver (induced dizziness)

C. General nursing assessments
  1. Patient history: Obtain medical, family, and medication history; ascertain degree of hearing problem and methods used to understand speech.
  2. Observation and physical examination
    a) Examine external ear and mastoid process for redness, swelling, pain on manipulation, excess cerumen, poor hygiene, drainage, and tenderness.
    b) Perform voice test by whispering a statement to patient as he/she covers 1 ear.
    c) Assist during diagnostic exam procedures.
  3. Diagnostic tests
    a) Otoscopic examination
      (1) Check for cerumen buildup; flush ear with warm water if necessary.
      (2) Tip patient's head away, grasp external ear firmly and pull upward, backward, and slightly outward.
      (3) Position speculum down and slightly forward in ear canal.

   (4) Examine ear canal, noting discharge, inflammation, deviations, and presence of foreign body; note position and color of eardrum.

  b) Air/bone conduction test

   (1) Place vibrating tuning fork stem on patient's mastoid process (bone conduction test).

   (2) When patient no longer hears sound, bring fork to front of pinna and ask if sound is heard (air conduction test).

  c) Miscellaneous tests of vestibular function

   (1) Test for falling: After assuring patient that nurse will prevent a fall, have him/her stand with feet together, arms hanging at sides, and eyes closed; normal response is slight sway.

   (2) Past pointing: Instruct seated patient to close eyes and point at nurse; nurse touches fingers with own index fingers for point of reference; after raising and lowering arms, patient is asked to return to reference point.

   (3) Gaze nystagmus assay: Examine patient's eyes for rapid spontaneous movements while he/she looks straight ahead, 30° to each side, upward, and downward.

   (4) Hallpike maneuver: Check for nystagmus when head of supine patient is rotated to side for 1 minute.

D. Nursing considerations associated with ear surgery

 1. Assist patient with all activities before surgery if vertigo is present, and alert physician if patient to be given local anesthetic is extremely anxious.

 2. After surgery, administer prophylactic antibiotics, if ordered.

 3. Change internal and/or external dressings, if ordered.

 4. Unless otherwise indicated, keep patient in flat position with operative ear up for 12 hours after surgery.

 5. Notify physician of postoperative headache, severe or sudden onset of pain, excess drainage, extreme dizziness, or fever.

 6. Wipe any discharge from ear with dry applicator; do not insert cotton plug into ear unless ordered.

 7. Instruct patient in proper technique for self-administration of ear medication and for changing ear dressing (if needed).

 8. Advise patient to avoid increased middle-ear pressure by not straining during defecation, avoiding air travel, and not drinking through a straw for 2–3 weeks; teach patient to blow nose by blowing 1 side at a time with the mouth open.

 9. Caution patient to reduce risk of infection by avoiding people with respiratory infections.

 10. Instruct patient to keep water out of the ear by not washing the hair or showering for 1 week.

E. Selected disorders

 1. Ear infections

  a) Definition: infection of the middle ear (otitis media) or mastoid process (mastoiditis)

b) Pathophysiology and etiology
    (1) Otitis media: upper respiratory infections spread from nose and throat to ear through eustachian tube, with children at special risk because their eustachian tubes are shorter and straighter
    (2) Mastoiditis: bone infection caused by acute or chronic otitis media

c) Symptoms
    (1) Acute otitis media: fever, ear noises, malaise, severe earache, diminished hearing
    (2) Chronic otitis media: chronic discharge from ear, reduced hearing, slight fever
    (3) Mastoiditis: pain or tenderness behind ear, fever, malaise, headache, symptoms of otitis media

d) Diagnostic evaluation
    (1) Acute otitis media: noting of symptoms, otoscopic examination of eardrum (appears red/bulging)
    (2) Chronic otitis media: same as for acute version, with added history of ear infections
    (3) Mastoiditis: recording of symptoms, palpation of mastoid bone, radiography, computed tomographic (CT) scan, magnetic resonance imaging (MRI)

e) Medical treatment
    (1) Acute otitis media: antibiotics, myringotomy, culture and sensitivity studies
    (2) Chronic otitis media and mastoiditis: antibiotics, radical mastoidectomy

f) Complications: hearing loss, vestibular disturbance

g) Essential nursing care for patients with ear infections
    (1) Nursing assessment: Obtain symptom, medical, and allergy history.
    (2) Nursing diagnoses
        (a) Pain related to inflammation and swelling
        (b) Sensory/perceptual alterations (auditory) related to obstruction of the external auditory canal
        (c) Potential for injury related to altered auditory perception
    (3) Nursing intervention
        (a) Apply heat locally for 20 minutes, 3 times a day using warm towels or heating pads.
        (b) Administer topical antibiotics, steroids, and analgesics as ordered; administer antivertigo agent such as dimenhydrinate if necessary.
        (c) Advise patient to take special precautions because of diminished hearing.

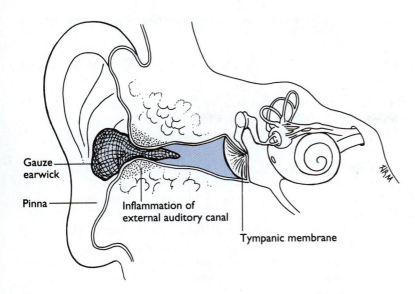

Labels on figure:
Gauze earwick
Pinna
Inflammation of external auditory canal
Tympanic membrane

Figure 11–2
Earwick for Instilling Antibiotics into External Auditory Canal

(4) Nursing evaluation
    (a) Patient states that pain is relieved.
    (b) Patient states that hearing has returned to normal.
    (c) Patient avoids injury associated with temporary hearing loss.

2. Ménière's disease
   a) Definition: an inner ear problem stemming from a dysfunctional labyrinth
   b) Pathophysiology and etiology
     (1) Pathophysiology: distortion of inner canal system by high levels of endolymphatic fluid; damage to vestibular system and dilated cochlear duct, causing hearing loss
     (2) Etiology: infections, allergic reactions, biochemical disturbances, vascular disturbance, psychologic factors, stress, heredity
   c) Symptoms: severe vertigo, tinnitus, nausea, and progressive sensorineural hearing loss in 1 ear that may last a few minutes to weeks
   d) Diagnostic evaluation: pure tone audiometry, noting of recruitment or diplacusis, CT scan, MRI, glucose tolerance tests, electronystagmography, auditory dehydration test
   e) Medical treatment: administration of antihistamines if allergy present; low-salt diet to reduce swelling; fluid limitation; avoidance of caffeine, alcohol, and smoking; bed rest; medication to suppress vestibular system, control nausea, and cause diuresis; destructive labyrinthectomy; endolymphatic subarachnoid shunt; endolymphatic system-mastoid shunt with valve implant
   f) Complications: trauma related to vertigo, hearing loss

  g) Essential nursing care for patients with Ménière's disease (see Client Teaching Checklist, "Home Care for Patients with Vertigo")

   (1) Nursing assessment: Obtain medical and symptom history.

   (2) Nursing diagnoses

    (a) Potential for injury related to vertigo

    (b) Auditory perception changes related to disease

    (c) Social isolation related to vertigo and hearing loss

   (3) Nursing intervention

    (a) Provide assistance when patient is out of bed; administer medication as ordered to control vertigo.

    (b) Urge patient to exercise special care because of hearing loss.

    (c) Encourage patient to continue as many normal activities and interactions as possible.

   (4) Nursing evaluation

    (a) Patient states understanding of how to prevent injury.

    (b) Patient copes with disorder and resumes usual social activities.

 3. Otosclerosis

  a) Definition: middle ear disease of labyrinthine capsule causing formation of abnormal spongy bone that immobilizes stapes

  b) Pathophysiology and etiology

   (1) Pathophysiology: stiffening of the stapes that interferes with its vibration, gradually affecting transmission of sound to inner ear

   (2) Etiology: heredity, exacerbated by pregnancy

✔ CLIENT TEACHING CHECKLIST ✔

Home Care for Patients with Vertigo

The following suggestions may help to limit the severity and frequency of vertigo attacks and help the patient prevent vertigo-related injury.

✔ Rest in a dark, quiet, uncluttered environment.

✔ Follow a low-salt diet, avoid smoking, and take prescribed medication.

✔ Avoid driving or potentially dangerous activities when vertigo attack is imminent.

✔ Learn symptoms of impending attack, including headache, increasing tinnitus, and feeling of fullness in affected ear.

✔ Move head slowly, and use walker or cane during attack.

✔ Learn and practice stress reduction techniques, including meditation, deep breathing, and directed muscle relaxation, which may reduce severity of attacks.

✔ Consider joining a support group.

c) Symptoms: progressive conductive hearing loss in both ears, beginning with lower frequencies; tinnitus
d) Diagnostic evaluation: otoscopic exam (to detect pink eardrum), tuning fork tests
e) Treatment: hearing aids, partial or complete stapedectomy
f) Complications: deafness, prolonged vertigo, facial nerve damage
g) Essential nursing care for patients with otosclerosis
   (1) Nursing assessment: Obtain medical and symptom history.
   (2) Nursing diagnoses
      (a) Auditory alterations related to changes in bony structures of middle ear
      (b) Potential for social isolation related to inability to communicate
   (3) Nursing intervention
      (a) Encourage use of hearing aids, writing paper, and computers.
      (b) Encourage social interaction, and provide information about support groups.
      (c) Advise patient who is planning to undergo stapedectomy to remove hearing aid 2 weeks before surgery to promote tissue integrity; follow standard nursing procedures for postoperative care of patient who has undergone ear surgery, as outlined in section II,D of this chapter; caution patient that improvement in hearing may not be noted for 6 weeks.
   (4) Nursing evaluation
      (a) Patient states that hearing loss is improved.
      (b) Patient uses hearing aids or other communication aids.
      (c) Patient resumes normal social activities.

1. The nurse is teaching Mr. George Makiko about the procedure for instilling atropine sulfate into the eye. The nurse tells the patient to tilt his head backward and incline it slightly to the outside during instillation, to press on the lacrimal sac immediately after instillation, and to continue to apply pressure for several minutes. This is done because systemic absorption of the medication from the nose and pharynx could cause:

   a. Tachycardia.
   b. Hypertension.
   c. Tetany.
   d. Bradypnea.

2. The nurse is counseling 65-year-old Ella Markowitz, who is newly diagnosed with glaucoma. In explaining the rationale for drug therapy, the nurse tells the patient that medication is necessary to:

   a. Increase intraocular pressure within the eye.
   b. Slow progression of optic nerve damage.
   c. Decrease the opacity of the lens.
   d. Reduce circulation of aqueous humor.

3. Ms. Markowitz states, "My glaucoma is not that severe, since I haven't had impaired vision or other problems. I understand that this medication therapy is temporary until my condition improves." The most appropriate nursing diagnosis for Ms. Markowitz would be:

   a. Sensory/perceptual alteration (visual) related to destruction of nerve fibers by increased intraocular pressure.
   b. Chronic pain related to increased intraocular pressure.
   c. Knowledge deficit related to need for lifelong treatment.
   d. Potential for injury related to reduced peripheral vision.

4. In discussing risk factors related to diabetic retinopathy with Sam Baker, a patient who has type II diabetes (non-insulin-dependent diabetes mellitus [NIDDM]), which of the following statements by the nurse would be least important?

   a. "Early diagnosis and treatment may reduce the risk of severe visual loss."
   b. "Controlling blood glucose levels is significant in controlling the progression of retinopathy."
   c. "Compliance with diet, medication, and exercise regimens will decrease your risk of retinopathy."
   d. "You are at increased risk of developing this complication if you have had diabetes a long time."

5. A nurse wearing gloves is attempting to remove the hard contact lenses of a patient who cannot remove them by himself. Which of the following describes the proper technique?

   a. Placing the index finger near the outer canthus of the eye and pulling gently toward the temporal area
   b. Positioning 1 thumb on the upper eyelid and 1 thumb on the lower eyelid and then gently separating the eyelids
   c. Gently placing the thumb and index finger directly on the eye and around the contact lens
   d. Placing the thumb of 1 hand on the upper eyelid and the index finger of 1 hand on the lower eyelid while squeezing gently

6. Which of the following pieces of information would be included in the nurse's teaching plan for a patient who has received an intraocular lens (IOL) implant?

   a. "You may resume your normal daily activities as tolerated."
   b. "You will no longer need to wear prescription eyeglasses."
   c. "You will need to wear eye shields at night for about 2 weeks."
   d. "Because pain medications may mask complications, they are not prescribed."

7. Ms. Ida Harrison, who is 62 years old, has undergone emergency surgery (scleral buckling procedure) for a retinal detachment of her right eye. Following surgery, Ms. Harrison should lie:

   a. On her unaffected side with her head slightly elevated.
   b. In a supine position with her head flat.
   c. Supine with her head positioned to the affected side.
   d. In Trendelenburg's position on her unaffected side.

8. The nurse continues to monitor Ms. Harrison for signs and symptoms of complications throughout her postoperative course. Which of the following would indicate late complications of retinal surgery?

   a. Purulent or excessive mucoid drainage
   b. Severe nausea and vomiting
   c. Cloudy vision and halos around objects
   d. Extrusion of silicone through the conjunctiva

9. Uveitis should be treated promptly, because scar formation can cause:

   a. Glaucoma.
   b. Hypertensive retinopathy.
   c. Cataracts.
   d. Corneal abrasions.

10. Ménière's disease is characterized by a triad of symptoms, including:

    a. Otalgia, progressive hearing loss, and facial paralysis.
    b. Ear pain, tenderness behind the ear, and headache.
    c. Vertigo with nausea and vomiting, tinnitus, and hearing loss.
    d. Otalgia, headache, and loss of appetite.

11. A hearing aid would be most likely to benefit a person who experiences hearing loss as the result of a deficiency that is primarily:

    a. Sensorineural.
    b. Conversion reactive.
    c. Conductive.
    d. Congenital.

12. The physician performs a myringotomy on 24-year-old Harry Toomey to treat a severe case of otitis media. The incision is made into his tympanic membrane to relieve pressure and to drain serous fluid from the:

    a. Middle ear behind the eardrum.
    b. Mastoid process.
    c. External auditory canal.
    d. Eustachian tube.

ANSWERS

1. **Correct answer is a.** Atropine is a cholinergic blocking agent that is also classified as a mydriatic. It blocks the effect of acetylcholine in the sphincter muscle of the iris and the accommodative muscle of the ciliary body, resulting in dilation of the pupil (mydriasis) and loss of accommodation for near vision. Atropine also blocks vagal impulses to the heart, causing an increase in the rate and speed of impulse conduction through the atrioventricular conducting system, thereby increasing heart rate. If pressure is not placed on the lacrimal gland after instillation of these eyedrops, a patient could experience tachycardia due to systemic absorption of the medication.

   b, c, and **d.** All are incorrect based on the explanation given in correct answer **a.** Atropine would not cause hypertension, tetany, or bradypnea.

2. **Correct answer is b.** Patients with glaucoma experience visual field loss due to optic nerve damage. This damage results from increased intraocular pressure when aqueous humor circulation is impaired.

   a. Glaucoma treatment is focused on decreasing intraocular pressure.
   c. Cataract therapy involves decreasing lens opacity.
   d. A treatment goal in glaucoma would be to increase the outflow circulation of aqueous humor, thereby decreasing intraocular pressure. Reducing circulation of aqueous humor would not be desirable.

3. **Correct answer is c.** Based on the information given, it is evident that Ms. Markowitz does not understand that glaucoma therapy must continue for the rest of her life. Although there is no cure for the disorder, it can usually be controlled with medication. The goal of treatment is to arrest progression of the disease or to slow it enough to maintain optimal vision throughout the patient's lifetime.

a, b, and **d.** All are incorrect based on both the information given in correct answer **c** and the patient's statement that she has not experienced other symptoms. Although sensory/perceptual alteration (visual) and potential for injury are priority diagnoses, it is most important at this time that the patient understand the need to comply with lifelong therapy.

4. **Correct answer is d.** Because Mr. Baker has type II diabetes mellitus, he is at lower risk for developing diabetic retinopathy than a patient with type I diabetes (insulin-dependent diabetes mellitus [IDDM]).

a, b, and **c.** Emphasizing early diagnosis and treatment, the control of blood glucose levels, and compliance with the diet, medication, and treatment regimens is important in teaching patients with either type of diabetes.

5. **Correct answer is b.** The nurse would properly remove the hard contact lens by separating the eyelids. If the lens does not drop out easily, it can be slid onto the sclera until a more experienced health care professional can remove it.

a, c, and **d.** These are all incorrect procedures that would not remove hard contact lenses safely.

6. **Correct answer is c.** In addition to wearing eye shields at night, during the day the patient should wear eyeglasses (or sunglasses in bright sunlight) to protect the eye.

a. Following an IOL implant, the patient's activities will be restricted. Areas of restriction include driving, lifting heavy objects, and sexual activity.
b. Patients will need to wear prescription eyeglasses for 6–8 weeks after surgery.
d. Although pain medications are prescribed, pain that is not relieved by the medication should be reported to the physician immediately.

7. **Correct answer is a.** The patient should lie on the unaffected side with her head slightly elevated to decrease the amount of edema. The position should be maintained so that a gas bubble that may be present in the eye can effectively tamponade the retinal break.

b and **c.** A supine position could cause the gas bubble to rise and push the iris forward, causing acute glaucoma in patients who have had the crystalline lens removed. In some patients, this position can also cause the bubble to rest against the crystalline lens, possibly causing cataract formation.
d. Lying in Trendelenburg's position on the unaffected side would not facilitate the goal of decreasing edema and could increase intraocular pressure.

8. **Correct answer is d.** A late complication after surgery to reattach the retina is extrusion of the buckling material or silicone through the conjunctiva.

a, b, and **c.** Abnormal drainage, nausea and vomiting, and visual disturbances are early complications of surgery to correct a retinal detachment.

9. **Correct answer is a.** In a patient with uveitis, failure to institute use of dilating drops immediately could impede aqueous humor outflow and cause an increase in intraocular pressure, resulting in glaucoma.

b, c, and **d.** Hypertensive retinopathy, cataracts, and corneal abrasions are not potential complications of uveitis.

10. **Correct answer is c.** A sense of pressure within the ear is a fourth symptom of Ménière's disease. Initially, if vertigo, tinnitus, and hearing loss are not present, a diagnosis of Ménière's disease is not made.

   a. Otalgia, progressive hearing loss, and facial paralysis are symptoms of chronic otitis media.
   b. Ear pain, tenderness behind the ear, and headache are symptoms of mastoiditis.
   d. Otalgia, headache, and loss of appetite are symptoms of acute otitis media, also known as purulent or suppurative otitis media.

11. **Correct answer is c.** Patients with conductive hearing loss often benefit greatly from a hearing aid, because correction of their problem requires only the amplification of sound.

   a. Patients with sensorineural (perceptive) hearing loss are less sensitive to sound than normal individuals. Although use of a hearing aid might be helpful, it is unlikely to be as beneficial as it is in patients with conductive hearing loss.
   b. A patient whose hearing loss is the result of a conversion reaction, a repressed emotion that becomes manifest through a physical symptom, is unlikely to benefit from a hearing aid. Psychotherapy would probably be the preferred treatment.
   d. A patient whose hearing impairment preceded the development of speech would be less likely to benefit from a hearing aid than one whose hearing loss occurred later in life.

12. **Correct answer is a.** The goal of a myringotomy is to relieve pressure and to drain serous or purulent fluid from the middle ear behind the eardrum. The procedure also relieves the patient's pain.

   b. Myringotomy is performed in conjunction with an open or closed mastoidectomy during an operative procedure for mastoiditis.
   c. The external auditory canal lies in front of the middle ear, where otitis media occurs. Serous or purulent fluid would drain out through this canal once the tympanic membrane has been punctured.
   d. The eustachian tube extends from the middle ear to the nasopharynx. The fluid buildup that occurs in otitis media lies behind the tympanic membrane.

12

Gastrointestinal Tract Function

OVERVIEW

I. Structure and function of gastrointestinal tract
A. Structure of gastrointestinal tract
B. Function of gastrointestinal tract

II. General diagnostic tests
A. Gastric analysis
B. Barium swallow
C. Barium enema
D. Endoscopy

III. General nursing assessments
A. Patient history
B. Observation and physical examination
C. Diagnostic tests

IV. Nursing considerations with selected therapies and techniques
A. Gastrointestinal intubation
B. Gastrostomy and tube feeding
C. Total parenteral nutrition
D. Esophageal surgery
E. Gastric surgery
F. Colostomy
G. Ileostomy

V. Selected disorders
A. Problems associated with digestion
B. Problems associated with absorption and elimination
C. Problems associated with nutrition

NURSING HIGHLIGHTS

1. Because the symptoms of different intestinal disorders are often similar, systematic use of the nursing process is essential in identifying appropriate nursing interventions.
2. The nurse must realize that treatment of physical problems associated with eating disorders is only the beginning of the patient's long-term process of emotional recovery.

GLOSSARY

basal gastric secretion test—type of gastric analysis used to measure hydrochloric acid secretion between meals

borborygmus—rumbling noise caused when gas is propelled through the intestines

chyme—creamy, semifluid material produced when food is digested in the stomach

fundoplication—surgical repair of hiatal hernia in which part of the stomach fundus is wrapped around the distal esophagus

gas bloat syndrome—usually temporary complication of fundoplication in which patient cannot voluntarily eructate (belch)

gastric acid stimulation test—type of gastric analysis in which a drug that stimulates gastric acid secretion is given to patient

herniorrhaphy—surgical repair of a hernia

Kock's ileostomy—surgical removal of colon, rectum, and anus, with anal closure, and construction of an intra-abdominal pouch from the terminal ileum; pouch is connected to a stoma that has a nipplelike valve, from which patient can drain stool

lumen—the channel within a tube (plural, lumina)

peristalsis—the wavelike movement by which the muscles of the alimentary canal propel material forward

peritoneum—the membrane that lines the wall of the abdominal and pelvic cavities

total proctocolectomy with permanent ileostomy—surgical removal of colon, rectum, and anus, with anal closure, and bringing of the end of the terminal ileum through the abdominal wall to form a stoma, or ostomy

ENHANCED OUTLINE

I. Structure and function of gastrointestinal tract

See text pages
_____

A. Structure of gastrointestinal tract
  1. Upper gastrointestinal (GI) tract: Structures include the mouth, pharynx, esophagus, and stomach.
  2. Lower GI tract: Structures include the small intestine (duodenum, jejunum, and ileum), colon, rectum, and anus.

B. Function of gastrointestinal tract
  1. Upper GI tract
     a) Food digestion begins in the mouth (action of saliva and ptyalin); food is propelled into stomach via pharynx and esophagus.
     b) Stomach liquifies food into chyme (gastric enzymes); absorbs small quantities of food (water, glucose); regulates flow of chyme into duodenum.
  2. Lower GI tract
     a) Small intestine completes digestion of food (chyme mixes with bile and pancreatic enzymes).
     b) Mucosal enzymes complete the process of digestion and nutrients are absorbed, while waste products and fluid proceed to the colon.
     c) The colon absorbs fluids; waste is then stored in the colon and rectum until it is expelled through the anus.

II. General diagnostic tests

See text pages
_____

A. Gastric analysis: measurement of stomach's secretion of hydrochloric acid and pepsin done from a sample of contents aspirated through a nasogastric tube; used to help diagnose pernicious anemia

B. Barium swallow
   1. Fluoroscopic or radiographic observation of barium moving down esophagus into stomach
   2. Used to identify pharyngeal or esophageal abnormalities, including tumors, strictures, varices, peptic ulcer, gastric tumors, and hiatal hernia
   3. Often combined with a small bowel follow-through

C. Barium enema: fluoroscopic or radiographic examination of rectum after instillation of barium

D. Endoscopy
   1. Definition and purpose: group of procedures that use a lighted endoscope to allow a direct view and some manipulation of part of GI tract
      a) When inserted orally, used to diagnose esophageal, gastric, duodenal, pancreatic, or bile duct abnormalities, including inflammatory, neoplastic, or infectious diseases
      b) When inserted through the rectum, used to diagnose disorders of colon
   2. Individual procedures: esophagoscopy; colonoscopy; gastroscopy; sigmoidoscopy (sigmoid colon, rectum, and anus); proctoscopy (rectum and anus); anoscopy (anus)

III. General nursing assessments

See text pages
_____

A. Patient history: Determine duration and suspected cause of symptoms, medical and family history, environment, diet, allergies, drugs taken, and weight history.

B. Observation and physical examination: Assess vital signs and check weight; examine skin, oral cavity, pharynx, tonsils, and anus; check stomach for tenderness; auscultate abdomen; assist during diagnostic exam procedures.

C. Diagnostic tests
   1. Gastric analysis
      a) Patient preparation: Keep patient "nothing by mouth" (NPO) for 12 hours before procedure; insert nasogastric (NG) tube.
      b) Basal gastric secretion: Attach NG tube to suctioning equipment; collect and measure contents every 15 minutes for 1 hour; label each sample with time and volume obtained.

c) Gastric acid stimulation: After basal gastric secretion test, give injection of pentagastrin, betazole (Histalog), or another drug that stimulates gastric acid secretion; 15 minutes after drug administration, collect and measure contents every 15 minutes for 1 hour; label each sample with time and volume obtained.

2. Barium swallow: Instruct patient to maintain low-residue diet for 2–3 days before procedure; keep patient NPO after midnight; caution patient against smoking on day of test; help patient assume necessary position(s); after procedure, assess abdomen for distention and bowel sounds; administer laxative; evaluate stools to make sure all barium is expelled; and if combined with small bowel follow-through, explain that patient will be returned to radiology department for additional films.

3. Barium enema: Advise patient to maintain low-residue diet for 1–3 days before test; administer clear liquids and laxatives on evening before test; keep patient NPO after midnight; administer cleansing enemas until returns are clear.

4. Endoscopy
   a) Upper GI: Keep patient NPO after midnight; administer a benzodiazepine to relax patient and atropine to dry secretions; remove any dentures; after procedure, keep patient NPO until gag reflex returns (2–4 hours); observe patient for bleeding, fever, or pain, which may indicate perforation of esophagus.
   b) Colonoscopy: Administer liquid diet for 24 hours before test; keep patient NPO after midnight; administer oral preparation to cleanse bowel on evening before procedure; help patient lie on left side with knees drawn up during procedure; observe patient for signs of bowel perforation.
   c) Sigmoidoscopy, proctoscopy, anoscopy: Maintain liquid diet for 24 hours before procedure; administer laxative, if ordered; administer cleaning or sodium biphosphate enema; help patient assume necessary position; after procedure, observe for signs of perforation; help with sitz bath.

IV. Nursing considerations with selected therapies and techniques

See text pages

A. Gastrointestinal intubation
   1. Purpose: to decompress intestinal tract by draining fluid and air and to provide nutrition and/or restore fluid and electrolyte balance by means of nasogastric (NG) tube or nasointestinal tube; nasointestinal tube often used for more severe intestinal obstructions
   2. Nasogastric (NG) tube for gastric decompression
      a) Type of tubing used: Salem sump and Anderson suction tubes, which sit distally in the stomach and are attached to low continuous suction
      b) Method of insertion and postinsertion patient care
         (1) Help patient assume sitting position, and place pillows behind shoulders.
         (2) Coat tube with water-soluble lubricant.

      (3) Determine length of tube to be inserted by measuring from bridge of patient's nose to earlobe to xiphoid process; use piece of tape to mark this length.

      (4) After identifying more patent nostril, gently pass tube into nasopharynx, asking patient to swallow repeatedly while tube is advanced.

      (5) Should resistance be encountered, gently rotate tube, aiming it downward and toward closer ear.

      (6) Should respiratory status change, withdraw tube immediately.

      (7) Confirm correct tube placement by aspirating sample of gastric contents, by auscultating with stethoscope over gastric area while air is inserted into tube with syringe, or by obtaining order for x-ray film.

      (8) Connect tube to intermittent or continuous low suction.

      (9) Using adhesive tape, secure tube to patient's nose.

      (10) Check patient's intake and output at least every 4 hours.

      (11) Monitor patient for nausea or vomiting and abdominal distention or fullness.

   3. Nasointestinal tube for decompression

     a) Type of tubing used: tubes that are longer than NG tubes, extend into small intestine, and have mercury-filled balloons at the end of a lumen to act like a bolus of food, advancing down the intestinal tract by stimulating peristalsis

      (1) Cantor or Harris tubes: tubes with mercury-filled balloons and suction ports within same lumen

      (2) Miller-Abbott tube: tube with separate lumina for mercury and for drainage

     b) Method of insertion and postinsertion patient care

      (1) Fill upper portion of balloon bag with mercury, and aspirate all air from bag before inserting Cantor or Harris tube.

      (2) Begin insertion as for NG tube.

      (3) Place patient on right side once tube has been inserted into esophagus.

      (4) Advance tube 2–4 inches at a time, if ordered, changing patient's position to facilitate passage.

      (5) Wait until tube has reached desired position before securing it with tape.

      (6) Allow drainage to occur by gravity as the tube advances; obtain physician's order to inject 10 ml of air, but do not irrigate with fluid.

      (7) Obtain order for x-ray films to confirm that tube has reached small intestine.

     (8) For Miller-Abbott tube, fill balloon lumen with mercury when tube reaches stomach; clamp and label lumen.

     (9) Attach suction lumen to low intermittent suction when tube reaches destination.

B. Gastrostomy and tube feeding
1. Weigh patient; prepare abdominal skin for surgery by cleaning it with povidone-iodine.
2. After surgery, report any signs of infection at operative site or fever; wash skin, and apply ointments to prevent irritation.
3. Confirm placement of NG tube via auscultation; monitor temperature, volume, and flow rate of feeding.
4. Administer 50 ml of water before and after each tube feeding, or every 4–6 hours with continuous feeding.
5. Assess patient for feeding intolerance, including bloating, urticaria, nausea, vomiting, diarrhea, and constipation.
6. Check residual gastric content before each feeding; delay feeding for 2 hours if amount is >150 ml; notify physician if problem persists for 4 hours.
7. For continuous feeding, hang fresh tube formula every 4 hours (unless using a closed, pre-filled system); change container and line every 24 hours.
8. Unless patient is being fed, keep catheter end of gastrostomy tube clamped; if drainage occurs around tube, protect skin with ostomy products; refer to enterostomal therapy nurse for skin care.
9. Weigh patient 3 times per week.
10. Report changes in elimination patterns.
11. Provide information on home care, including food preparation, proper catheter insertion techniques, and maintenance of weekly weight record.

C. Total parenteral nutrition (TPN)
1. Follow institution's protocol for IV therapy and "Universal Precautions" guidelines; prepare access site prior to insertion of catheter to be used for TPN delivery.
2. Observe patient for complications, including sepsis, air embolism, clotted catheter line, hyperglycemia, fluid overload, pneumothorax, and rebound hypoglycemia.
3. Monitor weight, intake and output, lab values, signs of infection at IV site, level of activity, and mobility.

D. Esophageal surgery
1. Observe patient for signs of breathing or swallowing problems.
2. Assess cutaneous suture line for redness, excess drainage, and other signs of infection; clean sutures once per shift with half-strength peroxide; and apply bacterial ointment after drying area.
3. Monitor IV hydration while patient is NPO and before tube feedings are begun; remind patient of NPO status when he/she is alert.
4. Observe nasogastric tube drainage for blood, checking to see that amount of blood gradually decreases; do not reposition or replace NG tube, since this can cause trauma and increase the risk of infection.

5. When tube feedings are begun, flush tube carefully with water after each feeding or medication administration; assess and document bowel sounds every shift until tube feedings are well tolerated.
6. When patient drinks fluids, observe for possible regurgitation of ingested fluid.
7. Encourage patient to suction or expectorate oral secretions instead of swallowing them.
8. To prevent reflux, elevate head of bed 30° when patient is at rest and 90° during each feeding and for 30 minutes afterward.

E. Gastric surgery
1. Before surgery, insert NG tube and connect it to suction to remove secretions and empty stomach.
2. During the immediate postoperative period, watch for signs and symptoms of acute gastric dilation, including hypotension, tachycardia, epigastric pain and fullness, hiccups, and gagging; reassure patient that symptoms will resolve upon insertion of NG tube or restoration of patency to clogged tube.
3. Frequently monitor patency of NG tube; ensure that no more than a minute amount of blood drains from tube and that there is no abdominal distention; do not reposition NG tube, since this may disrupt sutures and increase the risk of infection.
4. Maintain asepsis during procedures; inspect wound during dressing changes; administer antibiotics as ordered.
5. Observe for postsurgical complications (see Nurse Alert, "Warning Signs of Gastric Surgery Complications").
6. Watch for common problems that may arise in the postsurgical period.
   a) Absence of intrinsic factor, which can lead to pernicious anemia, occurs after removal of stomach because of folic acid, iron, and

---

! NURSE *ALERT* !

Warning Signs of Gastric Surgery Complications

- Change in vital signs
- Severe pain in legs, head, and chest
- Abdominal distention and rigidity
- Extreme restlessness and diaphoresis
- Excess bloody drainage from nasogastric tube, surgical dressing, or drain; unusual odor from drainage
- Breathing problems, increased respiratory rate, or cyanosis

---

vitamin B_{12} deficiency, impaired calcium metabolism, and decreased absorption of vitamin D and calcium; disorder can be corrected by administering vitamin B_{12}.

   b) Dumping syndrome is a postprandial problem that occurs after surgical bypass of the pylorus, when partially digested food rapidly enters the jejunum (see Nurse Alert, "Dumping Syndrome").

   c) Alkaline reflux gastritis, which occurs when the pylorus is bypassed or removed, is caused by the reflux of duodenal contents with bile acids into the remaining stomach, causing injury to the gastric mucosal barrier; symptoms include epigastric pain, nausea, and vomiting, which are aggravated by eating.

F. Colostomy
   1. Report sudden fever or fever >101°F, sudden pain, or abdominal tenderness.
   2. Check surgical dressing often; observe size and color of stoma.
   3. Measure fluid intake and output; observe patient for signs of dehydration and electrolyte imbalance.
   4. Check colostomy appliance often, and change it as needed; record amount, color, and consistency of fecal material.
   5. Clean skin around stoma each time appliance is changed; remove excess powder, ointment, or karaya gum.
   6. Be alert for the presence of postoperative complications, including signs of poor circulation to the stoma (necrotic tissue, heavy bleeding, or dull color) and signs of infection or excessive bleeding at the perineal wound.
   7. Provide information on caring for perineal wound and colostomy (see Client Teaching Checklist, "Home Colostomy Care").

! NURSE **ALERT** !

Dumping Syndrome

Dumping syndrome is a nutritional problem that sometimes occurs after a gastric resection in which the pylorus has been bypassed. It occurs when ingested food that has not been properly digested enters the jejunum rapidly. The nurse should provide the following information to at-risk patients.

- Early manifestations, which appear 5–30 minutes after a meal, include:
  —Vasomotor disturbances, including tachycardia, syncope, palpitations, vertigo, sweating, and the desire to lie down
  —Falling or rising pulse
- Late manifestations, which occur 2–3 hours after eating, consist of epigastric fullness, distention, abdominal cramping, diarrhea, nausea, occasional vomiting, borborygmus, and the desire to defecate.
- Dumping syndrome can be controlled or prevented by:
  —Eating small meals
  —Maintaining a high-protein, high-fat, low-carbohydrate diet
  —Taking pectin as a dry powder
  —Lying down after meals
  —Taking sedatives or antispasmodics to delay gastric emptying

G. Ileostomy
1. Collaborate with enterostomal therapist to prepare a thorough program of preoperative patient education, dealing, as appropriate, with total proctocolectomy with permanent ileostomy or with Kock's ileostomy.
2. Provide postoperative care, including care of the abdominal incision, ostomy, and/or perineal wound.
3. Measure fluid intake and output; observe patient for signs of dehydration and electrolyte imbalance; provide adequate parenteral fluid and electrolytes.
4. In patient with Kock's ileostomy, check indwelling catheter within pouch for patency.
5. When peristalsis returns, help patient with Kock's ileostomy with stoma intubation (every 2–4 hours at first).
6. Encourage patient to verbalize concerns about altered body image and to demonstrate self-care of ileostomy.

See text pages

_____

V. Selected disorders

A. Problems associated with digestion
1. Gastritis
a) Definition: acute or chronic inflammation of stomach mucosa (lining)

✔ CLIENT TEACHING CHECKLIST ✔

Home Colostomy Care

Explain the following guidelines to patients with colostomies.

✔ Be aware that size and color of stoma change with emotional state and level of activity.

✔ Eat a regular diet, but avoid gas-forming foods, such as onions, beans, cabbage, spinach, corn, cheese, eggs, highly seasoned foods, carbonated beverages, and coffee.

✔ Treat constipation by increasing amount of bulk foods and drinking extra water.

✔ Eliminate foods that may cause diarrhea, such as foods high in fiber, and contact physician if diarrhea persists >2 days.

✔ Eat slowly, and chew food well.

✔ Weigh yourself weekly, and contact physician in case of sudden weight loss.

✔ Irrigation is an option; discuss your particular situation with an enterostomal therapy nurse.

✔ If you are irrigating your colostomy, perform irrigation at the same time each day, preferably after a meal.

✔ Engage in normal activities and travel.

---

b) Pathophysiology and etiology
  (1) Pathophysiology: breakdown of stomach's protective mucosal barrier, aggravated by histamine release and cholinergic nerve stimulation and followed by diffusion of hydrochloric acid back into mucosa, injuring small blood vessels and causing hemorrhage, edema, and erosion of gastric lining
  (2) Etiology: poor diet, drugs, poisons, toxic chemicals, corrosives, infection, and food allergies (acute gastritis); stomach cancer, gastric ulcer, alcoholism, autoimmune response to stressors
c) Symptoms: epigastric fullness or pressure, anorexia, nausea or vomiting, diarrhea, fever, or epigastric abdominal pain; with severe gastritis, gastric bleeding
d) Diagnostic evaluation: patient history, gastroscopy, upper GI series
e) Medical treatment: fasting until symptoms subside, followed by clear liquids; IV fluids; medication to control nausea, diarrhea, and vomiting; emergency treatment for toxic reactions; for chronic gastritis, antacids and avoidance of aggravating foods or substances
f) Complications: pernicious anemia, hemorrhage, stomach cancer
g) Essential nursing care for patients with gastritis
  (1) Nursing assessment: Obtain patient history and perform physical assessment, checking especially for abdominal tenderness and dehydration.
  (2) Nursing diagnoses
    (a) Pain related to stomach irritation
    (b) Altered nutrition, less than body requirements, related to food intolerance
    (c) Fluid volume deficit related to vomiting or diarrhea
  (3) Nursing intervention
    (a) Administer analgesics, and encourage patient to avoid irritating foods and beverages.
    (b) Keep patient NPO until symptoms subside; then provide small, frequent, bland meals.
    (c) Monitor fluid intake and output; assess electrolyte values every 24 hours.
  (4) Nursing evaluation
    (a) Patient states that pain is reduced.
    (b) Patient maintains weight at ideal level.
    (c) Patient maintains fluid balance.
2. Peptic ulcer
  a) Definition: break in the mucosal lining of the part of the GI tract that comes in contact with hydrochloric acid and pepsin
  b) Pathophysiology and etiology
    (1) Pathophysiology: interruption in gastric mucosa due to back-diffusion of stomach acid or pyloric sphincter dysfunction (gastric ulcer); chronic break in duodenal mucosa extending through muscularis mucosa due to increased acid secretion (duodenal ulcer); multiple gastric erosions (stress ulcer)

(2) Etiology: infection with *Helicobacter pylori;* ingestion of aspirin, alcohol, or indomethacin (gastric ulcer); stressful situations or ingestion of foods that lead to a high level of gastric acid secretion (peptic ulcer); acute medical crisis or trauma (stress ulcer)

c) Symptoms: nausea, vomiting, back pain, bleeding, constipation, abdominal pain after meals that may be relieved by ingestion of protein foods

d) Diagnostic evaluation: medical history, upper GI series, gastroscopy, radiographic studies, gastric analysis, gastric washing; breath test or stool specimens (except for peptic ulcer)

e) Medical treatment

    (1) Dietary management per individual tolerance, usually including avoidance of highly seasoned foods

    (2) Drug therapy, including antibiotics, antacids to neutralize hydrochloric acid, and cholinergic blocking agents to decrease gastric motility and acid secretion

    (3) Avoidance of fatigue, stress, smoking, alcohol, and caffeine

f) Complications: hemorrhage, perforation, pyloric obstruction

g) Essential nursing care for patients with peptic ulcer

    (1) Nursing assessment: Obtain history; check for signs of anemia; examine stool for occult blood; palpate abdomen for tenderness.

    (2) Nursing diagnoses

        (a) Pain related to interruption in gastric mucosa

        (b) Knowledge deficit related to management of disease and prevention of recurrence

    (3) Nursing intervention

        (a) Administer medication as prescribed, and instruct patient on how to establish recommended meal patterns.

        (b) Monitor patient for potential complications.

        (c) Provide information about managing disorder and preventing its recurrence (see Client Teaching Checklist, "Home Care for the Patient with Peptic Ulcer").

    (4) Nursing evaluation

        (a) Patient states that pain is diminished or eliminated.

        (b) Patient experiences no complications.

        (c) Patient states an understanding of the role of diet, medication, and stress control in managing and preventing disease.

3. Stomach cancer

    a) Definition: malignant neoplasm or tumor found in stomach

    b) Pathophysiology and etiology

        (1) Pathophysiology: develop from stomach's mucous membrane in pyloric and antral areas

Home Care for the Patient with Peptic Ulcer

Explain the following guidelines to patients with peptic ulcers.

✔ Eat well-balanced meals at regular times, but avoid foods that cause discomfort or pain.
✔ Avoid caffeine and alcohol.
✔ Take prescribed medication, and avoid aspirin, baking soda, and laxatives.
✔ Get plenty of rest, and avoid stress.
✔ Watch for the following signs of complications:
— Hemorrhage: tarry, black, or sticky stools; bright red vomited blood; pallor; faintness; extreme thirst; profuse sweating
— Obstruction: fullness, distention, abdominal pain, nausea after eating, vomiting
— Perforation: sudden excruciating pain; profuse sweating; ashen, drawn face; rigid painful abdomen; rapid shallow breathing

(2) Etiology: heredity, chronic stomach inflammation, achlorhydria, gastric polyps, smoking, diet (excessive intake of smoked foods, lack of fruits and vegetables)
c) Symptoms: abdominal pain, anorexia, indigestion, dyspepsia, weight loss, constipation, anemia, nausea, vomiting, full feeling, occult blood in stool
d) Diagnostic evaluation: fluoroscopy, barium swallow, gastroscopy with biopsy, gastric analysis, and bone, liver, and CT scans
e) Medical treatment: partial or total gastrectomy, chemotherapy, radiation therapy
f) Complications: metastatic disease, hemorrhage
g) Essential nursing care for patients with stomach cancer
(1) Nursing assessment: Obtain history, including information about diet, smoking, and alcohol intake; perform physical exam, checking for tenderness or masses in stomach and other organs.
(2) Nursing diagnoses
(a) Pain related to presence of tumor
(b) Altered nutrition, less than body requirements, related to anorexia
(c) Knowledge deficit related to self-care and treatment
(3) Nursing intervention
(a) Administer analgesics as prescribed, usually patient-controlled analgesic (PCA), employing continuous IV therapy for severe pain.
(b) Provide small frequent feedings of bland foods.
(c) Administer parenteral vitamin B_{12} after total gastrectomy.
(d) Provide information about disease and treatment, including timetable for resumption of regular meals and normal activities.

         (e) Teach patient with total gastrectomy to use equipment and formula for tube feedings.

         (f) Provide information about dumping syndrome, the events caused by rapid entry of food from the stomach into the jejunum (see Nurse Alert, "Dumping Syndrome").

     (4) Nursing evaluation

         (a) Patient states that pain is reduced.

         (b) Patient attains optimum nutrition.

         (c) Patient states understanding of treatment and performs self-care activities.

B. Problems associated with absorption and elimination

    1. Severe diarrhea

      a) Definition: condition in which there is unusual frequency and consistency of bowel movements

      b) Pathophysiology and etiology

        (1) Pathophysiology: increased peristalsis, causing decreased amount of water absorption by large intestine

        (2) Etiology: infections, diverticulitis, food poisoning, uremia, stress, diet deficient in fiber, inflammatory bowel disease, irritable colon, intestinal obstruction, food allergies, laxative abuse, adverse drug effects, dumping syndrome, malabsorption

      c) Symptoms: frequent loose, watery, greasy stools; abdominal cramps; abdominal distention; intestinal rumbling; anorexia; thirst

      d) Diagnostic evaluation: patient history; stool examination for blood, parasites, and microorganisms; complete blood count (CBC), chemical profile; urinalysis; proctosigmoidoscopy; barium enema

      e) Medical treatment

        (1) Manage underlying disease.

        (2) Give oral fluids or oral glucose and electrolyte solution for mild cases.

        (3) Administer IV therapy to achieve rapid rehydration, especially in very young and elderly patients.

      f) Complications: electrolyte imbalance, dehydration, vitamin deficiency, perianal skin impairment

      g) Essential nursing care for patients with diarrhea

        (1) Nursing assessment

          (a) Obtain complete patient history and detailed information about bowel habits, abdominal pain, cramping, urgency, and stools.

          (b) Observe for signs of dehydration and electrolyte imbalance.

          (c) Examine anal area for redness and fissures.

          (d) Palpate abdomen for distention or masses; auscultate for bowel sounds.

    (2) Nursing diagnoses
        (a) Altered nutrition, less than body requirements, related to anorexia, diarrhea
        (b) Fluid volume deficit related to swift stool passage
        (c) Potential for impaired skin integrity related to frequent loose stools
    (3) Nursing intervention
        (a) Encourage patient to rest, drink plenty of liquids (excluding milk or beverages containing milk products, alcohol, or caffeine), and eat a bland diet.
        (b) Contact physician if there is sudden onset of acute abdominal pain, fever, or blood or excess mucus in stool.
        (c) Observe patient closely for dehydration and electrolyte imbalance; measure fluid intake and output; offer oral fluids often; administer IV fluids, if necessary.
        (d) Wash anal area after each bowel movement with soap and water, rinsing with clear water and thoroughly drying; apply ointment to prevent skin breakdown.
    (4) Nursing evaluation
        (a) Normal bowel elimination pattern is established.
        (b) Patient's nutritional needs are met.
        (c) Patient maintains normal fluid volume and electrolyte balance.
        (d) Patient's skin remains intact.
2. Constipation
  a) Definition: abnormal infrequency of defecation with abnormally hardened stools that pass painfully and with difficulty
  b) Pathophysiology and etiology
    (1) Pathophysiology: interference in the colon with mucosal transport, myoelectric activity, or the processes involved in defecation
    (2) Etiology: emotional stress, poor diet or bowel habits, drugs (especially narcotics), chronic laxative use, lack of exercise, inadequate fluid intake, underlying disease, lead poisoning, irritable bowel syndrome
  c) Symptoms: hard, dry, infrequent stools; diarrhea around an impaction; abdominal distention, rumbling, pain, and pressure; decreased appetite; headache; fatigue; indigestion
  d) Diagnostic evaluation: patient history, stool examination, rectal exam, sigmoidoscopy, barium enema, anorectal studies, lab tests
  e) Medical treatment
    (1) Correct any underlying medical disorder.
    (2) Instruct patient to drink abundant fluids and to eat a diet including plentiful raw fruits and vegetables and whole-grain breads and cereals.
    (3) Advise patient to allow for adequate rest periods, exercise, and time for evacuation.
  f) Complications: hemorrhoids, diverticulosis

g) Essential nursing care for patients with constipation
    (1) Nursing assessment
        (a) Obtain complete patient history and detailed information about bowel habits.
        (b) Examine anal area for redness and fissures.
        (c) Palpate abdomen for distention or masses; auscultate for bowel sounds.
        (d) Perform rectal exam to rule out impaction.
    (2) Nursing diagnoses
        (a) Constipation related to diet, decreased fluid intake, or decreased activity
        (b) Knowledge deficit related to preventive measures
    (3) Nursing intervention
        (a) Give stool softeners or bulk agents as indicated.
        (b) Encourage proper diet, fluid intake, and exercise.
        (c) Provide information about prevention and treatment.
        (d) Give senna with narcotics to decrease narcotic-induced constipation.
    (4) Nursing evaluation
        (a) Bowel elimination pattern is established.
        (b) Patient consumes sufficient fluids and maintains prescribed diet.
        (c) Patient states understanding of prevention and treatment factors.

3. Irritable bowel syndrome (IBS)
  a) Definition: digestive disorder characterized by intermittent abdominal pain and irregular bowel habits
  b) Pathophysiology and etiology
    (1) Pathophysiology: disturbed involuntary muscle movement in large intestine with no abnormality of intestinal structure
    (2) Etiology: stress, diet, anxiety, depression, fear, food, drugs, toxins, colonic distention
  c) Symptoms: bouts of diarrhea or constipation, cramps, abdominal pain, nausea, gas, bloating, fatigue, anxiety, headaches
  d) Diagnostic evaluation: patient history, barium enema, sigmoidoscopy
  e) Medical treatment: exercise; bulk-forming agents and antispasmodic drugs for constipation; antidiarrheal drugs and high-fiber diet for diarrhea
  f) Complication: dehydration
  g) Essential nursing care for patients with irritable bowel syndrome
    (1) Nursing assessment: Obtain patient history, including information about symptoms, diet, bowel habits, stressors, and weight; auscultate and palpate patient's abdomen; perform rectal exam.

  (2) Nursing diagnoses
    (a) Diarrhea and constipation related to changes in motility
    (b) Ineffective individual coping related to feelings of loss of control
    (c) Altered nutrition, less than body requirements, related to anorexia
  (3) Nursing intervention
    (a) Provide drug and diet therapy to alleviate symptoms.
    (b) Provide emotional support, and explain causes of disorder.
    (c) Encourage patient to exercise regularly and adhere to stress management program.
    (d) Encourage patient to eat 30–40 gm of fiber and to drink 8–10 cups of fluid daily.
  (4) Nursing evaluation
    (a) Patient experiences no further bouts of diarrhea or constipation.
    (b) Patient exhibits effective coping skills and understands how to control disorder through diet and stress management.
    (c) Patient's nutritional needs are met, using prescribed diet.
4. **Inflammatory bowel diseases** (Crohn's disease, ulcerative colitis, enteritis) (see Nurse Alerts, "Peritonitis," "Comparison of Crohn's Disease and Ulcerative Colitis")
  a) Definition
    (1) Crohn's disease (regional enteritis): chronic inflammatory disease that usually involves the terminal ileum but may affect any part of the GI tract
    (2) Ulcerative colitis: chronic inflammatory bowel disease of the colon

---

!   NURSE *ALERT*   !

Peritonitis

The nurse should be alert to the symptoms of peritonitis, inflammation of the lining of the abdominal cavity (peritoneum), which is characterized by edema, decreased circulatory volume, and decreased peristalsis. Peritonitis is a life-threatening disorder that can proceed to sepsis.

- Causes: Peritonitis can be caused by perforation of a peptic ulcer, bowel, or appendix; trauma; ruptured ectopic pregnancy; or infection during peritoneal dialysis.
- Symptoms: Symptoms include severe abdominal pain, tenderness, nausea, vomiting, fever, paralytic ileus, and boardlike abdomen; in the final stages, there is a rapid, thready pulse, distended abdomen, and a drop in body temperature.
- Diagnosis: Confirmation of suspected peritonitis in patients at risk for this disorder can be made by obtaining white blood cell (WBC) count and abdominal radiographs.
- Treatment: Treatment includes gastrointestinal decompression, replacement of fluids and electrolytes, and antibiotic and analgesic therapy.

(3) Enteritis: inflammation of mucous membranes of the intestines

b) Pathophysiology and etiology
  (1) Pathophysiology
    (a) Crohn's disease: thickening and edema of wall of terminal ileum
    (b) Ulcerative colitis: loss of surface epithelium due to inflammation; thickening and shortening of bowel
    (c) Enteritis: release by viral or bacterial organisms of enterotoxin, causing inflammation, intestinal malabsorption, and eventual intestinal destruction; increased GI motility, leading to rapid secretion of fluids and electrolytes into intestines

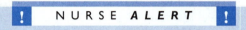

NURSE ALERT

Comparison of Crohn's Disease and Ulcerative Colitis

The following summary presents the usual course of the 2 disorders. Because the signs and symptoms of the diseases are often similar, diagnosis relies on endoscopy and biopsy.

Crohn's disease
- The disease usually begins in the terminal ileum but can occur anywhere in the GI tract.
- All bowel layers are involved.
- Patient produces 5–6 soft loose stools per day that are rarely bloody.
- Complications include fistulas and nutritional deficiencies.
- The disease has a prolonged variable course.
- Diarrhea tends not to be severe.
- Rectal involvement occurs in about 20% of cases.
- Perianal involvement is common.

Ulcerative colitis
- The disease is confined to the colon; it begins in the rectum and travels toward the cecum.
- The mucosa and submucosa are involved.
- Patient produces 10–20 liquid bloody stools per day.
- Complications include hemorrhage, perforation, fistulas, and nutritional deficiencies.
- Exacerbations tend to alternate with remissions.
- Severe diarrhea is common.
- Rectal involvement occurs in almost 100% of cases.
- Perianal involvement and fistulas are uncommon.
- Total colectomy with ileostomy is curative.

(2) Etiology
  (a) Crohn's disease and ulcerative colitis: unknown; may be associated with autoimmune dysfunction, stress, or microorganism; possible role of heredity in ulcerative colitis
  (b) Enteritis: bacterial or viral infection
c) Symptoms
  (1) Crohn's disease: abdominal pain, distention, diarrhea, fever, leukocytosis, weight loss, dehydration, electrolyte imbalance
  (2) Ulcerative colitis: severe bloody diarrhea, weight loss, fever, severe electrolyte imbalance, dehydration, anemia, cachexia, cramps, nausea and vomiting, weakness, incontinence
  (3) Enteritis: nausea and vomiting; bloody mucous stools for up to 5 days, fever to 105°F, and abdominal pain when due to *Shigella;* bloody foul-smelling stools for 7 days, fever to 105°F, and abdominal pain when caused by *Campylobacter;* diarrhea for up to 10 days when caused by *Escherichia coli;* watery diarrhea with rectal bleeding for up to 8 days when caused by rotavirus; diarrhea for 24–48 hours, myalgia, headache, and malaise when caused by epidemic viral gastroenteritis
d) Diagnostic evaluation
  (1) Crohn's disease and ulcerative colitis: symptom history, barium enema, stool samples to rule out infection or parasites, sigmoidoscopy, colonoscopy, proctoscopy
  (2) Enteritis: stool culture, Gram's stain
e) Medical treatment
  (1) Crohn's disease and ulcerative colitis: rest, stress relief, dietary modifications, parenteral therapy, drug therapy; surgery to correct intestinal blockage or perforation in Crohn's disease; colectomy with permanent ileostomy curative in ulcerative colitis
  (2) Enteritis: gastrointestinal decompression to drain intestinal contents and gas; replacement of fluids and electrolytes; antibiotic and analgesic therapy
f) Complications
  (1) Crohn's disease and ulcerative colitis: nutritional deficiencies; also hemorrhage, perforation, and fistulas
  (2) Enteritis: sepsis
g) Essential nursing care for patients with inflammatory bowel diseases
  (1) Nursing assessment: Obtain medical history; record all symptoms, including sequence in which they occurred; obtain description of stool; weigh patient; check for abdominal tenderness, pain, and distention.
  (2) Nursing diagnoses
    (a) Fluid volume deficit related to diarrhea or the inability to consume oral fluids
    (b) Altered nutrition, less than body requirements, related to rapid passage of food through bowel or to vomiting

             (c) Pain related to bowel inflammation

             (d) Potential for impaired skin integrity related to diarrhea

       (3) Nursing intervention

             (a) Monitor fluid intake and output; observe patient for signs of dehydration and electrolyte imbalance; provide clear fluids containing electrolytes, such as ginger ale; administer IV fluids, if necessary.

             (b) Encourage patient to eat small meals; note amount and type of food eaten.

             (c) Record detailed description of pain; administer drugs to slow peristalsis as prescribed; administer narcotic analgesics cautiously.

             (d) Inspect anal area for redness and fissures; apply ointment if necessary; wash with soap and water after defecation and dry thoroughly.

       (4) Nursing evaluation

             (a) Patient's diarrhea is minimized.

             (b) Patient drinks normal amount of fluids and shows no evidence of fluid and electrolyte imbalance.

             (c) Patient tolerates small feedings and gains or maintains weight.

             (d) Patient states that pain is controlled.

             (e) Patient's skin integrity is intact.

   5. Hemorrhoids

      a) Definition: varicose veins of the anus and rectum

      b) Pathophysiology and etiology

         (1) Pathophysiology: separation of veins from muscle, causing prolapse of hemorrhoidal vessels

         (2) Etiology: pregnancy, intra-abdominal tumors, chronic constipation, heredity, anal intercourse, portal hypertension

      c) Symptoms: pain, itching, soreness in anal area; bleeding

      d) Diagnostic evaluation: visual examination of anus, anoscopy, proctoscopy

      e) Medical treatment: avoidance of straining during defecation, avoidance of anal intercourse, sitz baths, analgesic ointments, high-fiber diet, laxatives, bed rest, infrared photocoagulation, bipolar diathermy, injections of sclerosing solution, hemorrhoidectomy

      f) Complications: hemorrhage, infection

      g) Essential nursing care for patients with hemorrhoids

         (1) Nursing assessment: Obtain complete history, including diet information and history of constipation or diarrhea; examine anal region.

      (2) Nursing diagnoses
         (a) Pain related to inflammation
         (b) Potential for infection related to ruptured veins
      (3) Nursing intervention
         (a) Administer anesthetic ointment as prescribed.
         (b) Instruct patient how to perform sitz baths.
         (c) Review diet and fluid intake recommendation with patient; provide a list of high-fiber foods.
         (d) For patient who has undergone hemorrhoidectomy, help him/her to assume side-lying position; keep fresh ice packs over dressing until anal packing is removed; use moist heat 3–4 times during first 12 postsurgical hours, placing ice pack on patient's head to prevent faintness if sitz baths are used; administer stool softener beginning on first postoperative day; give narcotic analgesic before first defecation, and remain with patient; monitor for urinary retention, and take measures to facilitate voiding, if needed; perform patient teaching, stressing importance of high-fluid, high-fiber diet.
      (4) Nursing evaluation
         (a) Patient states that pain is relieved.
         (b) Patient eats high-fiber diet and drinks adequate fluids.
6. Hernia
  a) Definition: protrusion of a bowel segment or other abdominal structure through a weakness in abdominal muscle wall, inguinal area, diaphragmatic hiatus, or scrotal sac
  b) Pathophysiology and etiology
      (1) Pathophysiology: formation of hernial sac by outpouching of peritoneum, including large or small intestine, omentum, or bladder
      (2) Etiology: congenital defects; obesity; weakened muscles, especially at previous surgical site; increased intra-abdominal pressure due to coughing or straining
  c) Symptoms: abdominal swelling while coughing, standing, or lifting; abdominal pain
  d) Diagnostic evaluation: physical exam, GI radiographs
  e) Medical treatment: herniorrhaphy or hernioplasty
  f) Complications: hernial strangulation
  g) Essential nursing care for patients with hernia
      (1) Nursing assessment: Obtain patient history; check abdominal region for swelling or tenderness.
      (2) Nursing diagnoses
         (a) Potential for injury related to possible strangulated hernia
         (b) Pain related to hernia
         (c) Potential for infection related to herniorrhaphy
      (3) Nursing intervention
         (a) Advise patient to avoid strenuous activities that may cause strangulated hernia during presurgical period; caution patient not to try to reduce an incarcerated abdominal hernia.

(b) After surgery, remind patient to avoid coughing; encourage deep breathing and frequent turning; use ice bag and scrotal support for patient who has had indirect inguinal hernia repair; encourage early ambulation if not contraindicated; monitor fluid intake and output carefully to identify problems with voiding; use methods to stimulate voiding, if needed; report inability to void to physician; stress importance of avoiding constipation and associated straining during recovery period.

(c) In patient who has had hiatal hernia repair (fundoplication), use incentive spirometers and chest physiotherapy to keep airway open; administer sufficient analgesic 30 minutes before chest physical therapy; carefully monitor NG tube for patency and stability; monitor fluid replacement to ensure that respiratory secretions remain thin; supervise first oral feedings, since temporary dysphagia is common; teach patient to eat smaller, more frequent meals, since capacity of stomach has been reduced by surgery; encourage patient with gas bloat syndrome to avoid gas-producing foods, carbonated beverages, and drinking through straw.

(4) Nursing evaluation

    (a) Patient avoids strangulated hernia.

    (b) Patient states that pain is controlled.

    (c) Evidence of infection is absent.

7. Colon or rectal cancer

    a) Definition: malignant disease of the colon or rectum

    b) Pathophysiology and etiology

        (1) Pathophysiology: neoplasm arising from epithelial lining of intestine, destroying normal tissues; possible obstruction due to occlusion of intestinal lumen by tumor

        (2) Etiology: diet abundant in fats, fried or broiled meats and fish, and refined carbohydrates without fiber; decreased bowel transit time; presence of inflammatory bowel disease or polyps

    c) Symptoms: change in bowel habits, occult blood in stool, anemia, abdominal pain, weight loss, narrowing of stool, feeling of incomplete emptying after defecation, bloody stool (rare)

    d) Diagnostic evaluation: barium enema, sigmoidoscopy, colonoscopy, proctosigmoidoscopy, occult blood in stool, carcinoembryonic antigen test

    e) Medical treatment: surgery, including partial colectomy with colostomy, colectomy with reanastomosis, or total proctocolectomy with ileostomy; radiation therapy; chemotherapy

f) Complications: metastatic disease, infections
g) Essential nursing care for patients with colon or rectal cancer
   (1) Nursing assessment: Obtain patient history; determine stool characteristics, and inspect them for blood; and auscultate and palpate abdomen.
   (2) Nursing diagnoses
       (a) Pain related to obstruction in intestine
       (b) Potential for injury related to possible metastasis
       (c) High risk for infection related to potential contamination during surgery
   (3) Nursing intervention
       (a) Administer analgesics as prescribed; offer back rubs, massage, and relaxation techniques.
       (b) Alert patient to signs and symptoms of metastatic disease.
       (c) Administer antibiotics as prescribed before surgery; cleanse bowel with laxatives, enemas, and colonic irrigation.
       (d) Examine wound for signs of complications; change dressings as needed.
       (e) Report fever >101°F to physician.
       (f) If patient has had colostomy or ileostomy, examine stoma for swelling, color, discharge, and bleeding; clean skin around stoma (see sections IV,F and IV,G of this chapter).
   (4) Nursing evaluation
       (a) Patient states that pain is reduced.
       (b) Patient states that anxiety regarding metastatic disease is reduced.
       (c) Patient acquires no postsurgical infection.

C. Problems associated with nutrition
   1. Eating disorders
      a) Definition
         (1) Anorexia nervosa: life-threatening condition of self-induced starvation occurring primarily in women <30 years old
         (2) Bulimia nervosa: eating disorder characterized by episodes of uncontrollable binge eating, usually followed by some form of purging behavior
      b) Pathophysiology and etiology
         (1) Pathophysiology: morbid eating patterns associated with cultural and environmental stressors or possible neurochemical disturbance
         (2) Etiology
             (a) Anorexia nervosa: etiology unclear, although considered a psychiatric disorder; associated with parental problems, anxiety, cultural emphasis on slimness, overwhelming stress, neurochemical imbalance
             (b) Bulimia nervosa: need for control; familial conflicts; poor self-discipline, self-esteem, and impulse control; mood swings; depression; anxiety

c) Symptoms
  (1) Both disorders: increased level of growth hormone, orthostatic hypotension, regressed breast development, abnormal liver function, hypercholesterolemia, amenorrhea, decreased sexual drive, pedal edema, loss of subcutaneous lipid layer, muscular weakness, decreased muscle mass, lanugo hair, constipation, low core temperature, anemia
  (2) Anorexia: extreme emaciation, bizarre preoccupation with eating, fear of being fat
  (3) Bulimia: gastrointestinal symptoms, calluses from digital pressure on abdomen, scars on dorsum of hand, tetany, erosion of tooth enamel caused by repeated vomiting
d) Diagnostic evaluation: medical history, physical exam, psychologic testing; for bulimia, electrocardiogram, upper and lower GI tract studies
e) Medical treatment: IV administration of fluids and electrolytes for patients with anorexia and for severely malnourished patients with bulimia, psychotherapy, group therapy, behavior modification, antidepressant administration (for bulimia)
f) Complications: renal impairment, cardiac dysrhythmias, seizures
g) Essential nursing care for patients with eating disorders
  (1) Nursing assessment
    (a) Obtain medical, allergy, diet, and eating pattern history.
    (b) Check weight, height, and vital signs.
    (c) Observe for tetany, edema, parotid gland tenderness or swelling, discolored tooth enamel, excess number of caries, and jaundice.
  (2) Nursing diagnoses
    (a) Altered nutrition, less than body requirements, related to eating disorder
    (b) Potential fluid volume deficit related to vomiting
    (c) Ineffective individual coping related to improper defense mechanisms
    (d) Altered family processes related to problems coping with patient's illness
  (3) Nursing intervention
    (a) Record food intake; frequently observe patient undergoing IV or nasogastric feedings to prevent removal of lines.
    (b) Observe patient for signs of dehydration and electrolyte imbalance.
    (c) Be accepting of patient, and try to provide opportunities for interaction with others.

      (d) Discuss possible causes of eating disorders and long- and short-term treatments with patient and family.

    (4) Nursing evaluation

      (a) Patient increases food intake and gains weight.

      (b) Patient's fluid and electrolyte imbalances are corrected.

      (c) Patient cooperates with treatment and begins to socialize.

      (d) Patient and family state understanding and acceptance of eating disorder and treatment.

2. Obesity

  a) Definition: body weight >20% in excess of recommended weight

  b) Pathophysiology and etiology

    (1) Pathophysiology: excessive number of fat deposits associated with caloric intake that exceeds metabolic demands

    (2) Etiology: heredity, individual body build, metabolism, presence of fat cells, psychosocial factors, eating and activity habits

  c) Symptoms: excess body weight

  d) Diagnostic evaluation: physical exam, measuring weight

  e) Medical treatment: diet and exercise programs, administration of appetite suppressants; lipectomy, jaw wiring, gastric stapling, bypass procedures for morbid obesity

  f) Complications: cardiovascular and musculoskeletal disorders, diabetes

  g) Essential nursing care for patients with obesity

    (1) Nursing assessment: Obtain medical, dietary, and weight history; weigh patient.

    (2) Nursing diagnoses

      (a) Activity intolerance related to obesity

      (b) Altered nutrition, more than body requirements, related to poor eating habits and/or insufficient activity

      (c) Constipation and diarrhea related to weight-loss products

      (d) Impaired social interaction related to poor self-concept

    (3) Nursing intervention

      (a) Encourage patient to increase activity, alternating between periods of activity and rest.

      (b) Instruct patient about prescribed diet.

      (c) Advise patient of the dangers associated with weight-loss products.

      (d) Keep record of bowel movements; encourage patient to eat foods that minimize constipation or diarrhea; report continuing problems to physician.

      (e) Provide emotional support, and encourage patient to resume normal social activities.

    (4) Nursing evaluation

      (a) Patient tolerates increased activity.

      (b) Patient adheres to a weight-loss diet.

      (c) Patient avoids potentially dangerous weight-loss products.

      (d) Patient has normal elimination pattern.

      (e) Patient socializes with others.

1. Rose Whelan is scheduled to have a barium enema in 3 days. Which meal choice indicates that Ms. Whelan has understood the dietary instructions to be followed in preparation for the exam?

   a. Baked chicken, baked potato, applesauce, and skim milk
   b. Tuna salad sandwich, apple, carrot sticks, and skim milk
   c. Prime rib, leafy green salad, rice, and de-caffeinated coffee
   d. Oatmeal with fresh strawberries, wheat toast, and tea

2. Abe Turner, 78 years old, is receiving total parenteral nutrition (TPN) prior to colon resection surgery. He asks why his blood sugar is measured 4 times a day. The nurse explains that blood sugar testing is necessary because:

   a. Mr. Turner's age places him at high risk for developing type II diabetes.
   b. TPN decreases pancreatic production of insulin, thereby increasing the risk that hypoglycemia will develop.
   c. TPN has a concentrated sugar content that may result in a hyperglycemic reaction.
   d. Diabetes is a major complication of TPN therapy, and it is important to monitor for hyperglycemia.

3. Which observation indicates a desired outcome of TPN therapy for Mr. Turner?

   a. He remains alert and oriented.
   b. He gains 2 lb in 1 week.
   c. His intake and output totals are equal.
   d. His blood glucose remains between 100 and 180 mg/dl.

4. Before administering an intermittent Osmolite tube feeding through a nasogastric (NG) tube, the nurse must:

   a. Assess for the presence of bowel sounds.
   b. Warm the Osmolite to 98°F.
   c. Flush the NG tube with 10 ml of water.
   d. Make sure that the patient's residuals are <50 ml.

5. Which observation indicates that nursing interventions taken to reduce a patient's peptic ulcer symptoms have been effective?

   a. The patient's weight remains within 5 lb of the desired weight.
   b. The patient takes ranitidine (Zantac) p.r.n. for increased gastric discomfort.
   c. The patient eats 2–3 large meals each day.
   d. The patient attends smoking-cessation classes.

6. Opal Yusepa, 72 years old, is receiving cimetidine (Tagamet) intravenously to reduce peptic ulcer symptoms. Which observation indicates an adverse reaction to Tagamet?

   a. Confusion
   b. Dyspnea
   c. Hot flashes
   d. Urticaria

7. Teaching of a client with Crohn's disease would include information about the need to monitor which blood value on a regular basis?

   a. Fasting blood sugar (FBS)
   b. Folic acid
   c. Lactate dehydrogenase (LDH)
   d. Serum creatinine

8. The primary causes of obstruction in long-standing Crohn's disease in which there have been repeated exacerbations of inflammation are:

   a. Volvulus and intussusception.
   b. Slowed peristalsis and strictures.
   c. Adhesions and narrowing of the lumen.
   d. Ulcerations and incarcerated bowel segments.

9. Kevin Connor, who is 19 years old, is scheduled to have a Kock's ileostomy. During preoperative teaching, Kevin asks the nurse, "Would you ever date a guy who had stool coming out of his stomach?" Which is the most appropriate response?

   a. "I've never really thought about it."
   b. "The ileostomy will help improve your health so that you can have dating experiences."
   c. "Yes, I would. I also understand why you would have concerns about dating."
   d. "Having the ileostomy seems to be a concern for you."

10. Teaching Kevin about ileostomy care would include information about:

    a. Applying a protective gel barrier to the skin around the stoma site daily.
    b. Fitting the collection appliance tightly around the stoma to prevent skin breakdown.
    c. Inserting a catheter into the stoma to drain the pouch when a sensation of fullness is felt.
    d. Irrigating the ileostomy twice daily with 60 ml of normal saline to flush stool out of the Kock's pouch.

11. Which of the following pain experiences would be consistent with a gastric ulcer?

    a. Pain that peaks 2–3 hours after eating
    b. Pain that diminishes after ingestion of food
    c. Pain that causes awakening between 1:00 and 2:00 A.M.
    d. Pain that is relieved by vomiting

12. Tarloh Hinopen had a Billroth's II resection several weeks ago and now reports having explosive diarrhea after eating. What might the nurse recommend to control this situation?

    a. Avoid taking fluids with meals.
    b. Eliminate sugars and fats from the diet.
    c. Follow a clear liquid diet for 3 days.
    d. Take 2 TUMS tablets before meals.

1. **Correct answer is a.** The patient should follow a low-residue diet for the 3 days prior to a barium enema. Acceptable foods include milk (2 glasses), juice, tea, coffee, eggs, cheese, broth, cream soups, cooked strained vegetables and fruits, refined breads, cooked cereals, strained oatmeal, potatoes, pasta, rice, and roasted, baked, or broiled meats (except pork). Forbidden foods include raw vegetables and fruits, whole-grain cereals and breads, waffles, and pancakes.

   b. Tuna salad, apples, and carrot sticks are inappropriate food choices for the patient.
   c. A green salad is an inappropriate food choice.
   d. Fresh strawberries and wheat toast are inappropriate food choices. The oatmeal would be appropriate only if it were strained.

2. **Correct answer is c.** Total parenteral nutrition (TPN) has a 10%–25% dextrose base. This highly concentrated sugar solution can result in hyperglycemia if pancreatic insulin output is insufficient. An external source of insulin may be needed to enable the patient to utilize TPN properly.

   a. Elderly persons are at higher risk for decreased pancreatic function and type II diabetes. However, a decrease in pancreatic function is age related, not related to TPN therapy by itself.
   b. TPN typically stimulates insulin production rather than suppressing it.
   d. Diabetes is not a complication of TPN therapy.

3. **Correct answer is b.** The purpose of TPN therapy is to correct protein and calorie malnutrition. Weight gain of 1–3 lb per week is desired. A more rapid weight gain, averaging 1 lb or more per day, would probably be related to fluid retention.

   a. Patients who are receiving TPN may have altered levels of consciousness.

c. Intake/output measures are not directly related to TPN therapy.

d. The recommended adjusted blood glucose range for patients >65 years of age is 60–140 mg/dl. The 100–180 mg/dl range cited in this answer is too high.

4. **Correct answer is a.** The following assessments must be made before the administration of tube feedings: Observe for abdominal distention, auscultate bowel sounds, check for tube patency and placement with air administration, check for residual from the last feeding, and ensure that the patient's head is elevated at least 30°.

b. Tube feedings are administered at room temperature (68°–72°F).

c. Tubes are flushed with 100–150 ml of water after the feeding but are not usually flushed beforehand.

d. Feedings are withheld if the patient's residuals are ≥100 ml. A residual of 50 ml would not prevent another feeding.

5. **Correct answer is a.** Stable weight in a patient with peptic ulcer disease indicates that he/she is not experiencing an acute episode of the disease. Absence of pain allows the ingestion of sufficient amounts of food to maintain proper nutrition.

b. If prescribed, ranitidine (Zantac) should be taken on a regular basis to control ulcer symptoms. It is typically taken at bedtime or twice daily when used for maintenance.

c. Patients with peptic ulcer disease should eat small meals frequently throughout the day.

d. Although attending smoking-cessation classes may be a valuable means of preventing future episodes of acute peptic ulceration, it does not measure the absence of peptic ulcer symptoms.

6. **Correct answer is a.** A significant adverse reaction to cimetidine (Tagamet) in elderly patients is pseudodementia of the delirium type. The initial and primary manifestation of delirium is confusion, which warrants the discontinuation of drug therapy. Since the majority of patients taking Tagamet are elderly, it is particularly important to bear this adverse effect in mind.

b, c, and **d.** Dyspnea, hot flashes, and urticaria are not expected adverse reactions to Tagamet.

7. **Correct answer is b.** Crohn's disease results in malabsorption of many nutrients. During quiescent periods of the disease, it is important to monitor the patient for adequate absorption of nutrients and stability of the inflammatory process. Blood tests typically monitored include analysis of serum albumin, folic acid and serum iron, hemoglobin, hematocrit, complete blood count with differential, erythrocyte sedimentation rate, and liver function.

a, c, and **d.** FBS, LDH, and serum creatinine levels would not typically be monitored in patients with Crohn's disease.

8. **Correct answer is c.** Crohn's disease is characterized by periods of remission and exacerbation. During the active phase, inflammation and ulceration are the main physiologic events; they result in narrowing of the lumen and formation of adhesions. The primary complications of Crohn's disease that must be monitored are sepsis, peritonitis, hemorrhage, and mechanical obstruction.

a. Volvulus and intussusception are not specific to Crohn's disease.

b. Peristalsis is increased, not slowed, in Crohn's disease.

d. The ulcerations associated with Crohn's disease cause adhesions and incarcerations to form.

9. **Correct answer is d.** The nurse uses therapeutic communication techniques to invite the patient to explore his concerns. Kevin has reached the developmental stage at

which intimate relationships are important. Because his body image and self-esteem are threatened by the upcoming surgery, it is reasonable for him to have concerns about how his altered personal appearance will be received by another person.

a and **c.** The nurse's statements that she had never thought about dating someone with an ileostomy or that she would be willing to date such a person do not invite the patient to explore his concerns.
b. Telling the patient that the surgery will improve his health, and thus make dating possible, is an example of false reassurance.

10. **Correct answer is c.** Kock's ileostomy is a procedure in which a reservoir to collect and retain stool is formed from a loop of the ileum. A nipple valve is created and is pulled through the stoma. This valve closes because of fluid pressure within the pouch. A large volume of liquid is continually being produced. The pouch, which holds 500–700 ml of fluid, must be drained several times a day. The patient needs to learn how to drain the pouch by inserting a urinary catheter into the nipple valve.

a and **b.** Because Kock's ileostomy is a continent ileostomy, it is not necessary for the patient to use protective gel or a collection appliance.
d. Irrigating a Kock's ileostomy is not part of routine care.

11. **Correct answer is d.** Gastric ulcer pain is typically relieved by vomiting. Ingestion of food makes symptoms worse, and pain tends to be most severe 30 minutes–1 hour after a meal.

a, b, and **c.** Pain that peaks 2–3 hours after eating, that causes awakening between 1:00 and 2:00 A.M., and that is reduced by ingestion of food is characteristic of duodenal ulcers.

12. **Correct answer is a.** Ms. Hinopen is experiencing dumping syndrome, a common condition that begins several weeks after Billroth's II resection (gastrojejunostomy) and lasts 6–12 months after the surgery. Methods that can be used to decrease gastric exit time and to limit the associated diarrhea include eating small amounts of food in 5–6 meals daily; not drinking fluids with meals; taking pectin powder with meals; eating in a semirecumbent position; ingesting a high-fat, high-protein, low-carbohydrate diet; and taking sedatives and antispasmodics.

b. Eliminating fats from the diet would not be appropriate. Consumption of a high-fat diet can help to decrease emptying time and the incidence of diarrhea.
c. Consuming a clear liquid diet would probably exacerbate dumping syndrome.
d. TUMS and other antacids have no role in the treatment of dumping syndrome, although sedatives and antispasmodics have been shown to be effective.

13

Hepatic, Biliary, and Pancreatic Function

OVERVIEW

I. Structure and function of liver, gallbladder, and pancreas
  A. Liver
  B. Gallbladder
  C. Pancreas

II. General diagnostic tests
  A. Laboratory tests
  B. Liver biopsy
  C. Computed tomography
  D. Endoscopic retrograde cholangiopancreatography
  E. Percutaneous transhepatic cholangiography

III. General nursing assessments
  A. Patient history
  B. Observation and physical examination
  C. Diagnostic tests

IV. Nursing considerations with selected therapies and techniques
  A. Paracentesis
  B. Peritoneovenous shunt
  C. Esophagogastric tamponade tube
  D. Liver transplant
  E. Gallbladder surgery
  F. Whipple's procedure

V. Selected disorders
  A. Jaundice
  B. Viral hepatitis
  C. Hepatic cirrhosis
  D. Hepatic carcinoma
  E. Cholelithiasis
  F. Pancreatitis
  G. Pancreatic carcinoma

NURSING HIGHLIGHTS

1. Because hepatic and pancreatic disturbances are often connected to lifestyle, the nurse must assess patient's lifestyle and learn how to explain the risks of harmful behaviors.

2. Because many patients with hepatic or pancreatic carcinomas have a poor prognosis, nurse must be prepared to provide patient and family with emotional support and information about sources of help in the community.

cholangitis—inflammation of a bile duct
cholecystectomy—removal of the gallbladder
cholecystography—roentgenography of the gallbladder
esophageal varices—distended veins of the esophagus that may become irritated and rupture
hepatorenal syndrome—progressive oliguric renal failure associated with hepatic failure, resulting in impaired kidneys with normal anatomy and morphology
spider telangiectasis—a vascular lesion that is formed by the dilation of a group of small blood vessels and that has the shape of limbs radiating from a central point

ENHANCED OUTLINE

I. Structure and function of liver, gallbladder, and pancreas

See text pages

_____

A. Liver
   1. Structure
      a) Overall: largest organ of body, located in upper right abdominal quadrant; has 2 lobes divided by falciform ligament, which attaches liver to diaphragm
      b) Lobes: made up of lobules with connective tissue cover
      c) Vasculature: platelike arrangement of liver cells radiating from central vein; small bile channels fitting between plates and emptying into terminal bile ducts, which merge into single hepatic duct
   2. Function
      a) Storage: stores several minerals and vitamins
      b) Protection: detoxifies potentially harmful compounds and produces phagocytic Kupffer's cells
      c) Metabolism: breaks down amino acids; synthesizes several plasma proteins; stores and releases glycogen; synthesizes, breaks down, and stores fatty acids and triglycerides
      d) Digestion: forms and secretes bile, essential for fat digestion in small intestine

B. Gallbladder
   1. Structure: pear-shaped bulbous sac attached to and located beneath the liver; has 3 parts—neck, body (main portion), and fundus (lower bulbous section); connected to the liver via hepatic ducts and to the duodenum via the cystic duct and common bile duct
   2. Function: concentrates and stores bile from liver; releases bile into duodenum via common bile duct when fat is present in small intestine

C. Pancreas
   1. Structure: smooth carrot-shaped organ divided into head (right extremity), body (main part), neck (constricted area), and tail (left narrow portion); releases enzymes into duodenum via common bile duct

2. Function: secretes enzymes necessary for digestion of carbohydrates, fat, and protein (exocrine pancreas); produces glucagon and insulin (endocrine pancreas, in islets of Langerhans)

II. General diagnostic tests

A. Laboratory tests
1. Procedures: analysis of prothrombin time, calcium, serum protein electrophoresis, aspartate aminotransferase (AST), alanine aminotransferase (ALT), lactate dehydrogenase (LDH), alkaline phosphatase, bilirubin, serum amylase, serum lipase, glucose (fasting), cholesterol
2. Purpose: to screen for possible hepatic, biliary, and pancreatic disease

B. Liver biopsy
1. Procedure: aspiration of liver tissue sample for histologic study
2. Purpose: to determine the presence of liver disease

C. Computed tomography (CT)
1. Definition: cross-sectional x-ray visualization used to detect tissue abnormalities and densities
2. Purpose: to indicate the presence of liver, gallbladder, or pancreatic disease

D. Endoscopic retrograde cholangiopancreatography (ERCP)
1. Definition: visual and radiographic exam of liver, gallbladder, and pancreas in which an endoscope with a fiberoptic instrument is advanced through the mouth and into the duodenum; catheter is inserted through the ampulla of Vater into the biliary tract and x-rays taken after the injection of contrast dye
2. Purpose: to detect the presence of liver, gallbladder, or pancreatic disease

E. Percutaneous transhepatic cholangiography (PTC)
1. Definition: x-ray of biliary duct system in which iodine dye is injected into liver
2. Purpose: to evaluate patients who experience jaundice and/or persistent upper abdominal pain, even after cholecystectomy

III. General nursing assessments

A. Patient history: symptoms, personal and family history, travel, diet, drugs taken, toxin exposure, alcohol abuse

B. Observation and physical examination
1. Measure height, weight, and triceps skinfold thickness.
2. Inspect and palpate mouth.
3. Inspect skin of neck, shoulders, and chest for spider telangiectases.

See text pages

See text pages

4. Inspect, auscultate, percuss, and palpate abdomen.
5. Assist during diagnostic procedures.

C. Diagnostic tests: nursing responsibilities
   1. Liver function tests: Explain purpose of test to patient, and take specimens.
   2. Liver biopsy
      a) After procedure, help patient turn to right side, place pillow under costal margin, and instruct him/her to maintain position for several hours.
      b) Record vital signs at 10–20 minute intervals; report any pulse rate increase, arterial pressure decrease, or pain.
   3. Computed tomography (CT)
      a) On night before procedure, do not permit food or fluid to be taken orally after midnight.
      b) Advise patient that procedure is painless, that CT equipment is large and often noisy, and that he/she will need to lie still and hold breath at different times throughout procedure.
   4. Endoscopic retrograde cholangiopancreatography (ERCP)
      a) Preprocedure nursing care
         (1) Withhold food or fluids (taken orally) after midnight.
         (2) Ask patient to remove dentures.
         (3) If prescribed, administer a relaxing agent, such as a benzodiazepine, as well as atropine to dry secretions.
         (4) Explain that patient will receive a local anesthetic to calm the gag reflex at the beginning of the procedure.
      b) Postprocedure nursing care
         (1) Assess vital signs every 15 minutes for 1 hour, every 30 minutes for the next 2 hours, and hourly thereafter for 4 hours.
         (2) Test for presence of gag reflex.
         (3) Do not give food or fluid orally until gag reflex returns, usually after 2–4 hours.
         (4) Assess patient for signs of cholangitis or perforation (fever, chills, hypotension, tachycardia, abdominal pain).
   5. Percutaneous transhepatic cholangiography (PTC)
      a) Ask patient about allergies to iodine or seafood before procedure.
      b) Confine patient to bed for 8 hours after procedure; frequently check vital signs during this period.
      c) Observe and report bleeding or swelling at injection site; abdominal distention or tenderness; and signs of septicemia, peritonitis, or bleeding.

IV. Nursing considerations with selected therapies and techniques

See text pages
_____

A. Paracentesis
   1. Purpose: to manage ascites by using large-bore needle to remove excess fluid from peritoneal cavity
   2. Nursing management
      a) Weigh patient, and mark and measure abdominal girth.
      b) Ask patient to void or to drain Foley catheter.

      c) Help patient maintain sitting position during procedure, and monitor vital signs every 15 minutes.

      d) Measure and describe collected fluid after procedure, and send it to laboratory for analysis.

      e) Apply dressing to puncture site after trocar catheter has been removed; assess site for drainage.

      f) Continue bed rest until patient's vital signs are stable.

B. Peritoneovenous shunt

   1. Purpose: to manage ascites by causing excess fluid from the abdominal cavity to drain into the venous system

   2. Nursing management

      a) Correct electrolyte imbalance and abnormal coagulation before surgery.

      b) Monitor for elevated blood pressure, especially elevated central venous pressure, after surgery.

      c) Auscultate lung sounds for presence of rales.

      d) If prescribed, administer a diuretic, such as furosemide (Lasix), to prevent pulmonary edema.

      e) Monitor urinary output, weight, and abdominal girth.

C. Esophagogastric tamponade tube

   1. Purpose: to treat GI and esophageal variceal hemorrhage related to hepatic cirrhosis by compressing vessels with a pair of balloons

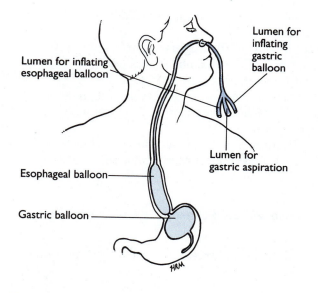

Lumen for inflating esophageal balloon

Lumen for inflating gastric balloon

Lumen for gastric aspiration

Esophageal balloon

Gastric balloon

Figure 13–1
Insertion of an Esophagogastric Tamponade Tube

2. Nursing management
   a) After labeling all lumina, assist physician with tube placement.
   b) Elevate head of bed while tube is in place.
   c) Apply gentle tension to tube, and apply gauze sponge around tube under patient's nose to prevent tissue necrosis.
   d) Provide oral care; maintain balloon pressures and volumes.
   e) Report blood pressure drop, heart rate increase, or sudden pain in the upper abdomen or back.

D. Liver transplant
   1. Purpose: to treat end-stage liver disease that has not responded to medical or other surgical intervention
   2. Nursing management
      a) Maintain strict asepsis.
      b) Monitor patient postoperatively for cardiovascular, pulmonary, renal, neurologic, and metabolic function.
      c) Report fever, blood oozing from catheter drain or incision site, or increased abdominal pain, distention, and rigidity.
      d) Provide patient education about medications to be taken and signs of rejection or infection.

E. Gallbladder surgery
   1. Purpose: to treat acute or chronic cholecystitis or cholelithiasis by removing the gallbladder through an abdominal incision or a laparoscope (which is associated with significantly fewer postoperative complications)
   2. Nursing management
      a) Teach patient about measures to take to prevent respiratory infections (see Nurse Alert, "Avoiding Respiratory Infections after Gallbladder Surgery").
      b) Place patient in low Fowler's position immediately after recovery from anesthesia.
      c) Inspect surgical wound at each dressing change, and report any sign of infection.
      d) Auscultate lungs daily, and encourage patient to practice techniques that prevent respiratory complications.
      e) Observe patient for leakage of bile into peritoneal cavity and for obstruction of bile drainage.
      f) Administer IV fluids as ordered; observe for electrolyte imbalance and dehydration.
      g) In patient who has undergone cholecystostomy or choledochostomy, fasten drainage tubing to dressings or to bottom sheet, with enough leeway that movement will not kink or dislodge it; when patient ambulates, place collection bag in bathrobe pocket or fasten it below waist or common duct level.
      h) Prior to discharge, instruct patient to avoid dietary fats for 6 weeks and to report signs of infection, inflammation, jaundice, dark urine, pale-colored stools, or pruritus to the physician.

F. Whipple's procedure
   1. Purpose: to treat pancreatic carcinoma by resecting proximal head of pancreas, duodenum, part of jejunum, part of stomach, and gallbladder, with anastomosis of pancreatic duct, common bile duct, and stomach to jejunum
   2. Nursing management
      a) Administer prescribed IV fluids or hyperalimentation before surgery.
      b) After surgery, assess pain frequently before and after analgesic administration; administer prescribed analgesic; and assist patient to assume comfortable position.
      c) Monitor nasogastric tube patency.
      d) Check suction gauge often, and observe amount and color of drained fluid.
      e) Maintain patient in semi-Fowler's position.
      f) Monitor patient for signs of fluid and electrolyte imbalance.

V. Selected disorders

See text pages
_____

A. Jaundice
   1. Definition: yellow discoloration of tissue caused by an abnormally high concentration of bilirubin in the blood

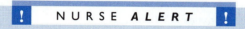

! NURSE ALERT !

Avoiding Respiratory Infections after Gallbladder Surgery

Patients who have had gallbladder surgery are at high risk for potentially serious respiratory complications due to muscle pain related to surgical manipulation of the diaphragm and the incision in the right subcostal area. To avoid these complications, nurse should:

- Anticipate patient's needs for analgesic, particularly in connection with increased activity and need for pulmonary toilet.
- Instruct patient to take sustained maximal inspirations and turn at least every 2 hours; encourage cough if secretions persist.
- Demonstrate how to use a pillow or folded bath blanket as a splinting device to reduce abdominal jarring during deep breathing and coughing.
- Explain that patient can expect to get out of bed on the first postsurgical day and maintain mobility thereafter.
- Because the patient who smokes is at special risk for postoperative atelectasis, caution against smoking during the presurgical period, and teach him/her to use a sustained maximal inspiration (SMI) device, such as an incentive spirometer.

2. Pathophysiology and etiology
   a) Pathophysiology: Jaundice is visible when bilirubin levels reach 3 mg/dl of blood (normal levels being 0.1–1.0 mg/dl).
   b) Etiology
      (1) Hemolytic jaundice: too much bilirubin produced for the liver to process, caused by excess hemolysis of red blood cells
      (2) Hepatocellular jaundice: internal liver disease preventing normal transformation of bile by liver cells and causing buildup of bilirubin
      (3) Obstructive jaundice: inability of bile to flow out of liver because of blocked bile ducts
3. Symptoms: yellow skin, mucous membranes, and sclerae; deep orange, frothy urine; light, clay-colored stools; pruritus; dyspepsia; elevated bilirubin and alkaline phosphatase levels
4. Diagnostic evaluation: laboratory tests of pigment type in blood, urine, and stool
5. Medical treatment: identification and treatment of underlying cause
6. Complications: depend on underlying disorder
7. Essential nursing care for patients with jaundice
   a) Nursing assessment: Obtain patient history, with emphasis on risk factors for liver, biliary, or pancreatic disease; take samples for lab tests.
   b) Nursing diagnoses: related to underlying cause
   c) Nursing intervention: related to underlying cause
   d) Nursing evaluation: related to underlying cause

B. Viral hepatitis
   1. Definition: an infectious, contagious liver disease caused by a group of viruses
   2. Pathophysiology and etiology
      a) Pathophysiology: metabolic dysfunction and decreased bile secretion and excretion due to parenchymal injury, progressing in severe cases to cirrhosis
      b) Etiology
         (1) Hepatitis A and E: person-to-person transmission by contact with virus in feces, saliva, or contaminated water and food; contaminated bedpans, rectal thermometers, or linen; contaminated blood (hepatitis A)
         (2) Hepatitis B and D: transfusion of infected blood or plasma, contaminated syringes and medical or dental equipment, sexual contact with infected person
         (3) Hepatitis C: contaminated blood, sexual contact with infected person
   3. Symptoms
      a) Prejaundice phase: nausea; vomiting; anorexia; fever; malaise; arthralgia; headache; enlarged liver, spleen, and lymph nodes; weight loss; rash; urticaria
      b) Jaundice phase: jaundice, pruritus, clay-colored stools, dark urine, fatigue, anorexia, right upper quadrant discomfort
      c) Postjaundice phase: liver enlargement, malaise, fatigue

4. Diagnostic evaluation: complement fixation, immune adherence, and radioimmunoassay tests
5. Medical treatment
    a) Confine patient to bed and serve small, low-fat or fat-free, well-balanced meals; provide vitamin and IV supplementation, if necessary.
    b) Avoid drug therapy until liver recovers.
6. Complications: hepatic coma, cirrhosis, fulminant hepatic failure
7. Essential nursing care for patients with viral hepatitis
    a) Nursing assessment
        (1) Assess symptoms, and inspect skin for jaundice.
        (2) Palpate right upper abdominal quadrant for liver tenderness and firmness.
    b) Nursing diagnoses
        (1) Altered nutrition, less than body requirements, related to nausea
        (2) High risk for infection due to contagious nature of disease
        (3) Activity intolerance related to malaise
    c) Nursing intervention
        (1) Provide small frequent meals; encourage patient to select appealing foods; administer antiemetics when vomiting is severe.
        (2) Provide care plan to reflect severity of symptoms.
        (3) Provide information on contagious nature of disease and follow-up home care.
    d) Nursing evaluation
        (1) Patient eats nutritious balanced diet.
        (2) Patient follows precautionary isolation measures and understands the communicable nature of the disease.
        (3) Patient obeys activity limits.

C. Hepatic cirrhosis
  1. Definition: chronic progressive liver disease that results in necrosis and scarring
  2. Pathophysiology and etiology
    a) Pathophysiology: necrosis of liver cells, which are gradually replaced by scar tissue
    b) Etiology
        (1) Laënnec's portal cirrhosis: surrounding of portal areas of liver with scar tissue; associated with heavy alcohol abuse, poor nutrition, and exposure to industrial solvents and chemicals
        (2) Postnecrotic cirrhosis: formation of broad bands of scar tissue resulting from acute viral hepatitis

(3) Biliary cirrhosis: chronic obstruction or infection of bile ducts due to an unknown cause
3. Symptoms: metabolic disorders, blood coagulation defects, fluid and electrolyte imbalances, decreased immunity, jaundice, ecchymosis, scant body hair, palmar erythema, cutaneous spider angiomata, ascites
4. Diagnostic evaluation
   a) Patient history with emphasis on behavioral risk factors and previous liver disease; physical exam
   b) Lab tests, including complete blood count, serum enzyme studies, bleeding/coagulation tests, serum albumin and globulin levels
   c) Liver biopsy, ultrasonography, computed tomography, magnetic resonance imaging, radioisotope scanning
5. Medical treatment
   a) Manage presenting symptoms.
   b) Administer vitamins and nutritional supplements to promote healing of liver cells and enhance general health.
   c) Administer potassium-sparing diuretics to decrease amount of ascites.
6. Complications: hepatic coma, bleeding esophageal varices, infection, ascites, portal hypertension, jaundice, hepatorenal syndrome
7. Essential nursing care for patients with hepatic cirrhosis
   a) Nursing assessment
      (1) Obtain patient history, including data on precipitating factors, alcohol use, and physical and mental changes.
      (2) Record weight, abdominal distention, GI bleeding, and bruising.
      (3) Assess for encephalopathy through interview and other interactions; determine orientation to time and place and ability to carry out family responsibilities and/or maintain employment.
   b) Nursing diagnoses
      (1) Fluid volume excess related to ascites
      (2) Activity intolerance related to debility
      (3) High risk for injury related to altered clotting mechanisms
      (4) Altered thought processes related to increased ammonia levels
   c) Nursing intervention
      (1) Assess patient for symptoms of epigastric fullness, weakness, restlessness, and hemorrhage.
      (2) Restrict salt and fluid intake; administer potassium-sparing diuretics as prescribed; record fluid intake and output.
      (3) Encourage patient to avoid further use of alcohol, narcotics, barbiturates, and acetaminophen, which are metabolized in the liver.
      (4) Offer small frequent meals, following instructions about protein restriction; administer antiemetics as prescribed.
      (5) Observe stool for color, amount, consistency, and presence of occult blood.

      (6) Advise patient to alternate between rest and activity; restrict visitors.

      (7) Take precautionary measures against hemorrhage, such as using padded side rails and applying pressure to injection sites; monitor patient for gastrointestinal bleeding; administer vitamin K as prescribed.

      (8) Restrict dietary protein intake and give small carbohydrate snacks; provide careful nursing surveillance; avoid barbiturates and narcotics; limit visitors; arouse patient periodically.

    d) Nursing evaluation

      (1) Patient has normal fluid volume.

      (2) Patient allows time for adequate rest periods.

      (3) Patient sustains no hemorrhagic injury.

      (4) Patient maintains skin integrity.

      (5) Patient maintains normal thought processes.

D. Hepatic carcinoma

  1. Definition: malignant tumor of the liver

  2. Pathophysiology and etiology

    a) Pathophysiology: rapidly growing tumor, due to degree of liver's vascularization, that may spread to lung, heart, kidneys, stomach, pancreas, lymph nodes, adrenals, and bone

    b) Etiology

      (1) Primary malignant tumors (rare in United States): linked to cirrhosis and hepatitis B, diet deficiencies, *Aspergillus* fungus

      (2) Secondary malignant (metastatic) tumors: spread from breast, lung, or GI tract

  3. Symptoms: weight loss, weakness, pain in upper right quadrant, sudden abdominal distention, anorexia, anemia

  4. Diagnostic evaluation: laboratory studies, needle biopsy, liver scanning, ultrasonography, CT, MRI

  5. Medical treatment

    a) Hepatic lobectomy, if carcinoma confined to 1 lobe

    b) Palliative treatment for metastatic disease, including radiation, chemotherapy (sometimes administered by implantable pump), hepatic artery ligation, percutaneous biliary drainage, hyperthermia

  6. Complications: chemotherapy-related toxicity, hemorrhage, sepsis

  7. Essential nursing care for patients with hepatic carcinoma

    a) Nursing assessment

      (1) Assess patient for signs of encroaching tumor, including jaundice, pruritus, and pain.

      (2) Inquire about family support structure to determine feasibility of in-home chemotherapy.

b) Nursing diagnoses
   (1) High risk of infection related to percutaneous biliary drainage
   (2) High risk of injury related to presence of implanted chemotherapy pump
c) Nursing intervention
   (1) Percutaneous biliary drainage
      (a) Alert patient and family to benefits of percutaneous biliary drainage and to its associated risks, including hemorrhage, sepsis, bile leakage, and reobstruction of biliary system due to debris in catheter.
      (b) After procedure, observe patient for fever and chills; bile drainage around catheter; changes in vital signs; and pain, pressure, jaundice, and pruritus, which may indicate biliary obstruction.
      (c) Prior to discharge, instruct patient and family in catheter care, and explain the signs of complications.
   (2) Chemotherapy
      (a) Instruct patient to be alert for complications associated with chemotherapy, including toxic reactions and infection due to presence of implanted pump.
      (b) Stress importance of follow-up visits to patient with pump.
      (c) Encourage patient to resume normal activities, with the exception of sports and other strenuous activities that may damage pump.
d) Nursing evaluation
   (1) Patient watches for sudden fever or other signs of infection.
   (2) Patient avoids sports or other activities that may damage implanted pump and cause bodily injury.

E. Cholelithiasis (gallstones)
   1. Definition: the most common disorder of the biliary tract, in which solid particles of bile form stones, inflaming gallbladder and often lodging in cystic duct
   2. Pathophysiology and etiology
      a) Pathophysiology: Pigment stones are formed by precipitation of unconjugated bile pigments; cholesterol stones are formed by supersaturation of bile with cholesterol.
      b) Etiology: obesity, middle age or advanced age; use of oral contraceptives, estrogens, and clofibrate; malabsorption of bile salts due to gastrointestinal disease
   3. Symptoms: epigastric distress, severe pain radiating to back or right shoulder, dark urine, grayish stools
   4. Diagnostic evaluation: symptom history, abdominal radiography, ultrasonography, radionuclide imaging, cholecystography, endoscopy, PTC, ERCP
   5. Medical treatment
      a) Rest, dietary restrictions, IV fluids, nasogastric suction, analgesic, antibiotics
      b) Medication to dissolve gallstones

        c) Extracorporeal shock wave lithotripsy, intracorporeal lithotripsy

        d) Surgery, including cholecystectomy, minicholecystectomy, laparoscopic or laser cholecystectomy, choledochostomy, percutaneous cholecystostomy

    6. Complications: hemorrhage, abscess or necrosis of gallbladder, peritonitis

    7. Essential nursing care for patients with cholelithiasis

        a) Nursing assessment

            (1) Obtain patient history, including information about symptoms, diet, and drug and tobacco use.

            (2) Perform physical exam, including palpation of abdomen and examination of skin and sclerae for jaundice.

        b) Nursing diagnoses

            (1) Anxiety related to symptoms, diagnosis, and disease

            (2) Pain related to presence of stones

            (3) Altered nutrition related to inadequate bile secretion

            (4) Potential for infection related to surgery

            (5) Knowledge deficit related to home care

        c) Nursing intervention

            (1) Explain treatment, diagnostic tests, and possible surgery; provide emotional support.

            (2) Administer narcotic analgesic as ordered; evaluate patient's response to medication; omit pain-causing food from diet.

            (3) Encourage patient to avoid intake of excess dietary fat.

            (4) Monitor vital signs every 4 hours; inspect surgical wound at dressing changes; report sudden fever and signs of infection.

            (5) Provide information on home care, including avoidance of dietary fat for 6 weeks; care of drainage system, if it is still in place, including reporting of any changes in drainage; medication regimen for prescribed anticholinergics, antispasmodics, and vitamins; and need to report jaundice, dark urine, pale-colored stools, pruritus, and signs of infection or inflammation to physician.

        d) Nursing evaluation

            (1) Patient's anxiety is relieved.

            (2) Patient states that pain is diminished or alleviated.

            (3) Patient eats balanced nutritious diet.

            (4) Patient exhibits no sign of infection.

            (5) Patient states understanding of diet and drug therapy and care of incision, drains, and T tube.

    F. Pancreatitis

        1. Definition: inflammatory process of the pancreas in which pancreatic enzymes, especially trypsin, destroy organ tissue

2. Pathophysiology and etiology
   a) Pathophysiology: obstruction of the flow of pancreatic juice by gallstones, spasm, and edema of the ampulla of Vater; activation of pancreatic enzymes causing autodigestion of the pancreas; chronic pancreatitis results in calcification and scarring
   b) Etiology: associated with biliary tract disease; alcohol abuse; hyperparathyroidism; ischemic vascular disease; hypercalcemia; hyperlipidemia; bacterial or viral infection; abdominal trauma; use of thiazide diuretics, oral contraceptives, and corticosteroids; heredity
3. Symptoms: severe abdominal pain, back pain, abdominal distention, nausea, vomiting, fever, mental confusion, jaundice, hyperglycemia
4. Diagnostic evaluation: serum amylase and lipase tests, CT, chest radiography
5. Medical treatment
   a) Pain relief and restoration of fluid and electrolyte balance; total parenteral nutrition in severe cases
   b) Administration of pancreatic enzyme, insulin, anticholinergic drugs, and antacids
   c) Avoidance of alcohol, caffeine, and high-fat foods
   d) Endoscopic placement of biliary drains
6. Complications: fluid and electrolyte imbalances, hypotension, peritonitis, shock, anoxia
7. Essential nursing care for patients with pancreatitis
   a) Nursing assessment
      (1) Obtain history, focusing on nature of abdominal pain.
      (2) Palpate abdomen for pain, distention, and rigidity.
      (3) Obtain stool and urine samples for laboratory evaluation.
   b) Nursing diagnoses
      (1) Pain related to pancreatic inflammation
      (2) Ineffective breathing pattern related to pleural effusion
   c) Nursing intervention
      (1) Administer prescribed analgesics, and report failure of pain relief.
      (2) Measure gastric secretions every 8 hours, recording color, consistency, and amount.
      (3) Maintain patient in semi-Fowler's position; encourage him/her to cough and deep breathe.
      (4) In patient with biliary drain or stents in the pancreatic duct, assess for patency of drainage system; monitor for signs of inflammation and infection; monitor on a continuing basis for decreased pain and increased weight gain.
   d) Nursing evaluation
      (1) Patient states that pain has been relieved.
      (2) Patient experiences improved breathing function.

G. Pancreatic carcinoma
   1. Definition: tumor of the pancreas, usually an adenocarcinoma
   2. Pathophysiology and etiology
      a) Pathophysiology: originating from pancreatic ductal system cells and found in the head (most common), body, or tail of pancreas

b) Etiology: associated with cigarette smoking, alcohol abuse, high-fat diet, exposure to environmental toxins or industrial chemicals

3. Symptoms: abdominal pain, jaundice, severe anorexia, weight loss (often sudden), diabetes (occasional)

4. Diagnostic evaluation

    a) Lab studies: elevation of serum amylase, alkaline phosphatase, and bilirubin levels; elevated carcinoembryonic antigen levels in 80%–90% of patients with pancreatic carcinoma

    b) CT, ultrasonography, radiography, needle biopsy, surgical exploration, percutaneous transhepatic cholangiography

5. Medical treatment

    a) Surgery (Whipple's procedure)

    b) Palliative measures, including radiation, chemotherapy, pain management, and nutritional support

6. Complications: hemorrhage, vascular collapse, hepatorenal failure

7. Essential nursing care for patients with pancreatic carcinoma

    a) Nursing assessment

        (1) Inquire about history of diabetes and pancreatitis, smoking, exposure to industrial carcinogens, duration of jaundice, and presence of abdominal or referred pain.

        (2) Palpate liver, gallbladder, and pancreas.

    b) Nursing diagnoses

        (1) Pain related to tumor progression

        (2) Fluid volume deficit related to extensive surgical procedure

        (3) Altered nutrition, less than body requirements, related to anorexia

        (4) Impaired skin integrity related to jaundice

    c) Nursing intervention

        (1) Administer narcotic analgesics, and provide comfort measures for side effects of chemotherapy, including use of water-soluble lubricant around external nares and provision of oral hygiene and gargling solutions.

        (2) Maintain fluid and electrolyte balance in patient recovering from Whipple's procedure.

        (3) Administer parenteral fluids, electrolytes, and nutrients as prescribed; monitor serum glucose level, and observe patient for signs of hypoglycemia and hyperglycemia; check skin and other tissues for breakdown related to malnutrition.

        (4) Maintain patient with enteral feedings when intestinal function permits.

        (5) Use bath oil rather than soap to bathe patient, and apply prescription ointments when appropriate.

d) Nursing evaluation
   (1) Patient states that pain and discomfort are diminished.
   (2) Patient maintains adequate hydration.
   (3) Patient receives sufficient nutritional support.
   (4) Patient's pruritus is relieved.

1. Ms. Coreto is admitted to the hospital for a diagnostic work-up for cholelithiasis. Which sign is the nurse most likely to observe?

   a. Vague left upper quadrant pain 2 hours after eating

   b. Abdominal distention following ingestion of fatty foods

   c. Acute pain radiating to the back or upper right shoulder after meals

   d. Feeling of fullness and nausea immediately after eating

2. Ms. Coreto asks why her skin is so yellow. Which response by the nurse most accurately addresses this question?

   a. A stone blocking the common bile duct causes bile to be absorbed and circulated in the blood, causing the yellow color.

   b. Inflammation of the liver causes red blood cells to break down and to release a substance that turns the skin yellow.

   c. After excess production of cholesterol by the liver plugs acini channels, bile is absorbed by the skin.

   d. Increased amounts of bile secreted by the gallbladder react with melanin in the skin to produce the yellow color.

3. Ms. Coreto experiences an episode of biliary colic. Which of the following medications would the nurse give to reduce her discomfort?

   a. Diazepam (Valium), 5 mg intramuscularly

   b. Meperidine hydrochloride (Demerol), 75 mg intramuscularly

   c. Acetaminophen with codeine (Tylenol #3), 625 mg rectally

   d. Morphine sulfate, 2 mg intramuscularly

4. Germaine Randolph underwent endoscopic retrograde cholangiopancreatography (ERCP) this morning and is now requesting some ice. Which action does the nurse take?

   a. Consult the physician for permission to give the ice.

   b. Check for gag and swallow reflexes.

   c. Offer oral care and apply lip moisturizer.

   d. Give the ice as requested and monitor the patient's swallowing.

5. Ms. Orr is being discharged to home with dietary management instructions for cholecystitis. Which meal choice indicates that the patient understands the prescribed diet?

   a. Grilled hamburger, french fries, and iced tea

   b. Western omelet, Canadian bacon, and decaffeinated coffee

   c. Baked fish, rice, cooked green beans, and skim milk

   d. Lettuce, broccoli, and cucumber salad with fat-free dressing

6. Cholecystitis can interfere with the absorption of vitamin:

   a. C.

   b. B_6.

   c. B_{12}.

   d. K.

7. Which laboratory value would be observed with acute pancreatitis?

   a. Increased thyroid-stimulating hormone (TSH) level

   b. Increased fasting blood sugar (FBS)

   c. Decreased erythrocyte sedimentation rate (ESR)

   d. Decreased white blood cell (WBC) count

8. A patient with acute pancreatitis has a Salem sump nasogastric (NG) tube attached to low continuous suction. What is the reason for the NG tube?

   a. It prevents digestive juices from exiting the stomach, thereby decreasing stimulation of the pancreas.

   b. It suctions the excess bile being produced, thereby reducing direct irritation of the pancreas.

c. It prevents excess fluids from entering the site of inflammation, thereby preventing a small bowel obstruction.

d. It removes excess air and fluid from the duodenum, thereby preventing pancreatic inflammation.

9. The nurse suspects that a patient with diabetes is experiencing ketoacidosis. What manifestations is the nurse observing?

   a. Tachycardia and pale, moist skin
   b. Hypertension and dry mucous membranes
   c. Hypotension and dry, hot, flushed skin
   d. Bradycardia and dry, pale mucous membranes

10. Ms. Bernice Mason, a patient with diabetes, reports that she is feeling nervous and has double vision. What is the nurse's *first* action?

    a. Give a glass of orange juice.
    b. Elevate the head of the bed.
    c. Check the patient's blood sugar level.
    d. Give 4 units of regular insulin stat.

11. Ella James, 56 years old, is diagnosed as having type II diabetes (NIDDM). What information would the nurse share with her?

    a. The beta cells of her pancreas no longer produce insulin to mediate glucose metabolism.
    b. She will need to monitor her blood sugar 4 times a day and to take insulin.
    c. She should be able to manage her blood sugar levels through dietary modifications.
    d. She will need to avoid aerobic exercise, since this contributes to complications.

12. Steve Matsko, who has liver disease, is being discharged to home. Which medication does the nurse teach him to avoid?

    a. Acetaminophen (Tylenol)
    b. Vitamin K
    c. Triamterene (Dyazide)
    d. Docusate sodium (Colace)

---

1. **Correct answer is c.** Pain in cholelithiasis varies according to the following factors: size and location of the stone (obstructing or nonobstructing), degree and extent of inflammation, and whether the stone is stationary or moving. There may be a vague feeling of midepigastric discomfort, or there may be acute spastic pain originating in the right upper quadrant that radiates to the back and right shoulder.

   a. Left quadrant pain 2 hours after eating is characteristic of duodenal ulcer.
   b. Although the patient may report a feeling of fullness, bloating, and increased flatulence, especially after eating a fatty meal, the nurse does not typically observe distention.
   d. Symptoms of fullness and nausea immediately after eating are associated with gastritis and hiatal hernia.

2. **Correct answer is a.** Jaundice in cholelithiasis occurs when the flow of bile from the liver is obstructed by a stone in the common bile duct. Bile is absorbed into circulation and is excreted by the skin, giving it a yellow color. Jaundice is first noted in the sclera.

   b, c, and d. Jaundice in cholelithiasis is not caused by inflammation of the liver, excess cholesterol production, or increased secretion of bile by the gallbladder.

3. **Correct answer is b.** The primary drugs given to control the pain associated with biliary colic are meperidine hydrochloride (Demerol) for its analgesic action and propantheline bromide (Pro-Banthine) for its antispasmodic action. Prochlorperazine (Compazine) is given for associated nausea.

   a, c, and d. Diazepam (Valium), acetaminophen (Tylenol), and morphine sulfate would not be given to alleviate the pain of biliary colic. In fact, morphine can increase spastic activity of smooth muscles, resulting in increased pain.

4. Correct answer is b. The throat of the patient is anesthetized for passage of the scope for endoscopic retrograde cholangiopancreatography. Food and fluids may be given upon the return of the gag and swallow reflexes. The nurse assesses for gag and swallow prior to the administration of food and fluids.

a, c, and **d.** Ice can be given as soon as the nurse determines that the gag and swallow reflexes have returned.

5. Correct answer is c. Dietary modifications for persons with cholecystitis include the reduction or elimination of cholesterol, fat, and gas-forming foods. Fatty cuts of red meats, pork, fried foods, gas-forming vegetables (e.g., broccoli, cauliflower, cucumbers, and legumes), eggs, and whole milk should be avoided.

a. The hamburger and french fries would be inappropriate foods because of their high fat content.
b. The western omelet and Canadian bacon would be inappropriate foods because of their high fat and cholesterol content.
d. A salad containing broccoli and cucumbers would be inappropriate because of the gas-forming properties of these vegetables.

6. Correct answer is d. The absorption of fat-soluble vitamins (A, D, E, and K) is typically impaired in cholecystitis.

a, b, and **c.** Absorption of vitamins C, B_6, and B_{12} would not be affected, because these are water-soluble vitamins.

7. Correct answer is b. Inflammation of the pancreas interferes with its exocrine and endocrine functions, resulting in decreased release of enzymes and insulin. With decreased production and release of insulin, blood sugar values become elevated. An exogenous source of insulin is usually needed to control blood sugar during acute pancreatitis.

a. TSH is unrelated to pancreatic function.
c and **d.** ESR level and WBC count would be increased with pancreatitis.

8. Correct answer is a. The primary purpose of nasogastric (NG) suctioning during an acute episode of pancreatitis is to prevent gastric juice from passing into the duodenum and stimulating the pancreas to produce and excrete digestive enzymes. This allows the pancreas to rest, resulting in decreased inflammation.

b and **d.** The highest concentrations of bile are in the duodenum. A Salem sump is a gastric tube, and therefore it does not pass through the pylorus into the duodenum to suction duodenal fluid. A Miller-Abbott tube suctions intestinal contents.
c. The anatomic location of the pancreas precludes inflammation in this area from leading to small bowel obstruction.

9. Correct answer is c. Diabetic ketoacidosis (DKA) is an emergency situation that occurs in type I diabetes. The nurse must recognize the signs of DKA in its early stages to prevent the patient from entering into a coma. High blood glucose level (>400 mg/dl) results in increased thirst, nausea, vomiting, abdominal pain, fatigue, polyuria to anuria, elevated temperature, signs of dehydration, flushed face, rapid and thready pulse, and hypotension.

a, b, and **d.** Tachycardia combined with pale and moist skin, hypertension, and bradycardia are not signs of DKA.

10. Correct answer is c. The nurse's first action should always be to collect sufficient data to determine the most appropriate follow-up actions. Determining the blood sugar level will help to distinguish between hyper- and hypoglycemia.

a, b, and **d.** The appropriateness of giving a glass of orange juice, elevating the head of the bed, and giving 4 units of regular insulin could only be determined by evaluating the results of the blood sugar test.

11. Correct answer is c. The 2 primary factors associated with the development of type II diabetes (non-insulin-dependent diabetes mellitus [NIDDM]) are aging and obesity. It is believed that obesity interferes with the binding of insulin at cell receptors, thus interfering with the adequate utilization of available circulating insulin. The first line of treatment in type II diabetes is therefore weight loss and dietary modification.

a. Pancreatic cells continue to produce insulin in type II diabetes.
b. Type I, not type II, diabetes mellitus is insulin dependent.
d. Aerobic exercise is beneficial, since it aids in weight reduction and better blood glucose utilization.

12. **Correct answer is a.** Tylenol is hepatotoxic, and the reduction of liver function associated with liver disease can result in an increase in its toxic effects, which can precipitate advanced cirrhosis.

b, c, and **d.** Vitamin K, triamterene (Dyazide), and docusate sodium (Colace) are not hepatotoxic. In fact, vitamin K should be taken in prescribed amounts to prevent the bleeding tendencies that are associated with liver disease.

14

Endocrine System Function

OVERVIEW

I. Structure and function of endocrine system
A. Structure
B. Function

II. General diagnostic tests
A. Radioimmunoassay
B. Urine tests
C. Glucose tests
D. Thyroid scan

III. General nursing assessments
A. Patient history
B. Observation and physical examination
C. Diagnostic tests

IV. Nursing considerations with selected therapies and techniques
A. Thyroid surgery
B. Adrenalectomy

V. Selected disorders
A. Pituitary gland dysfunction
B. Thyroid gland dysfunction
C. Parathyroid dysfunction
D. Adrenal gland dysfunction
E. Diabetes mellitus

NURSING HIGHLIGHTS

1. Nursing interventions for patients with endocrine disorders are geared toward preventing complications, teaching patients about their disease and treatment regimen, and helping patients adapt to lifestyle changes.
2. Nurses play a vital role in helping patients with diabetes and their families understand the disease and its management, including daily treatment regimens and means to prevent and treat acute and long-term complications.

GLOSSARY

reactive hypoglycemia—a response to excessive insulin production, usually occurring after a carbohydrate meal has been eaten
tetany—tonic muscular spasm caused by severe hypocalcemia
thyroid storm—life-threatening disorder caused by metabolic insults in patient with untreated or poorly controlled hyperthyroidism; characterized by sudden onset, high fever, tachycardia, and delirium

I. Structure and function of endocrine system

See text pages
_____

A. Structure: pituitary, thyroid, parathyroid, thymus, and adrenal glands; islets of Langerhans in pancreas; ovaries or testicles; hormones produced by these glands

B. Function: glandular secretion of hormones, which help to regulate organ function, into bloodstream

II. General diagnostic tests

See text pages
_____

A. Radioimmunoassay: determines function of gland by assessing competition between labeled amounts of hormone and unlabeled hormone from the plasma or serum for binding sites on an antibody

B. Urine tests: measure amount of a specific hormone in a 24-hour urine collection to determine function of 1 or more glands

C. Glucose tests
   1. Fasting blood sugar: screening test for diabetes mellitus; diabetes indicated by glucose level >140 mg/dl on >1 occasion
   2. Random plasma glucose levels: screening test for diabetes mellitus; diabetes indicated by glucose level >200 mg/dl on >1 occasion
   3. Oral glucose tolerance test (OGTT): detects diabetes when a screening test has abnormal results; diabetes indicated by glucose level from a 2-hour sample >200 mg/dl
   4. Glycosylated hemoglobin test: determination of average blood glucose level over 2–3 months to determine degree of glucose control in diabetes; sustained periods of increased glucose level associated with elevated levels of glycosylated hemoglobins

D. Thyroid scan (radioactive iodine uptake [RAIU] test): evaluation of position, size, and function of thyroid gland by measuring uptake of orally administered radioactive iodine (^{123}I); normal thyroid uptake 5%–35% of administered dose; hypothyroidism indicated by lesser uptake, hyperthyroidism by greater uptake

III. General nursing assessments

See text pages
_____

A. Patient history: medical, family, drug, diet, allergy

B. Observation and physical examination
   1. Assess weight, height, vital signs, and physical and emotional status.
   2. Inspect skin for oiliness, dryness, ecchymosis, pigment, and wounds.
   3. Check eyes for bulging, protrusion, and puffiness.
   4. Inspect neck and extremities for swelling and tremors; palpate thyroid gland.
   5. Note patient's attitude and mental status.
   6. Assist during diagnostic procedures.

C. Diagnostic tests: nursing responsibilities
   1. Radioimmunoassay: Explain purpose, and draw blood.
   2. Urine tests of hormone levels (24-hour collection): Explain purpose; remind patient that test is for exactly 24 hours; caution patient not to discard preservative from container, to handle container carefully because solution may be caustic, and to avoid taking unnecessary medications.
   3. Glucose tests: Explain purpose and any fasting procedures; give glucose load; and take samples.
   4. Thyroid scan (radioactive iodine uptake [RAIU] test): Explain purpose; reassure patient that half-life of ^{123}I is short; instruct patient to discontinue iodine-containing medication 1 week before scan; confirm that pregnancy has been ruled out; ensure that no other procedure using iodine as contrast medium has been done during 4 preceding weeks; administer iodine by mouth.

IV. Nursing considerations with selected therapies and techniques

See text pages

A. Thyroid surgery
   1. Purpose: to treat hyperthyroidism (subtotal thyroidectomy) or malignancy (total thyroidectomy)
   2. Nursing management
     a) Before surgery, show patient how to support head when sitting up.
     b) After surgery, place patient in semi-Fowler's position with pillows under head, neck, and shoulders.
     c) Observe patient for postoperative respiratory obstruction; monitor receipt of humidified oxygen, if ordered.
     d) Inspect dressing and sides and back of neck for bleeding or excessive drainage.
     e) Ask patient to speak every 2–4 hours to detect possible laryngeal nerve injury.
     f) Notify physician if patient experiences tetany, fever, rapid pulse, cardiac dysrhythmia, vomiting, restlessness, or delirium.
     g) If patient has undergone complete thyroidectomy, be particularly attentive to signs of parathyroid damage, which manifests as tetany (hyperirritability of nerves, hand and foot spasms, and muscular twitching); explain use of postsurgical ^{131}I ablation if purpose of surgery was removal of radiosensitive malignancy; discuss thyroid hormone administration regimen.

B. Adrenalectomy
   1. Purpose: to remove pheochromocytoma, to treat Cushing's syndrome, or to control recurrent carcinoma of the prostate or breast

2. Nursing management
   a) Observe patient for signs of acute adrenal crisis, including hemorrhage, atelectasis, and pneumothorax (see Nurse Alert, "Acute Adrenal Crisis").
   b) Inspect incision during dressing changes, and report redness, swelling, or purulent drainage.
   c) Encourage deep breathing, coughing, and leg exercises; provide firm support when patient turns.
   d) In patient who has had bilateral adrenalectomy, administer adrenocortical hormones to compensate for sudden reduction in level of natural hormones.

V. Selected disorders

A. Pituitary gland dysfunction
   1. Definition: Over- or undersecretion of pituitary gland hormones
   2. Pathophysiology and etiology
      a) Pathophysiology
         (1) Oversecretion (hyperpituitarism): usually involves growth hormone or adrenocorticotropic hormone (ACTH, causing Cushing's disease)
         (2) Undersecretion (panhypopituitarism): involves all anterior pituitary hormones, causing thyroid, adrenal cortex, and gonads to atrophy
         (3) Posterior lobe dysfunction: deficiency of antidiuretic hormone (ADH), leading to diabetes insipidus
      b) Etiology: oversecretion caused by hormone-secreting adenomas or hypothalamic dysfunction; undersecretion caused by pituitary tumors, radiation, infections, trauma, or infiltrative processes; posterior lobe dysfunction caused by head trauma, brain tumor, or pituitary gland irradiation

See text pages
_____

! NURSE *ALERT* !

Acute Adrenal Crisis

Acute adrenal crisis may occur in patients who have undergone adrenal surgery or who have suddenly stopped taking corticosteroids. A physician must be notified immediately if any of the following symptoms appear:
- Nausea, vomiting, diarrhea, abdominal pain
- Anorexia
- Headache
- Hypotension
- Restlessness
- Fever

Without proper treatment, including administration of corticosteroids and antibiotics, patient will progress to adrenal shock and death.

3. Symptoms
   a) Hyperpituitarism (gigantism when occurring before puberty, acromegaly when occurring after puberty): large features; large lower jaw; thick lips; bulging forehead; bulbous nose; large hands and feet; partial blindness; enlarged heart, liver, and spleen; muscle weakness; painful joints; impotency in males; amenorrhea, increased facial hair, and deep voice in females; excessive height (with gigantism)
   b) Panhypopituitarism: atrophied gonads and genitalia, hypothyroidism, Addison's disease, premature aging
   c) Diabetes insipidus: copious dilute urine, constant thirst, weakness, anorexia, weight loss
4. Diagnostic evaluation: skull radiography, MRI, or CT scan for hyperpituitarism; lab tests (of thyroid, sex hormones, and corticosteroid) for panhypopituitarism; fluid deprivation test for diabetes insipidus
5. Medical treatment: surgical removal of pituitary gland or destruction of pituitary gland by radiation for hyperpituitarism; substitute hormones of glands usually stimulated by pituitary for panhypopituitarism; vasopressin for diabetes insipidus
6. Complications: blindness, coma
7. Essential nursing care for patients with pituitary gland dysfunction
   a) Nursing assessment: Obtain patient history, including information on symptoms and drugs taken; perform physical exam; note general appearance.
   b) Nursing diagnoses
      (1) Body image disturbance related to hyperpituitarism
      (2) Pain related to musculoskeletal changes
      (3) Altered nutrition, less than body requirements, related to anorexia
      (4) Sexual dysfunction related to sex hormone loss
   c) Nursing intervention
      (1) Explain which changes in appearance can be controlled with treatment; suggest counseling when appropriate.
      (2) Administer mild analgesic as ordered.
      (3) Weigh patient weekly; recommend eating 4–6 meals per day.
      (4) Refer patient with sexual dysfunction to appropriate resource personnel.
      (5) For patient who has had hypophysectomy (removal of the pituitary gland) through the transsphenoidal approach, assess visual acuity at regular intervals; monitor urine specific gravity to check for diabetes insipidus; administer prescribed antibiotics, analgesics, corticosteroids, and agents to control diabetes insipidus; raise head of bed to decrease pressure on sella turcica and to promote normal drainage; caution patient

against engaging in activities that raise intracranial pressure (ICP), including bending over or straining during elimination; provide oral care at least every 4 hours; use humidifier to keep mucous membranes moist.

    d) Nursing evaluation

        (1) Patient reports improved body image.

        (2) Patient states that pain has been relieved.

        (3) Patient eats nutritious diet, and weight remains stable.

        (4) Patient reports satisfactory sexual performance.

B. Thyroid gland dysfunction

  1. Definition: excessive or insufficient thyroid hormone secretion; benign or malignant tumor

  2. Pathophysiology and etiology

    a) Pathophysiology

        (1) Hyperthyroidism: metabolic rate increase

        (2) Hypothyroidism: metabolic rate decrease originating within thyroid (primary hypothyroidism) or pituitary (secondary hypothyroidism)

        (3) Thyroid tumors: commonly occur as follicular adenoma (benign) or papillary carcinoma (malignant)

    b) Etiology: hyperthyroidism caused by circulating immunoglobulins, related to shock or stress; hypothyroidism caused by autoimmune thyroiditis; thyroid tumors caused by previous radiation therapy for childhood disorders, including tonsil enlargement and acne

  3. Symptoms

    a) Hyperthyroidism: restlessness, excitability, agitation, tremors, diarrhea, bulging eyes, neck swelling, tachycardia, hypertension, warm moist skin, irregular menses, heat intolerance, fever, weight loss

    b) Hypothyroidism: anorexia, bradycardia, hypotension, lethargy, fatigue, thick hard nails, coarse hair, heavy menses, fertility problems, low sperm count

    c) Thyroid tumors: neck swelling

  4. Diagnostic evaluation

    a) Hyper- and hypothyroidism: history, symptoms, physical exam, protein-bound iodine (PBI) analysis, thyroid function tests, ultrasonography, thyroid scanning, radioactive iodine uptake (RAIU) test

    b) Thyroid tumors: lesion biopsy, RAIU test

  5. Medical treatment

    a) Hyperthyroidism: medication, including propylthiouracil and thimazole; radioactive iodine; subtotal thyroidectomy

    b) Hypothyroidism: replacement thyroid hormones

    c) Thyroid tumors: thyroidectomy, neck dissection, hormone replacement therapy

  6. Complications: myocardial infarction in response to therapy in extreme hypothyroidism; relapse or permanent hypothyroidism, thyroid storm in hyperthyroidism

7. Essential nursing care for patients with thyroid gland dysfunction
   a) Nursing assessment: Obtain complete patient history; check vital signs, weight, and overt symptoms; palpate thyroid, manipulating it gently to reduce risk of stimulating sudden release of thyroid hormones.
   b) Nursing diagnoses
      (1) Altered nutrition, less than body requirements, related to hypermetabolic state
      (2) Altered nutrition, more than body requirements, related to hypometabolic state
      (3) Activity intolerance related to thyroid hormone hyposecretion
      (4) Ineffective individual coping related to emotional instability
   c) Nursing intervention
      (1) Provide 4–6 high-calorie meals per day for patient with hyperthyroidism.
      (2) Provide low-calorie diet for patient with hypothyroidism.
      (3) Assist with activities of daily living; urge patient to alternate between tasks and rest periods.
      (4) Reassure patient with hyperthyroidism that emotional symptoms will subside as disorder is controlled; minimize stressful experiences for hospitalized patients; be conscious of decreased attention span when providing information about therapeutic regimen; reassure patient that most changes in appearance will disappear after treatment.
   d) Nursing evaluation
      (1) Patient eats well-balanced diet and maintains stable weight.
      (2) Patient conserves energy through advance planning of daily tasks.
      (3) Patient states understanding of the effects of the disorder on emotions and interpersonal relationships.

C. Parathyroid dysfunction
   1. Definition: overproduction or underproduction of parathyroid hormone
   2. Pathophysiology and etiology
      a) Pathophysiology: increased urinary excretion of phosphorus and loss of calcium from bones, which become demineralized, in hyperparathyroidism; decreased level of calcium and increased level of phosphorus in blood with hypoparathyroidism
      b) Etiology
         (1) Hyperparathyroidism: benign adenoma in 1 parathyroid gland, hyperplasia of all 4 glands, heredity, radiation therapy to neck
         (2) Hypoparathyroidism: trauma, surgical removal of parathyroid gland during thyroidectomy

3. Symptoms
   a) Hyperparathyroidism: kidney stones, renal disease, muscle weakness, fatigue, apathy, nausea or vomiting, constipation, cardiac dysrhythmia, excess blood level of calcium
   b) Hypoparathyroidism: tetany, numbness, tingling, muscle cramping, cyanosis, convulsions
4. Diagnostic evaluation
   a) Hyperparathyroidism: elevated serum calcium level, low serum phosphorus and parathyroid hormone levels, skeletal radiograph to show bone demineralization or bone tumors (in advanced cases)
   b) Hypoparathyroidism: low level of serum calcium, elevated serum phosphorus level, tetany
5. Medical treatment: surgical removal of hypertrophied gland for hyperparathyroidism; administration of IV calcium gluconate and mechanical ventilation for hypoparathyroidism
6. Complication: hypercalcemic crisis in hyperparathyroidism
7. Nursing management for patients with parathyroid dysfunction
   a) Nursing assessment
      (1) Inquire about family history of bone disease, kidney stones, ulcer disease, or endocrine disorders and use of thiazide diuretics or vitamin D.
      (2) Check for waxy skin pallor and bone deformities of back and extremities.
      (3) Check and monitor for signs and symptoms of tetany by eliciting positive Trousseau's sign or Chvostek's sign.
         (a) Positive Trousseau's sign: induction of carpopedal spasm by occluding blood flow to arm for 3 minutes with blood pressure cuff
         (b) Positive Chvostek's sign: induction of twitching of the mouth, eye, and nose by tapping over facial nerve immediately in front of parotid gland
   b) Nursing diagnoses
      (1) High risk for injury related to osteoporosis
      (2) Altered urinary elimination related to renal calculi formation
   c) Nursing intervention
      (1) Encourage patient with hyperparathyroidism to increase fluid intake, especially of cranberry juice (which can lower urinary pH), prior to surgical removal of abnormal parathyroid tissue; observe for symptoms of renal calculi.
      (2) Limit foods high in calcium and phosphorus in patient with hyperparathyroidism.
      (3) Provide high-calcium, low-phosphorus diet and oral calcium salt tablets for patient with hypoparathyroidism; administer aluminum hydroxide gel or aluminum carbonate after meals.
      (4) Minimize tetany in patient with hypoparathyroidism by keeping him or her in quiet, draft-free, dim room.
   d) Nursing evaluation
      (1) Patient avoids activities that may cause skeletal injury.

(2) Patient consumes adequate amount of fluids, normally the equivalent of 8–10 glasses per day.

D. Adrenal gland dysfunction
   1. Definition: deficiency (Addison's disease) or excess (Cushing's syndrome) of corticosteroid hormones normally produced by adrenal cortex; usually benign tumor of adrenal cortex (pheochromocytoma)
   2. Pathophysiology and etiology
      a) Pathophysiology
         (1) Addison's disease (primary adrenal cortical insufficiency): defects associated with loss of mineralocorticoid and glucocorticoid action
         (2) Cushing's syndrome (adrenal cortical hyperfunction): loss of normal diurnal rhythms; alterations of nitrogen, carbohydrate, and mineral metabolism
         (3) Pheochromocytoma: production of excess catecholamines

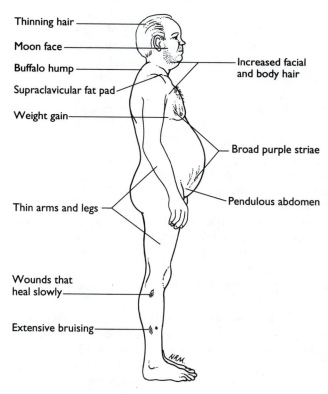

Figure 14–1
Features of Cushing's Syndrome

b) Etiology
    (1) Addison's disease: bilateral adrenalectomy, infection, hypopituitarism, steroids
    (2) Cushing's syndrome: pituitary or adrenal adenoma, lung or GI tract tumor, therapeutic use of glucocorticoids or ACTH
    (3) Pheochromocytoma: unknown; inherited disorders such as neurofibromatosis

3. Symptoms
  a) Addison's disease: increased excretion of sodium, phosphorus retention, weakness, fatigue, hypotension, hypothermia, dizziness, weight loss, anorexia, nervousness, depression, hypoglycemia, dark pigmentation
  b) Cushing's syndrome: wasted muscles, weakness, diabetes mellitus, moon face, buffalo hump, thin skin, ruddy face, infections, bruising, backache, sodium and water retention, edema, hypertension, psychosis, hirsutism, amenorrhea
  c) Pheochromocytoma: hypertension, tremor, nervousness, sweating, headache, nausea and vomiting, hyperglycemia, polyuria

4. Diagnostic evaluation
  a) Addison's disease: notation of symptoms, adrenal function test, analysis of serum sodium and potassium levels, glucose tolerance test
  b) Cushing's syndrome: observation of physical changes; urinalysis; sodium, potassium, and glucose level determination; abdominal radiography; CT; MRI; IV pyelography
  c) Pheochromocytoma: urinalysis, CT, MRI, ultrasonography, aortography, retrograde pyelography

5. Medical treatment
  a) Addison's disease: corticosteroids (secondary disease), hormone replacement
  b) Cushing's syndrome: radiation therapy and pituitary tumor removal for adrenal hyperplasia; slow withdrawal of corticosteroids for drug-induced disease
  c) Pheochromocytoma: surgical removal of tumor

6. Complication: acute adrenal crisis

7. Essential nursing care for patients with adrenal gland dysfunction
  a) Nursing assessment: Obtain history; check vital signs; evaluate patient for activity tolerance and electrolyte imbalance.
  b) Nursing diagnoses
    (1) Activity intolerance related to fatigue
    (2) Altered nutrition, less than body requirements, related to nausea or anorexia
    (3) High risk for infection related to altered inflammatory response
  c) Nursing intervention
    (1) Encourage rest periods between activities.
    (2) Weigh patient with Addison's disease daily; encourage well-balanced meals; watch for signs of hypoglycemia.
    (3) Urge patient with Cushing's syndrome to avoid injury; be alert for signs of infection.

    d) Nursing evaluation
       (1) Patient performs all activities of daily living.
       (2) Patient with Addison's disease eats prescribed diet.
       (3) Patient with Cushing's syndrome sustains no injuries and develops no infection.

E. Diabetes mellitus
  1. Definition: metabolic disorder of the pancreas in which insulin insufficiency causes glucose intolerance
  2. Pathophysiology and etiology
    a) Pathophysiology: type I, insulin-dependent diabetes mellitus (IDDM), associated with deficient insulin production, disruption of glycolytic pathway, and malfunction of insulin receptor sites; type II, non-insulin-dependent diabetes mellitus (NIDDM), associated with defective binding of insulin to proper cell membrane receptor
    b) Etiology: type I, autoimmune destruction of beta cells; type II, obesity and decreased exercise
  3. Symptoms: increased hunger, weight loss, excess thirst and urination, fatigue, weakness
  4. Diagnostic evaluation: glucose tolerance test, urinalysis, blood glucose tests
  5. Medical treatment: insulin injections for IDDM; oral hypoglycemic drugs for NIDDM; weight control; diet; exercise
  6. Complications: hyperglycemia and hypoglycemia (acute); coronary artery disease leading to myocardial infarction; cerebrovascular disease leading to stroke; peripheral vascular disease leading to chronic dermal ulcers; retinopathy; nephropathy; sensorimotor neuropathy of extremities; autonomic neuropathy of GI, cardiovascular, or genitourinary system
  7. Essential nursing care for patients with diabetes mellitus
    a) Nursing assessment: Obtain full history, including information on ongoing treatment for known diabetes, and assess peripheral pulse, skin changes at injection sites (especially when patient receives pork or beef insulin rather than human insulin), temperature of extremities, sensation loss, visual acuity, muscle atrophy, and weakness.
    b) Nursing diagnoses
       (1) Knowledge deficit about self-care skills
       (2) Anxiety related to fear of diabetic complications
       (3) Altered nutrition, more than body requirements, related to failure to follow diet and exercise plan
       (4) Impaired skin integrity related to decreased tissue perfusion or infection
       (5) Potential for injury related to circulatory problems

c) Nursing intervention
  (1) Encourage patient to follow practices that promote health and prevent injury, such as adhering to prescribed diet, getting sufficient exercise, taking scrupulous care of the feet, inspecting skin daily, checking temperature of bath water before use, and applying heating devices carefully.
  (2) Teach patient to use an appropriate method for self-monitoring of blood glucose (SMBG).
  (3) Teach patient about the type(s) of insulin prescribed for his/her diabetes (i.e., time course, concentration, and species); teach patient to inject self-injectable insulin; when appropriate, teach patient complex insulin regimen that will achieve maximum control of blood glucose level.
  (4) Do the following for hypoglycemia (insulin reaction).
    (a) Teach patient and family about causes, symptoms, and prevention of hypoglycemia; instruct patient to consume 10–15 g of a fast-acting sugar, followed by a snack, if hypoglycemia occurs.
    (b) Administer subcutaneous or intramuscular injection of 1 mg of glucagon to patient who is unconscious or unable to swallow; administer simple sugar, followed by snack, when patient regains consciousness.
    (c) Treat severe hypoglycemia in a hospitalized patient by IV administration of 50% dextrose in water (D-50).
  (5) Do the following for diabetic ketoacidosis (DKA or hyperglycemia).
    (a) Teach patient and family about causes, symptoms, and prevention of DKA.
    (b) Maintain tissue perfusion in patient with DKA by administering 0.9% normal saline at very high rate for 2–3 hours; continue rehydration with 0.45% normal saline at moderate to high rates for several hours; monitor vital signs, respiratory status, and intake and output frequently.
    (c) Replenish lost potassium in patient with DKA by infusion of up to 40 mEq per hour of potassium with IV fluids; monitor potassium levels every 2–4 hours to ensure that hyperkalemia is not present.
    (d) Treat acidosis in patient with DKA with IV infusion of insulin at a slow, continuous rate, such as 5 units per hour; measure blood glucose values hourly; add dextrose to IV fluids when levels reach 250–300 mg/dl.
d) Nursing evaluation
  (1) Patient demonstrates self-care skills.
  (2) Patient states understanding of common diabetic complications and their management.
  (3) Patient eats prescribed diet.
  (4) Patient maintains intact skin.
  (5) Patient avoids injury.

1. Irma Johns, 56 years old, reports that she has felt fatigued and slow for the past month. She has gained 7 lb in 3 weeks despite a report of not eating. Which question would the nurse consider asking the patient next?

   a. "Are you losing clumps of hair when you brush your hair?"

   b. "Do you frequently feel cold when other people in the same room are comfortable?"

   c. "Have you experienced any tremors of your arms or hands?"

   d. "Have you noticed any visual blurring or dizzy spells?"

2. The nurse would most likely observe Irma's skin to be:

   a. Dry and thick.

   b. Bruised and red.

   c. Velvety and smooth.

   d. Shiny and edematous.

3. Marie Barnes is scheduled to undergo thyroidectomy tomorrow. While preparing the patient for surgery, the nurse should:

   a. Caution Ms. Barnes not to try to speak until the day after surgery to prevent damage to the recurrent laryngeal nerve.

   b. Urge Ms. Barnes to cough at least every 2 hours to mobilize respiratory secretions.

   c. Advise Ms. Barnes that she will need to lie flat in bed for 1 day after surgery to prevent hemorrhage and damage to the muscles of her neck or her surgical incision.

   d. Teach the patient to assume a sitting position by supporting the back of her head with her arms and hands.

4. Bertha Kastner has been admitted for the treatment of severe hyperthyroidism. To increase her comfort, it would be appropriate to:

   a. Make sure her room remains at 68°–72°F.

   b. Change her gown and bedding frequently.

   c. Offer warm liquids, such as tea, cocoa, and broth.

   d. Locate her as close to the nursing station as possible so that the nurse can offer reassurance frequently.

5. Marge White underwent thyroidectomy 12 hours ago. Which finding by the nurse would be the greatest cause for concern?

   a. Small amount of blood at the back of Ms. White's neck

   b. Hoarseness

   c. Tingling and numbness of the patient's extremities

   d. Shoulder pain

6. A patient asks the nurse how the doctor can tell if she has been cheating on her diabetic diet. Which response gives the patient the most accurate information?

   a. "Glucose binds to hemoglobin to form a product that reflects what blood sugar levels have been over the past 2–3 months."

   b. "Glucose is excreted in the urine in amounts that reflect the level of hyperglycemia over the past 2 months."

   c. "Hemoglobin binds to red blood cells (RBCs) when blood glucose level is high. A diabetic control index (glycosylated hemoglobin or Hgb A_{1c}) measures the rate of binding over 3–4 months. The result indicates your dietary compliance."

   d. "An insulin-to-blood-glucose ratio can be measured from a sample of blood. A low insulin-to-glucose value indicates hyperglycemia of 2 or more months' duration."

7. James Kraska, who is 64 years old, reports that he is constantly thirsty and needs to urinate repeatedly. He says that his frequent trips to the bathroom embarrass him at work and keep him from getting a good night's sleep. He also comments that although he

had never had a problem previously maintaining his desired weight, he now has little appetite and has lost 11 lb. Given this information, which question by the nurse would be most appropriate?

a. "How much fluid would you estimate that you drink every day?"
b. "Is there a history of diabetes mellitus in your family?"
c. "What does your urine look like?"
d. "Have you ever had a problem with your prostate gland?"

8. David Altman, who has type I diabetes mellitus, is experiencing nausea and vomiting. Which action indicates that he understands the "sick day rules" for diabetes management?

a. Taking $2/3$ of his normal insulin dose
b. Abandoning his normal meal timing in favor of getting an extended period of sleep
c. Drinking nondietetic ginger ale
d. Monitoring his blood glucose every 6 hours

9. Marina Stockman, who is 26 years old, has just been diagnosed with type I diabetes mellitus in a case of Maturity Onset Diabetes of the Young (MODY). She tells the nurse, "I make my living as an artist, and I'm terrified that I'll lose my sight." The nurse's best response would be:

a. "Although most diabetic patients will eventually develop some retinopathy, serious visual problems can usually be avoided if you follow your treatment program carefully."
b. "Even if you were to experience a severe hemorrhage, a vitrectomy would restore your sight."
c. "Because there is a good chance that you will eventually lose much of your sight, you may want to think about an alternate career. Would you like me to refer you to a career counselor?"
d. "Laser photocoagulation therapy has become so sophisticated that you needn't worry about losing your vision."

10. Augusta Rodriguez has recently been diagnosed with adrenal hypofunction. In teaching her about the management of her condition, the nurse would be likely to tell her to:

a. Avoid putting salt on food or eating prepared foods that contain salt.
b. Take the prescribed fludrocortisone (Florinef) for no more than 3 months, since serious side effects may result from extended use.
c. Take dietary precautions to guard against the anemia that may result from the abnormally heavy menstrual flow associated with the disorder.
d. Avoid stressors, including cold, elective surgery, and extreme exertion.

11. Alice Potter, who is 56 years old, reports that she is chronically tired, bruises easily, and has developed 2 serious infections as a result of minor cuts from kitchen knives. During the course of Ms. Potter's physical assessment, the nurse notes the presence of supraclavicular fat pads and reddish-purple striae on her abdomen and thighs. On the basis of these data, which diagnostic test(s) would be most appropriate for Ms. Potter?

a. Fluid deprivation test
b. Urine testing to measure levels of free cortisol and adrenal metabolites of cortisol and androgens
c. Hormone assays for tri-iodothyronine, thyroxine, testosterone, and estradiol
d. Serum parathyroid hormone (PTH), calcium, and phosphorus level measurements and urinary cyclic adenosine monophosphate (cAMP) evaluations

ANSWERS

1. **Correct answer is b.** The data presented about Ms. Johns could indicate a physical or a psychologic problem. In performing an assessment, the nurse completes a review of systems that considers physical problems

first. Asking questions in the physical realm allows time for the nurse to establish a rapport with the patient and some degree of trust before moving into the more sensitive area of psychologic questioning. Hypothyroidism has the common presentation of fatigue, slowness, and weight gain. Intolerance to cold is characteristic of hypothyroidism.

a and **c.** Loss of hair in clumps and tremors are characteristic of hyperthyroidism.
d. Visual blurring and dizzy spells are not related to thyroid dysfunction.

2. **Correct answer is a.** The skin is dry, dull, coarse (thick), and pale in hypothyroidism. It is easily bruised.

b and **d.** Skin that is bruised and red or shiny and edematous is not associated with thyroid dysfunction.
c. Velvety smooth skin is observed in hyperthyroidism.

3. **Correct answer is d.** The nurse teaches Ms. Barnes to assume a sitting position by supporting the back of her head with her arms and linked hands. This technique protects the surgical incision and neck muscles and reduces the risk of hemorrhage.

a. As part of the postsurgical assessment, the patient will be asked to say a few words to make sure that the recurrent laryngeal nerve, which is responsible for speech, has not been damaged. The voice will be assessed for pitch, tone, and the presence of hoarseness. Talking during the immediate postsurgical period should ideally be kept to a minimum.
b. Ms. Barnes should refrain from coughing during the immediate postsurgical period, because doing so could damage her incision and possibly lead to hemorrhage.
c. Although the patient can sit up after surgery, the nurse must teach her to support her head with her hands while assuming a sitting position. The patient should also be encouraged to deep breathe and do leg exercises.

4. **Correct answer is b.** Because some patients with severe hyperthyroidism experience marked diaphoresis, it may be necessary to change their clothing and bedding frequently.

a. A room that is maintained at 68°–72°F may be too warm for a patient with hyperthyroidism.
c. Although offering warm liquids would serve as a comfort measure for a patient with hypothyroidism, the patient with hyperthyroidism should be offered cool drinks.
d. Although it is true that a patient with hyperthyroidism may be anxious and in need of frequent reassurance, a location near the nursing station would probably be too noisy for her. A quiet environment is important to reduce the anxiety associated with hyperthyroidism.

5. **Correct answer is c.** Tingling of the extremities, numbness, and muscle cramps are signs of tetany, a postoperative complication of thyroidectomy that is caused by a low concentration of calcium following accidental injury to or removal of the parathyroid glands. Because tetany can cause laryngospasm, intravenous administration of calcium must be begun immediately.

a. After thyroidectomy, it is common for a small amount of blood to ooze to the back of the patient's neck. The nurse should check the front and back of the neck dressing frequently and notify the physician immediately if severe bleeding occurs.
b. Moderate hoarseness usually occurs after thyroidectomy. Severe hoarseness or other changes in the patient's voice, which may indicate that the recurrent laryngeal nerve has been damaged during surgery, should be reported to the physician.
d. The patient typically experiences shoulder and neck pain after thyroidectomy. Administering analgesic, keeping the patient in a semi-Fowler's position, having the patient shrug the shoulders, and placing pillows under the patient's head, neck, and shoulders can relieve this pain.

6. **Correct answer is a.** Glycosylated hemoglobin (Hgb A_{1C}) analysis is the test used to measure blood glucose concentration over time. The red blood cell combines with glucose to form glycohemoglobin. The amount of glycosylated hemoglobin that is produced is in direct proportion to the degree of hyperglycemia. Normal levels range from 4.0%–7.0%.

b, c, and **d.** Decreased TSH, increased Hgb AC, and decreased T4 levels would not indicate whether the patient is following her diabetic diet.

7. **Correct answer is c.** Intense thirst, constant urination, anorexia, and weight loss are signs of diabetes insipidus. In this disorder, which is caused by reduced antidiuretic hormone (ADH) secretion, the patient may produce up to 20 L of extremely pale, dilute, clear urine each day. Although urinary frequency and nocturia are signs of many disorders, including cystitis and benign prostatic hypertrophy (BPH), the amount, color, and clarity of the urine produced by a patient with diabetes insipidus are distinctive.

a. Determining how much fluid Mr. Kraska actually drinks every day would be a useful part of the assessment process, but establishing the color and clarity of his urine is more important.
b. The patient's complaint about thirst might be suggestive of diabetes mellitus, but the marked urinary frequency that he is experiencing suggests a different problem. In addition, although Mr. Kraska's age puts him at some risk for type II diabetes mellitus, the fact that he has no history of obesity offsets that risk factor to some degree.
d. Although urinary frequency and nocturia may signal prostate disorders, such as BPH, the patient's constant thirst suggests the presence of another disorder.

8. **Correct answer is c.** While he is experiencing vomiting, Mr. Altman should consume small, frequent portions of carbohydrates, including juices and regular (nondietetic) sodas.

a. Mr. Altman should take his normal insulin dose unless his physician has previously prescribed a "sick day" dose for him.
b. Although Mr. Altman should try to get extra rest, he should also follow his normal meal plan. If he cannot follow this routine because of stomach upset, he should eat small portions of soft foods (such as regular gelatin or custard) 6–8 times a day. If vomiting or diarrhea persists, he should take liquids every 30 minutes–1 hour and contact his physician.
d. Mr. Altman should monitor his blood glucose and urine ketone levels every 3–4 hours, not every 6 hours.

9. **Correct answer is a.** Although up to 90% of patients with diabetes develop some degree of retinopathy within 5–15 years of diagnosis, few will experience visual impairment as a result of these changes. In most cases, careful control of blood glucose levels can prevent serious loss of vision.

b. In vitrectomy, vitreous fluid that is mixed with blood is removed and is replaced with saline or another liquid. Although this procedure usually restores some degree of useful vision, near-normal vision is rarely attained.
c. Although patients with type I diabetes mellitus may experience impaired vision or vision loss as a result of retinopathy, cataracts, and lens changes, good management of blood glucose levels can usually prevent serious visual impairment. Thus, this response is excessively pessimistic.
d. Although laser photocoagulation therapy has been shown to reduce the rate of progression to blindness in patients with diabetic retinopathy, it does not repair damage that has already occurred, and its overall effectiveness is still under investigation. The best means of preserving vision in patients with type I diabetes is careful blood glucose management.

10. **Correct answer is d.** Patients with adrenal hypofunction may develop acute adrenal crisis, a life-threatening condition, when they are subject to stress.

a. In patients with adrenal hypofunction, salt deprivation can trigger acute adrenal crisis. Most patients with this condition crave salt.

b. Although corticosteroids may have serious adverse effects, patients with adrenal hypofunction must take corticosteroid medication for the rest of their lives. Patients should be cautioned not to skip doses of their medication, since acute adrenal crisis may result.

c. Adrenal hypofunction is usually associated with scanty, not heavy, menstrual flow.

11. **Correct answer is b.** Ms. Potter's medical history and assessment suggest that she may have Cushing's syndrome (hypercortisolism). The definitive diagnostic test for this disorder measures the levels of free cortisol and the adrenal metabolites of cortisol and androgens (17-hydroxycorticosteroids and 17-ketosteroids).

a. The fluid deprivation test is especially useful in establishing a diagnosis of diabetes insipidus.

c. Hormone assays for tri-iodothyronine and thyroxine (secreted by the thyroid) and for testosterone and estradiol (secreted by the gonads) are usually conducted when hypopituitarism is suspected.

d. Serum PTH, calcium, and phosphorus measurements and urinary cyclic adenosine monophosphate (cAMP) evaluations are usually undertaken when hyperparathyroidism is suspected.

15

Reproductive and Sexual Function

OVERVIEW

I. Structure and function of reproductive system
A. Female reproductive system
B. Male reproductive system

II. General diagnostic tests
A. Breast examinations
B. Pap smears
C. Endoscopic examinations
D. Testicular examination
E. Needle biopsy of prostate

III. General nursing assessments
A. Patient history
B. Observation and physical examination
C. Diagnostic tests

IV. Nursing considerations with selected therapies and techniques
A. Uterectomy
B. Mastectomy
C. Reconstructive breast surgery
D. Vulvectomy
E. Prostatectomy
F. Testicular surgery

V. Selected disorders
A. Benign tumor
B. Cancer
C. Disorders of menstruation
D. Endometriosis
E. Vaginal disorders

NURSING HIGHLIGHTS

1. An important role for the nurse is to provide information on healthy reproductive alternatives, practices, and behaviors for patients and to be conscious of cultural issues that relate to sexuality.
2. The nurse must exhibit an open nonjudgmental attitude if the patient is to feel comfortable discussing personal issues dealing with reproductive health.
3. Because patients with a reproductive system disorder are often anxious, distressed, and embarrassed due to the private nature of reproduction and sexuality, they require sensitive, empathetic nursing care.

GLOSSARY

Cullen's sign—blue discoloration of skin around umbilicus, a late sign of intraperitoneal hemorrhage

Homans' sign—discomfort behind knee after dorsiflexion of foot, due to thrombosis of calf veins

panhysterectomy—total abdominal uterectomy and bilateral salpingectomy, with abdominal removal of uterus, ovaries, and fallopian tubes

salpingectomy—removal of a fallopian tube

tubal ligation—procedure by which female is sterilized by occlusion of fallopian tubes to prevent passage of ovum

ENHANCED OUTLINE

See text pages
_____

I. Structure and function of reproductive system

A. Female reproductive system
  1. External structures (mons pubis, labia majora and minora, clitoris, and perineum): tissues that protect underlying structures and provide sexual arousal and excitement
  2. Internal structures
     a) Vagina: canal that receives penis during intercourse, acts as channel for menstrual flow, and serves as passageway for fetus during delivery
     b) Uterus: hollow muscular organ in which fertilized ovum becomes embedded and fetus is nourished
     c) Fallopian tubes: pair of slender tubes that connect uterus to site near ovaries and provide duct between ovaries and uterus for transport of ova and sperm; usual site for fertilization of ovum
     d) Ovaries: almond-shaped organs that develop and release ova and produce sex hormones (estrogen, progesterone, androgens, and relaxin) necessary for normal female growth

B. Male reproductive system
  1. External structures
     a) Penis: organ used for intercourse and urination
     b) Scrotum: thin sac suspended below pubic bone behind penis; protects testes, epididymides, and vasa deferentia in cooler atmosphere than that provided within body
  2. Internal structures
     a) Testes: suspended in scrotum by spermatic cord, which also covers epididymis and part of vas deferens; produce sperm and testosterone

b) Epididymis: part of duct that transports sperm from testes to urethra
c) Vas deferens: 1 of 2 tubes that continue from each epididymis, merging with seminal vesicle duct to form ejaculatory duct at base of prostate gland
d) Seminal vesicles: paired glands located behind bladder that secrete most of penile ejaculate; duct from seminal vesicles joins vas deferens, forming ejaculatory duct
e) Prostate gland: large gland behind bladder that secretes part of seminal fluid

II. General diagnostic tests

See text pages
_____

A. Breast examinations
1. Professional examination: detects breast disease by means of taking breast history, making visual exam, and palpating each breast
2. Breast thermography: detects breast cancer, abscess, or fibrocystic breast disease with the use of infrared film and camera to photograph breasts and detect hot spots
3. Xeroradiography: detects abnormal breast lesions with the use of pictures produced by photoelectric process
4. Breast biopsy
   a) Incisional biopsy: surgery to remove 1 or more sections of tissue, which are examined microscopically while patient remains anesthetized
   b) Excisional biopsy: removal of entire lesion for examination, with patient discharged before results are determined
   c) Aspiration biopsy: outpatient procedure that uses needle and syringe to obtain sample of suspicious tissue with patient under local anesthesia

B. Pap smears: detect precancerous and cancerous conditions by examination of cervical cells obtained by scraping or aspiration

C. Endoscopic examinations
   a) Culdoscopy: diagnoses ectopic pregnancy and pelvic masses by insertion of culdoscope through incision in vaginal cul-de-sac in order to view uterus, broad ligaments, and fallopian tubes
   b) Laparoscopy: used in ectopic pregnancy, tubal ligation, ovarian biopsy, pelvic tumors, and pelvic inflammatory disease; enables dilation and curettage and pelvic exam to be carried out with patient under general anesthesia
   c) Colposcopy: visualizes cervix and vagina by means of speculum inserted into vagina

D. Testicular examination: detects tumors by means of testicle palpation

E. Needle biopsy of prostate: diagnoses prostatic cancer by retrieval of cells for histologic study

See text pages
_____

III. General nursing assessments

A. Patient history: description of overall health; family history; drug and allergy history; information on symptoms; data on prior tests, treatment, and surgery related to reproductive system; for female patients, pregnancy and abortion history, age at onset and description of menses, and age at menopause, if applicable

B. Observation and physical examination
   1. Female: gynecologic (pelvic) exam, breast exam
   2. Male: examination of external genitalia, palpation of testes, rectal exam of prostate

C. Diagnostic tests: nursing responsibilities
   1. Breast examinations
      a) Professional examination: Take breast history, visually examine breasts for symmetry, size, and skin and nipple changes; palpate each breast.
      b) Mammography: Advise patient not to use creams, powders, or deodorant on breasts or underarms, since such preparations may contain aluminum; ascertain that patient is not pregnant.
      c) Xeroradiography: Advise patient not to use creams, powders, or deodorant on breasts or underarms, since such preparations may contain aluminum; ascertain that patient is not pregnant.
      d) Breast biopsy: Advise patient to control postoperative pain with analgesics; to assess site of incision for bleeding and edema; to wear supportive bra continuously for 1 week after procedure; to avoid cold temperatures; and to expect area around biopsy site to be numb for 2–3 months.
   2. Pap smears
      a) Advise patient not to douche, use vaginal medications or deodorants, or have sexual intercourse for 24 hours before test.
      b) Help patient assume lithotomy position, and encourage apprehensive patient to use relaxation techniques.
      c) Through vaginal speculum, use wooden spatula to take scraping of exfoliated cells from cervix, endocervix, and vaginal pool.
      d) Transfer specimens to glass slide, and apply fixative.
      e) Provide patient with perineal pad to protect clothing from cervical bleeding.
   3. Endoscopic examinations
      a) Culdoscopy: Help patient assume and maintain knee-chest position; caution her that she may experience severe shoulder pain upon first sitting up; advise her to refrain from sexual intercourse and douching for 2 weeks after procedure.

b) Laparoscopy: Caution patient to expect mild discomfort at incision site and referred shoulder pain; instruct patient to observe wound for signs of infection or hematoma and to shower rather than bathe until incision has healed.

c) Colposcopy: Caution patient not to douche or use other vaginal preparations before procedure; help her assume lithotomy position; after procedure, provide her with supplies to clean perineum and a perineal pad to absorb dye or discharge.

4. Testicular examination: Have patient stand or lie down; locate each testis, and examine it for shape, size, symmetry, tenderness, consistency, and presence of nodules.

5. Needle biopsy of prostate: Administer cleaning enema and prophylactic antibiotic before transrectal biopsy; report any signs of infection or septic shock; advise patient to take all prophylactic antibiotics.

IV. Nursing considerations with selected therapies and techniques

See text pages

A. Uterectomy (formerly hysterectomy)
1. Administer preoperative douches, enema, and antibiotics; shave area.
2. Follow the following procedures for patients who have had abdominal uterectomy.
   a) Perform standard follow-up care as for patients who have had abdominal surgery.
   b) Assess vaginal bleeding, and report flow greater than that needed to saturate 1 pad in 4 hours.
   c) Check abdominal incision for intactness; assess abdominal bleeding at incision site, and report anything greater than a small amount.
   d) Provide Foley catheter care for 24–48 hours.
   e) Provide analgesics or heating pad for pain.
3. Follow the following procedures for patients who have had vaginal uterectomy.
   a) Assess vaginal bleeding, and report flow greater than that needed to saturate 1 pad in 4 hours.
   b) Provide Foley or suprapubic catheter care.
   c) Provide perineal care, including use of sitz baths, heat lamps, or ice packs.
4. If catheter is not already in place, realize that catheterization may be necessary if patient has not voided 8 hours after surgery.
5. Test for Homans' sign, which detects the presence of thrombophlebitis in the lower extremities, every shift; promote peripheral circulation by encouraging leg exercises and applying antiembolic stockings.
6. Be aware that depression, perceived loss of femininity, and decreased libido may occur after uterectomy; give patient the opportunity to verbalize fears; provide emotional support; refer her to sources of counseling, if appropriate.
7. Provide patient education (see Client Teaching Checklist, "Home Care for the Uterectomy Patient").

B. Mastectomy
1. Monitor vital signs every 30–60 minutes after surgery; take blood pressure and pulse on side that did not undergo surgery.
2. Check dressing and drainage set-up (e.g., Hemovac, Jackson-Pratt) every 30 minutes for the first several hours, and note color, amount, consistency, and odor of drainage; maintain patency of tube and of self-contained suction.
3. Assist awakening patient as she discovers extent of surgery.
4. Prevent lymphedema by placing pillow under arm on affected side so that arm is elevated above breast level.
5. Ensure that analgesic is adequate to provide pain relief, and encourage deep breathing and movement.
6. Check hands for signs of circulation problems.
7. Report temperature >101°F or foul-smelling drainage, pockets of swelling, redness, or suture line breaks at operative site.
8. Be sensitive to patient's body image and self-concept; provide guidance, support, and education to patient and her family.
9. Discuss and demonstrate exercises that will secure complete range of shoulder motion after surgery.
10. Provide information for home self-care (see Client Teaching Checklist, "Home Care for the Mastectomy Patient").

✔ CLIENT TEACHING CHECKLIST ✔

Home Care for the Uterectomy Patient

Explain the following guidelines to patients who have undergone uterectomy.

✔ Avoid heavy lifting, vigorous activities, sexual intercourse, douching, and tampon use until physician permits.
✔ Avoid sitting in 1 position for long periods.
✔ Take prescribed medication, and report any adverse drug effects.
✔ Clean incision as directed.
✔ Drink abundant fluids to avoid constipation and straining at stool.
✔ Contact physician if you experience:
— Fever
— Redness, swelling, pain, or drainage at incision site
— Vaginal bleeding or foul-smelling vaginal discharge
— Pain in chest, abdomen, or legs
— Constipation

Home Care for the Mastectomy Patient

Explain the following guidelines to patients who have undergone mastectomy.

✔ Wash affected area with washcloth and soap.
✔ Do not apply ointments to incision unless they have been approved by physician.
✔ Be aware that incision may be painful for several months and that slight swelling of the arm should disappear as function returns.
✔ Perform prescribed exercises during radiation therapy and chemotherapy.
✔ Avoid injury, injections, blood work, excess heat, and sun exposure on the affected arm.
✔ Contact physician immediately if you have:
— Fever or chills
— Drainage from, or separation of, incision
— Increased redness around the incision
— Sudden fatigue or weight loss
— Anorexia
— Infected hand

C. Reconstructive breast surgery
   1. Provide information about surgery and outcomes before procedure, stressing that optimal appearance may not occur for 6 months.
   2. Position patient on nonoperative side; avoid pressure due to gowns, dressings, and sheets.
   3. Elevate head of bed 30° and flex knees to lessen tension on abdominal incision.
   4. Assess circulation; report mottling, low skin temperature, or drainage >50 ml per hour.
   5. Check incision and flap for signs of infection (redness, odor, or drainage) or poor perfusion (blanching or decreased capillary refill).

D. Vulvectomy
   1. Shave operative site, insert indwelling urethral catheter and IV line, and administer enema.
   2. Measure fluid intake and output after surgery; check catheter patency.
   3. Change patient's position frequently, bending the upper leg and supporting it with pillows; keep patient in semirecumbent position to relieve pressure on sutures.
   4. Inspect surgical site for signs of infection several times a day.
   5. Report fever >101°F, chills, chest pain, cough, or fluid output <500 ml per day.

E. Prostatectomy
   1. Follow these procedures for patients who have had transurethral resection of the prostate (TURP): Connect catheter to closed continuous bladder irrigation system, and label each drainage container; check

catheter for patency every 1–4 hours; observe drainage from catheter, being alert for presence of clots; provide appropriate level of analgesic for pain relief as ordered; monitor rate of continuous irrigation every hour; and be alert for presence of urethral stricture, as evidenced by dysuria, straining, or weak urinary stream.

2. Follow these procedures for patients who have had suprapubic prostatectomy: Take standard postsurgical precautions for abdominal surgery; check abdominal dressings every 2 hours; provide appropriate level of analgesic for pain relief as ordered; be attentive to signs of shock and hemorrhage; and provide scrupulous aseptic care to area around suprapubic tube.

3. Follow these procedures for patients who have had perineal prostatectomy: Provide appropriate level of analgesic for pain relief as ordered; avoid use of enemas, rectal thermometers, and rectal tubes; be aware that urinary leakage may occur around wound for several days after catheter is removed; use pads to absorb urinary drainage; be alert for signs and symptoms of infection; and provide foam rubber ring to decrease discomfort when sitting.

4. Administer smooth-muscle relaxant medication as ordered for bladder spasms; apply warm compresses or give sitz baths for symptomatic relief.

5. Encourage patients to discuss their fears regarding possible impotence or sexual dysfunction; provide emotional support to patient and family.

F. Testicular surgery (orchiectomy)
1. Insert IV line and indwelling urethral catheter; administer enema.
2. Check IV line for extravasation or infiltration of IV fluid; report any sudden change in pulse rate or blood pressure.
3. Check patient for signs and symptoms of shock.
4. Check incision for drainage and signs of infection.
5. Provide patient education on home care (see Client Teaching Checklist, "Home Care for the Orchiectomy Patient").

See text pages
_____

V. Selected disorders

A. Benign tumor (fibroid, uterine leiomyoma, benign prostatic hypertrophy [see section V,G of Chapter 16])
1. Definition: myoma growing in uterine wall
2. Pathophysiology and etiology
   a) Pathophysiology: develops initially from myometrium; may be intramural, submucosal, or subserosal
   b) Etiology: unknown, but may be stimulated by estrogen
3. Symptoms: excess menstrual bleeding, pressure in pelvic region, dysmenorrhea, anemia, malaise

Home Care for the Orchiectomy Patient

Explain the following guidelines to patients who have undergone orchiectomy.

✔ Drink plenty of fluids, and eat nourishing meals.
✔ Get enough rest.
✔ Avoid heavy lifting.
✔ Wash incision with warm soap and water.
✔ Follow medication regimen, and do not take nonprescription drugs unless approved by physician.
✔ Perform self-exam of remaining testicle every month.
✔ Contact physician if you experience:
— Redness, drainage, pain, or swelling at incision
— Fever or chills
— Adverse drug reactions
— Weight loss or anorexia

4. Diagnostic evaluation: notation of symptoms, pelvic exam, Pap smear
5. Medical treatment: observation if asymptomatic, with re-exam every 3–6 months and Pap smear every 6–12 months; dilation and curettage (D&C) if abnormal bleeding occurs; myomectomy to remove tumor but preserve uterus; uterectomy if severe symptoms occur
6. Complications: infertility, anemia, pulmonary embolism or thromboembolism following surgery, depression
7. Essential nursing care for patients with benign tumors
   a) Nursing assessment: Inquire about abnormal bleeding, feeling of pelvic pressure, and urinary frequency or retention; undertake abdominal, vaginal, and rectal examination.
   b) Nursing diagnoses
      (1) Anxiety related to uncertain diagnosis
      (2) Pain related to benign tumor
   c) Nursing intervention
      (1) Provide patient with detailed information about the methods used to diagnose and treat benign tumors.
      (2) Reassure patient, who may have exaggerated fears about effects of uterectomy.
      (3) Encourage participation of patient's spouse or sexual partner in preoperative teaching.
      (4) Assess patient after surgery for excessive bleeding from vagina or at incision site.
      (5) Minimize postoperative pain with prescribed analgesic and heating pad.
   d) Nursing evaluation
      (1) Patient states that anxiety is diminished.
      (2) Patient states that pain is relieved.

B. Cancer (ovarian, uterine, cervical, breast, prostate, testicular)
  1. Definition: malignant condition of the reproductive system
  2. Pathophysiology and etiology
    a) Ovarian
      (1) Pathophysiology: rapidly growing, fast-spreading epithelial tumor, usually a serous adenocarcinoma
      (2) Etiology: unknown; associated with family history of breast or ovarian cancer; personal history of breast, colon, or endometrial cancer; smoking, high-fat diet, alcohol, or use of talcum powder on perineal area
    b) Uterine (cancer of the endometrium)
      (1) Pathophysiology: endometrial tumor, usually an adenocarcinoma, of the fundus or corpus of the uterus
      (2) Etiology: associated with estrogen replacement therapy, obesity, nulliparity, late menopause (after age 52), Caucasian race, and diabetes
    c) Cervical
      (1) Pathophysiology: squamous cell carcinoma or, less frequently, adenocarcinoma that begins *in situ* and becomes invasive after 10–15 years
      (2) Etiology: associated with multiple sex partners, early pregnancies, early age at first intercourse, chronic infection, smoking, and exposure to diethylstilbestrol (DES) *in utero*
    d) Breast
      (1) Pathophysiology: Early breast tumors originate *in situ* and, if undetected, spread to chest wall, lymph nodes, lungs, liver, bone, and brain.
      (2) Etiology: associated with breast cancer in first-degree relatives; high-fat diet; early menses; nulliparity or first pregnancy after age 30; previous x-ray treatment; malignancies of uterus, ovary, or colon; obesity; alcohol use; atypical hyperplasia
    e) Prostate
      (1) Pathophysiology: development of tumor in outer zone of the prostate, usually in elderly men; spread by blood and lymphatics to pelvic lymph nodes and bone (especially pelvis and hips)
      (2) Etiology: associated with high dietary fat intake, cytomegalovirus, and herpes virus type 2
    f) Testicular
      (1) Pathophysiology: development of tumors from sperm-producing germ cells (germinal tumors) or other structures in the testes (nongerminal tumors)

(2) Etiology: unknown, but associated with cryptorchidism and history of trauma or infection

3. Symptoms
    a) Ovarian: irregular menses, increasing premenstrual tension, menorrhagia with breast tenderness, early menopause, abdominal discomfort, dyspepsia, pelvic pressure, urinary frequency, flatulence, fullness after light meal, increasing abdominal size
    b) Uterine: bleeding after menopause, menorrhagia before menopause, pain
    c) Cervical: bleeding, leukorrhea, pain, pressure on bladder or bowel, bloody and foul-smelling discharge, wasting
    d) Breast: palpated mass, bloody discharge from nipple, skin dimpling, retraction of nipple, difference in breast sizes
    e) Prostate: nodule in posterior lobe farthest from urethra, frequent urination, nocturia, dysuria, back pain, pain down leg
    f) Testicular: presence of testicular mass; scrotal or testicular enlargement; heaviness, pain, dragging, or pulling sensation in groin or scrotum

4. Diagnostic evaluation
    a) Ovarian: no early screening test; seldom detected by pelvic exam or imaging; may be heralded by hydrothorax
    b) Uterine: endometrial smears, D&C tissue examination
    c) Cervical: Pap smear, biopsy, radiography, D&C, CT, lymphangiography, MRI, IVP, barium x-ray, colposcopy
    d) Breast: self-examination, mammography, ultrasonography, biopsy
    e) Prostate: rectal exam, radiography, serum acid phosphatase determination, prostate specific antigen, prostatic acid phosphatase, bone scanning, MRI, renal function tests, biopsy and microscopic exam of tissue
    f) Testicular: testicular examination and self-examination, elevated levels of alpha-fetoprotein (AFP) and beta subunit of human chorionic gonadotropin (hCG-beta), radiography, inguinal orchiectomy

5. Medical treatment
    a) Ovarian: surgery, chemotherapy, radiation, use of intraperitoneal radioisotopes, hormonal regulation (with tamoxifen)
    b) Uterine: uterectomy, radiation, radium implant, chemotherapy with progestins
    c) Cervical: surgery, radiation, chemotherapy
    d) Breast: surgery, radiation, chemotherapy
    e) Prostate: radical perineal prostatectomy, chemotherapy, chordotomy, radiation therapy
    f) Testicular: orchiectomy, radical retroperitoneal lymph node dissection, radiation, chemotherapy

6. Complications: metastatic disease; severe infection associated with immunosuppressive therapy

7. Essential nursing care for patients with cancer of the reproductive system: See Chapter 5.

C. Disorders of menstruation
    1. Definition: dysfunction associated with the menstrual cycle
    2. Pathophysiology and etiology
      a) Premenstrual syndrome
        (1) Pathophysiology: combination of symptoms experienced by some women before onset of menstruation
        (2) Etiology: progesterone deficit or estrogen excess in the luteal phase (probable)
      b) Amenorrhea
        (1) Pathophysiology: absence of menstrual flow as a result of a disturbance in the interplay between hypothalamic, pituitary, ovarian, and endometrial functions
        (2) Etiology: emotional stress, endocrine imbalance or tumor, wasting disease, strenuous exercise; normal occurrence after menopause, during pregnancy, and often during lactation
      c) Dysmenorrhea
        (1) Pathophysiology: spasmodic lower abdominal pain, often radiating to the lower back and thighs, that may last 12–48 hours
        (2) Etiology: excess prostaglandin production; exacerbated by stress and anxiety; possible symptom of endometriosis, displaced uterus, narrowing cervix, or pelvic inflammatory disease
      d) Menorrhagia
        (1) Pathophysiology: excessive bleeding during normal menstrual period
        (2) Etiology: endocrine imbalance, fibroid tumors, stress, abnormal blood coagulation, ovarian cysts, uterine polyps
    3. Symptoms
      a) Premenstrual syndrome: weight gain; nervousness; irritability; anxiety; personality changes; mood swings; headache; crying spells; depression; abdominal bloating; fatigue, breast pain, tenderness, or enlargement; low back pain; cravings for sweets; binge eating; swelling of ankles, feet, and hands; increased physical activity
      b) Amenorrhea: lack of blood flow during normal menstrual cycle
      c) Dysmenorrhea: pain, lower abdominal cramps
      d) Menorrhagia: heavy menstrual flow
    4. Diagnostic evaluation: symptom history, pelvic exam; for menorrhagia, D&C, endometrial biopsy, lab tests
    5. Medical treatment
      a) Premenstrual syndrome: salt-restricted diet, diuretics, analgesics, natural or synthetic progesterones, prostaglandin inhibitors (ibuprofen or naproxen sodium [Anaprox])
      b) Amenorrhea: correction of underlying cause, unless condition results from pregnancy or menopause

        c) Dysmenorrhea: mild analgesics (especially prostaglandin inhibitors); treatment of underlying cause, if any

        d) Menorrhagia: D&C to stop bleeding; treatment of underlying condition

   6. Complication: anemia (with menorrhagia)

   7. Essential nursing care for patients with disorders of menstruation

        a) Nursing assessment: Obtain patient history, including reproductive and symptom history; ask about diet, level of exercise, and exposure to stress.

        b) Nursing diagnoses

           (1) Anxiety related to disorder of menstruation

           (2) Pain related to dysmenorrhea

           (3) High risk for injury related to anemia (in menorrhagia)

        c) Nursing intervention

           (1) Explain to patient what is known about disorders of menstruation and the dietary, behavioral, and medical means of eliminating or controlling disorder.

           (2) Discuss with patient with dysmenorrhea options for pain control, including analgesics and relaxation techniques.

           (3) Advise patient with menorrhagia about the importance of eating a well-balanced diet and about the possible short-term use of nutritional supplements until condition is reversed.

        d) Nursing evaluation

           (1) Patient states that anxiety is relieved.

           (2) Patient states that pain is controlled.

           (3) Patient states that anemia is corrected.

D. Endometriosis

   1. Definition: a benign lesion in which endometrial tissue grows outside the uterus, often on the ovaries or in the pelvic cavity

   2. Pathophysiology and etiology

        a) Pathophysiology: flowing back of endometrial tissue through fallopian tubes during menstruation, with subsequent implantation on pelvic structures; transport of endometrial glands through vascular and lymphatic systems to other locations; spontaneous development of endometrial tissue outside uterus

        b) Etiology: unknown; associated with nulliparity, family history of endometriosis, age of 30–50 years

   3. Symptoms: lower abdominal pain, dysmenorrhea, menorrhagia, sterility, pelvic tenderness, dyspareunia, pain on defecation, painful intercourse

   4. Diagnostic evaluation: symptom history, pelvic exam, laparoscopy, ultrasonography, blood tests to rule out pelvic inflammatory disease

   5. Medical treatment

        a) Hormone treatments to keep patient in nonbleeding phase of menstrual cycle

        b) Surgery to remove cysts and as much ectopic tissue as possible without interfering with childbearing ability

        c) Panhysterectomy for extensive disease

   6. Complication: infertility

7. Essential nursing care for patients with endometriosis
    a) Nursing assessment: Obtain patient history, including reproductive and menstrual history.
    b) Nursing diagnoses
        (1) Pain related to excess bleeding of endometrial tissue
        (2) Decisional conflict related to uncertainty of choice of treatment
    c) Nursing intervention
        (1) Administer analgesic if ordered; note that aspirin is contraindicated in conditions associated with excessive bleeding.
        (2) Encourage bed rest and warm sitz baths.
        (3) Provide emotional support.
        (4) Provide information about disease; stress importance of following treatment regimen and seeking regular gynecologic care.
        (5) Discuss the feasibility of alternatives to uterectomy in patients with severe endometriosis.
    d) Nursing evaluation
        (1) Patient states that pain is lessened or relieved.
        (2) Patient makes a decision about treatment.

E. Vaginal disorders
    1. Definition: an abnormal opening into the vagina or an infection of the lower genital tract
    2. Pathophysiology and etiology
        a) Vaginal fistula
            (1) Pathophysiology: abnormal opening between ureter and vagina (ureterovaginal), between bladder and vagina (vesicovaginal), or between rectum and vagina (rectovaginal)
            (2) Etiology: congenital defect; surgical or obstetric trauma; cancer; irradiation for pelvic cancer; rectovaginal fistula a complication of ulcerative colitis
        b) Vaginitis
            (1) Pathophysiology: inflammation of lower genital tract associated with hormonal or bacterial imbalance in the vagina; common sources of infection *Candida albicans, Trichomonas vaginalis, Gardnerella vaginalis*
            (2) Etiology: insertion of foreign objects into vagina, chemical irritation, antibiotics
    3. Symptoms
        a) Vaginal fistula: urine leakage or infection with ureterovaginal or vesicovaginal fistulas; discharge of feces and gas through vagina with rectovaginal fistula
        b) Vaginitis: discharge, itching
    4. Diagnostic evaluation: physical exam with speculum and dye for vaginal fistula; pelvic exam and lab tests of vaginal smears for vaginitis

5. Medical treatment
   a) Vaginal fistula: surgery after inflammation and edema have disappeared; sitz baths in inoperable cases
   b) Vaginitis: application of yogurt or *Lactobacillus* culture with use of antibiotics
6. Complication: severe infection
7. Essential nursing care for patients with vaginal disorders
   a) Nursing assessment: Obtain symptom, medical, drug, allergy, and reproductive history, as well as information about previous treatment for reproductive disorders.
   b) Nursing diagnoses
      (1) Anxiety related to leaking urine or feces (vaginal fistula)
      (2) Chronic pain related to infection (vaginitis)
   c) Nursing intervention
      (1) Vaginal fistula: Change soiled linens; give analgesic and warm sitz bath; provide information on minimizing problems associated with disorder (see Client Teaching Checklist, "Home Care for Patients with Vaginal Fistula").
      (2) Vaginitis: Administer prescribed antibiotic, and caution patient to take all medication; stress good health habits to prevent recurrence: wearing of cotton underwear, avoiding strong douches and tight pants, and wiping with toilet paper from front to back after defecation.
   d) Nursing evaluation
      (1) Patient states that anxiety is reduced.
      (2) Patient states that pain is controlled.

✔ CLIENT TEACHING CHECKLIST ✔

Home Care for Patients with Vaginal Fistula

Explain the following procedures to patients with vaginal fistula.

✔ Keep perineal area clean and dry.
✔ Avoid perfume and scented sprays, powders, and lotions.
✔ Use a thin dusting of cornstarch if you wish, but wash it off if area becomes wet with urine or feces.
✔ Avoid heavy lifting.
✔ Change soiled clothes.
✔ Wear incontinence briefs to eliminate odors.
✔ Use commercial room deodorizer.
✔ Cover mattresses and chairs with plastic; wash plastic daily with soapy water.
✔ Contact physician if you experience:
— Pain or discomfort
— Fever or chills
— Cloudy urine

1. The nurse informs Maria that one diagnostic test performed during the pelvic examination is the Pap (Papanicolaou) test. She further explains that this test identifies cancer by:

    a. Obtaining direct smears from the endometrium.

    b. Aspirating or scraping vaginal secretions from the posterior fornix.

    c. Excising an inverted cone of tissue from the cervix.

    d. Painting the cervix with aqueous iodine solution.

2. Mammography is a breast-imaging diagnostic test that is useful in detecting nonpalpable, hidden lesions of the breast. Which of the following statements about the test would be appropriate for use in patient teaching?

    a. "The test may identify abnormal breast masses smaller than 1 cm."

    b. "The test requires the injection of a contrast medium prior to the test."

    c. "The test is not as effective in studying 'fatty' breasts."

    d. "The test can identify any lesions detectable on clinical examination."

3. The nurse is assessing 39-year-old Henrietta Gross for risk factors that may contribute to the development of premenstrual syndrome (PMS). Which of the following statements by the patient would be of greatest significance in her assessment?

    a. "I have cereal for breakfast and a salad for lunch every day."

    b. "My job affords me the greatest personal satisfaction."

    c. "My day is complete so long as I can drink my coffee."

    d. "I smoked 1 pack of cigarettes per day until I quit last year."

4. The nurse subsequently identifies which of the following as an appropriate nursing diagnosis for Ms. Gross?

    a. Anxiety related to the effects of PMS

    b. Ineffective individual and family coping related to the effects of PMS

    c. Potential for violence against family members related to symptoms of PMS

    d. Knowledge deficit related to the causes and treatment of PMS

5. The nurse is assessing 36-year-old Angela Venturino, who missed her menstrual period 2 weeks ago. Based on her symptoms, the nurse suspects that Ms. Venturino is experiencing early clinical manifestations of an ectopic pregnancy. Which of the following symptoms is the patient likely to be experiencing?

    a. Slight bleeding and sharp, colicky pain

    b. Nausea and vomiting associated with agonizing pain

    c. Generalized abdominal pain radiating to the neck and shoulders

    d. Difficulty in breathing and a rapid, thready pulse

6. Based on the nurse's assessment of Ms. Venturino, a priority nursing diagnosis for her would be:

    a. High risk for injury related to physiologic shock.

    b. Anxiety related to termination of pregnancy.

    c. Pain related to progression of ectopic pregnancy.

    d. Anticipatory grieving related to impending loss of pregnancy.

7. The nurse is teaching a patient who has undergone surgery for repair of a rectovaginal fistula. Which of the following points should be included in the teaching plan?

    a. Diet should include high-fiber foods.

    b. Normal activities may be resumed as desired.

c. Douching and use of enemas should be avoided for several months.

d. Beverages high in vitamin C are beneficial.

8. Which of the following women would be considered to be at greatest risk of developing endometriosis?

a. A 35-year-old multiparous woman

b. A 50-year-old multiparous post-menopausal woman

c. A 29-year-old nulliparous woman

d. A 30-year-old woman, gravida II, para I

9. The nurse is taking a health history on Ms. Maggie Ruschak, who is 45 years old. Which of the following statements by the patient indicates that she should be further evaluated for ovarian cancer?

a. "I have noted recent vaginal bleeding and a foul-smelling discharge."

b. "I am experiencing urinary incontinence and back pain."

c. "I frequently have a feeling of fullness even after light meals."

d. "There is an itchy lesion on my vulva."

10. The nurse is caring for 72-year-old Norman Gantz after a suprapubic prostatectomy. When assessing Mr. Gantz during the first 24 hours after surgery, the nurse would find which signs or symptoms of greatest significance in identifying possible complications?

a. The catheter bag contains numerous bright red, viscous clots.

b. The patient complains of flank pain within the first 8 hours.

c. Minimal swelling is noted above the pubic area.

d. The suprapubic dressing has a few patches of bloody drainage.

11. A nursing intervention that would be most likely to decrease Mr. Gantz's pain is:

a. To encourage him to sit rather than to ambulate.

b. To clamp his urinary catheter at intervals.

c. To administer antispasmodics as ordered by the physician.

d. To increase the traction on the urinary catheter.

12. Which of the following interventions should the nurse include when planning future teaching for a patient who is scheduled for an orchiectomy?

a. Assure the patient that testicular self-examination (TSE) will not be necessary after surgery.

b. Identify alternate methods of meeting the patient's reproductive needs.

c. Discuss erectile impotence as a potential complication.

d. Inform the patient that he may resume his normal activities as desired after surgery.

ANSWERS

1. **Correct answer is b.** The Pap (Papanicolaou) test is performed to detect cervical cancer. Secretions are aspirated or scraped from the posterior fornix, and a smear is transferred to a glass slide. The cytologic smear is then examined by a pathologist and is classified according to the presence or absence of atypical, abnormal, or malignant cells.

a. Endometrial (aspiration) smears provide a more accurate means of cytologic diagnosis by examining tissue directly from the endometrium.

c. A cone biopsy is an excision of a small piece of tissue that is performed when the results of the Pap test are suspicious.

d. In a Schiller's test, a long cotton-tipped swab is used to paint the cervix with an aqueous iodine solution. The cervix is abnormal if the tissues do not stain brown, and the test would then be considered positive.

2. **Correct answer is a.** A mammogram can detect abnormal masses as small as 1 cm, before they would be apparent during clinical examination.

b. No contrast medium is injected prior to the mammogram procedure, which is noninvasive.

c. Mammography is more effective in studying "fatty" breasts.

d. Mammography does not detect some lesions that are noted during clinical examination.

3. **Correct answer is c.** The patient's statement about coffee suggests that she ingests a large amount of caffeine throughout the day. Excessive caffeine intake has been implicated as a factor in PMS.

a. Increasing dietary intake of magnesium-rich foods, such as whole grains and green vegetables, may decrease the symptoms of PMS.

b. Although stress can aggravate the symptoms of PMS, this patient does not appear to find her job stressful.

d. Restriction of smoking may decrease PMS symptoms, but since this patient stopped smoking a year ago, it is not a current risk factor.

4. **Correct answer is d.** Since it is apparent that the patient does not realize that caffeine can precipitate or aggravate her symptoms, she has a knowledge deficit.

a, b, and **c.** Although these are appropriate diagnoses for patients with PMS, they do not apply in this case.

5. **Correct answer is a.** Early signs of an ectopic pregnancy include a delay in menstruation, followed by slight bleeding or spotting. Other symptoms include a vague soreness on the affected side and sharp, colicky pains.

b, c, and **d.** Nausea and vomiting, severe pain (including pain that radiates to the neck and shoulders), difficulty in breathing, and a rapid, thready pulse are signs of tubal rupture, a complication of untreated ectopic pregnancy.

6. **Correct answer is c.** A priority nursing diagnosis for Ms. Venturino would be pain. Since her condition has not progressed to a tubal rupture, she would not be exhibiting signs of physiologic shock.

a, b, and **d.** High risk for injury, anxiety, and anticipatory grieving are all incorrect, based on the explanation given in correct answer **c.**

7. **Correct answer is d.** Healing of tissues is promoted by increasing dietary intake of both vitamin C and protein.

a. Healing of a rectovaginal fistula will be promoted if the patient consumes a low-residue diet.

b. Patients should avoid heavy lifting.

c. Clients are encouraged to douche and use enemas. These measures promote healing of the tissues by ensuring cleanliness.

8. **Correct answer is c.** The incidence of endometriosis is highest in nulliparous women 25–35 years of age. There is also a predisposition to this condition in women who have close relatives with endometriosis.

a, b, and **d.** All are incorrect, based on the explanation given in correct answer **c.**

9. **Correct answer is c.** Early, insidious signs of ovarian cancer include gastrointestinal symptoms, such as abdominal discomfort, indigestion, flatulence, and a feeling of fullness after even light meals.

a. Leukorrhea (vaginal discharge) and irregular bleeding are signs of early cervical cancer.

b. Urinary incontinence and back pain are symptoms of a cystocele, a downward displacement of the bladder toward the vaginal orifice.

d. Chronic pruritus is a common symptom of vulvular cancer.

10. **Correct answer is a.** Following a radical prostatectomy, the most common immediate complications are bleeding and shock.

Urinary drainage should change from red-dish pink to clear-to-light pink within 24 hours after surgery. Bright red bleeding with increased viscosity and numerous clots indicates arterial bleeding. Arterial hemor-rhage usually requires surgical intervention.

b. Flank pain may be caused by bladder spasms or kidney problems. Bladder spasms can cause bleeding and clot retention, which are not immediate life-threatening complications.

c. Absence of swelling above the pubic area would be considered normal, since swelling indicates an overdistended bladder.

d. A urinary drainage bag containing pink-to amber-colored urine would be a normal finding after prostatectomy.

11. **Correct answer is c.** Antispasmodics or-dered by the physician would be adminis-tered to control pain related to bladder spasms. If uncontrolled, these spasms may lead to clot retention.

a. The patient should be encouraged to ambulate rather than to sit for long periods of time, since sitting can increase intra-abdominal pressure. Increased pressure can cause pain and bleeding.

b. Clamping of the catheter will cause an obstruction that can produce distention of the prostatic capsule and resultant hemorrhage.

d. Increasing the traction on the urinary catheter so that the balloon applies pressure to the prostatic fossa is a technique used to control venous bleeding.

12. **Correct answer is b.** The patient who is about to undergo an orchiectomy should be informed that alterations in reproductive function may occur and that methods such as sperm storage may be used to meet later reproductive needs.

a. The patient will still need to perform tes-ticular self-examination after orchiectomy so that metastasis or new primary tumors can be detected.

c. The orchiectomy should not affect the client's libido or ability to achieve an erec-tion and orgasm. Retroperitoneal lymph node dissection (RPLND) may affect ejacula-tory function.

d. Patients' activities are generally re-stricted for about 1 week after orchiectomy. Lifting more than 20 lb and climbing stairs are prohibited.

16

Urinary and Renal Function

OVERVIEW

I. Structure and function of urinary system
A. Kidneys
B. Ureters
C. Urinary bladder
D. Urethra

II. General diagnostic tests
A. Urinalysis
B. Renal function tests
C. Imaging studies
D. Urinary tract disorder tests
E. Intravenous pyelography

III. General nursing assessments
A. Patient history
B. Observation and physical examination
C. Diagnostic tests

IV. Nursing considerations with selected therapies and techniques
A. Bladder catheterization
B. Renal dialysis
C. Kidney surgery

V. Selected disorders
A. Urinary tract infection
B. Acute glomerulonephritis
C. Acute renal failure
D. Chronic renal failure
E. Obstructions
F. Bladder cancer
G. Prostate disorders

NURSING HIGHLIGHTS

1. The nurse treating a patient with a renal disorder must understand the physical, social, cultural, psychologic, and economic problems that this patient may be experiencing.
2. One of the greatest challenges for the nurse is helping a patient with chronic renal failure to lead a fulfilling life despite restrictions imposed by the disorder and its treatment.

GLOSSARY

anuria—suppression of urine formation by the kidney
calculus—abnormal concretion, usually composed of mineral salts, within the body (plural, calculi)

cystectomy—bladder excision or resection

glomeruli—globular tufts of capillaries in the kidney

nocturia—excessive urination at night

oliguria—decreased urine secretion in relation to fluid intake

proteinuria—excessive serum proteins in the urine

urinary meatus—opening of the urethra on the body surface, through which urine is expelled

ENHANCED OUTLINE

I. Structure and function of urinary system

See text pages
_____

A. Kidneys
   1. Structure: Kidneys are located in retroperitoneal space on either side of vertebral column; outer layer consists of fibrous tissue called *renal capsule;* middle layer consists of *parenchyma,* the functional tissue of kidney; innermost area is the *renal pelvis,* which funnels urine from parenchyma to ureter; basic structural unit is the *nephron.*
   2. Function: maintain internal homeostasis by removing nitrogenous wastes, regulating fluid, electrolyte, and acid-base balance, and regulating blood pressure; have role in red blood cell production by secretion of erythropoietin (EPO)

B. Ureters
   1. Structure: hollow tubes that connect renal pelvis to urinary bladder
   2. Function: propel urine from renal pelvis to urinary bladder

C. Urinary bladder
   1. Structure: muscular sac in posterior peritoneal cavity near pelvic floor
   2. Function: provides site for temporary storage of urine

D. Urethra
   1. Structure: narrow tube stretching from bladder to meatus lined with mucous membrane and epithelial cells
   2. Function: serves as conduit for elimination of urine from body

II. General diagnostic tests

See text pages
_____

A. Urinalysis: detects kidney disorders, electrolyte imbalance, and overall health problems through study of chemical content of urine

B. Renal function tests: measure renal efficiency by analysis of such values as creatinine clearance, blood urea nitrogen (BUN), serum electrolytes, and urine specific gravity

C. Imaging studies: detect renal or urinary disease by showing size, shape, and position of structures, with use of such techniques as CT scanning and ultrasonography

D. Urinary tract disorder tests
   1. Cystoscopy: detects bladder disease by means of magnified visual examination of bladder interior with cystoscope
   2. Retrograde pyelography: detects upper urinary tract bleeding or other disorder by means of insertion of radiopaque ureteral catheter (using a cystoscope) into pelvis of each kidney

E. Intravenous pyelography (IVP; sometimes called excretory urography): examines kidneys, ureters, and bladder after IV administration of contrast medium

See text pages

_____

III. General nursing assessments

A. Patient history: Inquire about symptoms, overall health, and drug, allergy, and family history; depending on symptoms, ask about work history, other exposure to toxic chemicals, history of childhood diseases, and history of urinary function.

B. Observation and physical examination
   1. Check patient for signs of electrolyte or fluid imbalance.
   2. Obtain height and weight; assess for periorbital edema, edema of the extremities, cardiac failure symptoms, and mental changes.
   3. Inspect abdomen and flank regions; auscultate aorta and renal arteries for presence of bruit; palpate all abdominal quadrants; perform percussion of abdominal region.
   4. Assist during diagnostic procedures.

C. Diagnostic tests: nursing responsibilities
   1. Urinalysis
      a) Voided urine: Ask patient to provide specimen of first urine voided in morning and to refrigerate specimen if he/she will be delayed in delivering it.
      b) Clean-catch specimen: Instruct male and female patients about respective self-cleaning procedures; ask patients to void briefly into toilet and then into container.
   2. Renal function tests: Instruct patient in appropriate urine collection technique; draw blood samples when needed.
   3. Imaging studies: Administer laxative or enema on evening before procedure; allow nothing by mouth after midnight.
   4. Urinary tract disorder tests: Serve light evening meal, and then place on NPO restrictions; prepare bowel with laxative or enema; help patient assume lithotomy position; monitor patient after procedure for signs of bleeding and infection.
   5. Intravenous pyelography: Ask patient whether he/she has a history of iodine sensitivity; administer laxative and enema, if ordered; follow

radiologist's instructions about food and fluid intake prior to procedure; administer IV fluid to patient instructed to avoid oral fluids; administer IV mannitol (Osmitrol) to patient at risk for acute renal failure after administration of contrast medium; after procedure, monitor patient for change in renal function; encourage oral fluid intake or administer parenteral fluids.

IV. Nursing considerations with selected therapies and techniques

See text pages

_____

A. Bladder catheterization
1. Always use sterile technique.
2. Before inserting indwelling catheter, test balloon by filling it with solution in prefilled syringe, then withdraw solution into same syringe.
3. Clean urinary meatus thoroughly before inserting catheter.
4. Lubricate catheter with sterile water-soluble lubricant; when urine returns, insert catheter up to bifurcation of balloon and main lumen to make sure the balloon is in the bladder, not the urethra, when it is inflated; inflate balloon with solution, then pull back on catheter until slight resistance is noted.
5. Connect catheter to sterile closed drainage system.
6. Change indwelling urethral catheters as physician directs.
7. Never reinsert indwelling urethral catheter that becomes dislodged; replace with new sterile catheter.

B. Renal dialysis
1. Hemodialysis
   a) Take vital signs, and weigh patient; do not give intramuscular injections for 2–4 hours after dialysis.
   b) During and immediately after dialysis, observe patient for bleeding, cardiac dysrhythmias, headache, muscle cramps, nausea, vomiting, hypotension, fever, diaphoresis, chest pain, anxiety, and restlessness.
   c) Check external shunt for patency; ensure that extremity in which shunt is implanted is warm with normal coloration; frequently evaluate shunt site for thrill or bruit; do not take blood pressure measurements in shunted arm; observe shunt site for signs of infection.
   d) Check internal arteriovenous (AV) fistula for correct functioning; assess for adequate circulation in the fistula and in distal part of extremity; check fistula for bruit or thrill; do not take blood pressure measurements in arm with fistula; do not use fistula to administer IV fluids; be alert for common complications, including thrombosis, infection, aneurysm formation, and ischemia.
   e) Educate patient about special orders for restricted diet, including adjustment or restriction of protein, sodium, potassium, and fluid intake.
   f) Closely monitor drug levels in patients; be especially alert to levels of cardiac glycosides, antidysrhythmic agents, antihypertensives, and antibiotics.

2. Peritoneal dialysis
   a) Draw blood for analysis of BUN, serum creatinine, and serum electrolytes; take vital signs and weight.
   b) Maintain fluid infusion and drainage during dialysis; ensure that correct amount of heparin has been added to dialysate bag; and if performing manual dialysis, initiate dialysate infusion and time infusion, dwell time, and outflow.
   c) Monitor blood pressure and pulse every 15 minutes during first exchange; monitor temperature every 4 hours; monitor heart rhythm for dysrhythmia.
   d) After procedure, take vital signs every 1–2 hours; check abdomen for tenderness and rigidity; measure fluid intake and output; observe patient for electrolyte imbalance; monitor weight.
   e) Be alert for any signs or symptoms of peritonitis.
C. Kidney surgery
   1. Administer analgesic and antibiotic as ordered before procedure.
   2. Check ureteral and urethral catheters for drainage after surgery; record color and amount of urine from each catheter; report sudden decrease in urine output or unusual bleeding.
   3. Report abnormal vital signs, restlessness, or sudden onset of flank pain.
   4. Monitor urinary pattern for possible retention after catheter removal.
   5. Evaluate pain, and administer narcotic analgesic as ordered.

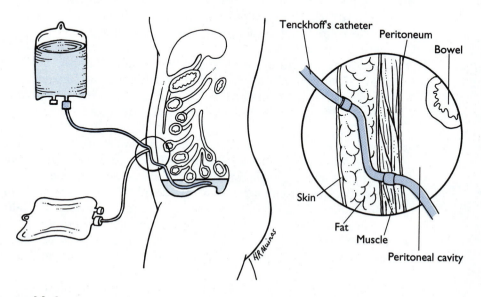

Figure 16–1
Peritoneal Dialysis with Implanted Abdominal Catheter

6. Check dressing every 1–2 hours on first day, every 3–4 hours thereafter; maintain aseptic technique, and report any signs of infection.
7. Encourage postoperative exercise regimen every 2 hours.

V. Selected disorders

See text pages
_____

A. Urinary tract infection (UTI)
1. Definition: infection of the upper or lower urinary tract
   a) Cystitis (lower UTI): inflammation of the urinary bladder
   b) Pyelonephritis (upper UTI): inflammation of kidney substance and pelvis
2. Pathophysiology and etiology
   a) Cystitis
      (1) Pathophysiology: infection of the urinary bladder (lower UTI)
      (2) Etiology: ascending urethral infection due to contaminated urologic instruments, fecal contamination, indwelling catheters, or sexual intercourse; common in women because of shortness of female urethra; may be secondary to infected prostate, epididymitis, or bladder stones in men
   b) Pyelonephritis
      (1) Pathophysiology: infection of renal parenchyma and collecting system lining (upper UTI)
      (2) Etiology: pregnancy, diabetes, ascending infection from bladder
3. Symptoms
   a) Cystitis: urgency, frequency, painful urination, perineal and suprapubic pain, hematuria, chills, or fever
   b) Pyelonephritis: kidney (lower back) pain, chills, fever, malaise, frequency, burning urination, leukocytosis, bacteria and white blood cells in urine (with acute form); asymptomatic or low-grade fever with vague GI complaints, anemia, hypertension, kidney stones, headache, poor appetite, thirst, weight loss (with chronic form)
4. Diagnostic evaluation
   a) Cystitis: patient history, physical exam, urinalysis (microscopic exam, culture and sensitivity studies)
   b) Pyelonephritis: urinalysis, cystoscopy, retrograde pyelography
5. Medical treatment
   a) Cystitis: correction of contributing factors; antimicrobial therapy (usually with sulfonamide); removal of partial obstruction, if present
   b) Pyelonephritis: symptomatic treatment, antimicrobial therapy, fluids (for acute form); antimicrobial therapy, removal of urinary tract obstruction, nephrectomy (for chronic form)
6. Complications: severe deterioration in renal function, uremia (with pyelonephritis)
7. Essential nursing care for patients with urinary tract infections
   a) Nursing assessment: Obtain history, including voiding pattern; review diagnostic test results.

      b) Nursing diagnoses
         (1) Pain related to bladder and urethral inflammation
         (2) Hyperthermia related to urinary tract infection
         (3) Activity intolerance related to chronic renal disease (pyelonephritis)
      c) Nursing intervention
         (1) Administer prescribed antibiotics.
         (2) Give analgesics and sitz baths to control pain.
         (3) Administer antipyretics to reduce fever.
         (4) Encourage patient with chronic pyelonephritis to space activities to provide rest periods.
         (5) Encourage fluid intake.
      d) Nursing evaluation
         (1) Patient states that pain is controlled.
         (2) Patient's temperature returns to normal.
         (3) Episodes of fatigue are eliminated.

B. Acute glomerulonephritis
  1. Definition: a type of nephritis most often found in children and young adults, characterized by inflammation of the glomeruli
  2. Pathophysiology and etiology
    a) Pathophysiology: inflammation of the glomeruli
    b) Etiology: host response to upper respiratory infection (especially Group A streptococcus)
  3. Symptoms: nausea, malaise, headache, edema, facial puffiness, pain and tenderness over kidneys, poor appetite, nocturia, oliguria, anuria, hematuria, irritability, shortness of breath, visual disturbances, nosebleeds, anemia
  4. Diagnostic evaluation: symptom history; examination of dark, smoky, bloody urine; laboratory findings, including proteinuria and elevated antistreptolysin-O titer; BUN, serum creatinine, serum potassium, and erythrocyte sedimentation rate measurement; decreased hemoglobin level
  5. Medical treatment: bed rest, fluids, sodium-restricted diet high in carbohydrates, antibiotics, diuretics, antihypertensives
  6. Complications: convulsions, congestive heart failure
  7. Essential nursing care for patients with acute glomerulonephritis (see section V,A,7 of this chapter)

C. Acute renal failure
  1. Definition: sudden dramatic reduction in kidney function
  2. Pathophysiology and etiology
    a) Pathophysiology: reduction in glomerular filtration, renal ischemia, and tubular damage

    b) Etiology: renal artery thrombosis, severe burns, prolonged severe hypotension, blood transfusion reactions, severe infection, crushing injuries, nephrotoxic substances, decreased renal perfusion

3. Symptoms
    a) Phases of acute renal failure
        (1) Period of oliguria: urinary volume <400–600 ml per 24 hours; increase in serum concentration of urea, creatinine, uric acid, organic acids, magnesium, and potassium; lasts about 10 days
        (2) Period of diuresis: gradual increase in urinary output, indicating recovery of glomerular filtration
        (3) Period of recovery: gradual improvement of renal function, taking 3–12 months; recovery normally followed by permanent reduction in glomerular filtration rate and in ability to concentrate urine
    b) Principal clinical manifestations: oliguria, anuria, hypertension, rising BUN and creatinine levels, anorexia, nausea, vomiting, diarrhea, pruritus, lethargy, hyperkalemia, hypertension, edema, anemia

4. Diagnostic evaluation: symptom and medical history; evaluation of BUN, serum creatinine, electrolyte levels, and creatinine clearance

5. Medical treatment
    a) Treatment of underlying cause
    b) Dialysis to prevent complications of uremia
    c) Correction of acidosis and electrolyte and fluid imbalance, especially hyperkalemia
    d) Administration of mannitol, furosemide, or ethacrynic acid to initiate diuresis and to prevent or minimize further renal failure
    e) Dietary therapy, including restriction of dietary proteins to 1 g/kg during oliguric phase to minimize protein breakdown and prevent accumulation of toxic waste products; high volume of carbohydrates; restriction of foods and fluids containing potassium, including bananas and citrus fruits and juices; total parenteral nutrition, if required

6. Complications: renal function loss, chronic renal failure, anemia

7. Essential nursing care for patients with acute renal failure
    a) Nursing assessment
        (1) Obtain patient's medical, symptom, drug, allergy, and diet history.
        (2) Assess physical appearance; record vital signs, weight, and skin color; check edema; appraise cognition; describe urine.
    b) Nursing diagnoses
        (1) Altered nutrition, less than body requirements, related to anorexia and nausea or vomiting
        (2) Fluid volume excess and electrolyte imbalance related to decreased urine output
        (3) Knowledge deficit related to follow-up care
    c) Nursing intervention
        (1) Weigh patient daily; provide small frequent meals; provide favorite foods within dietary restrictions.

(2) Evaluate patient's ability to perform self-care activities; allow enough time to carry out activities, including rest periods.

(3) Closely monitor patient for signs of infection; inspect skin daily for breakdown; maintain aseptic technique when inserting catheter or IV line; prohibit contact with infected people.

(4) Administer fluids as ordered, and measure intake and output each hour.

(5) Provide information on home care (see Client Teaching Checklist, "Home Care for Patients with Renal Failure").

d) Nursing evaluation

(1) Patient eats prescribed diet and restricts intake of fluids; nausea and vomiting are reduced.

(2) Patient exhibits no sign of infection.

(3) Patient states understanding of self-care.

✔ **CLIENT TEACHING CHECKLIST** ✔

Home Care for Patients with Renal Failure

Explain the following guidelines to patients with renal failure.

✔ Follow recommended diet (don't use salt substitutes); limit fluids as prescribed.

✔ Take medication as prescribed; don't use nonprescription drugs without approval.

✔ Record fluid intake and output.

✔ Avoid exposure to infection.

✔ Monitor blood pressure and pulse.

✔ Keep skin clean and dry; shower daily; avoid scratching; use lotion or cream for itching.

✔ Remove all detergents when laundering clothes and towels by using extra rinse cycle; avoid using harsh detergents.

✔ Keep record of daily weights.

✔ Avoid heavy exercise; take frequent rest breaks.

✔ Report any of the following:

— Slow decrease in or cessation of urination

— Weight gain or loss of >5 lb

— Chills and fever

— Sore throat

— Cough

— Bloody urine

— Easy bleeding or bruising

— Lethargy, extreme fatigue

— Persistent headache

— Nausea or vomiting, diarrhea

D. Chronic renal failure
  1. Definition: slow progressive decrease in kidney function
  2. Pathophysiology and etiology
     a) Pathophysiology: characterized by worsening electrolyte imbalances and accumulation of nitrogenous wastes, leading to slowing of mental processes; without dialysis, progresses to uremia
     b) Etiology: polycystic kidney disease, urinary tract obstruction, kidney stones, glomerulonephritis, chronic pyelonephritis, renal tumors, disseminated lupus erythematosus, nephropathy of diabetes mellitus
  3. Symptoms: lethargy, headache, anorexia, dry mouth (early stage); pruritus, dry skin, metallic taste in mouth, uremic breath odor, diarrhea, constipation, edema, anemia, abnormal bleeding, muscle cramps, mental changes, rising BUN and serum creatinine levels, hyponatremia, hypernatremia, acidosis, hypertension, vomiting, dry and scaly skin (middle stage); oliguria or anuria, mental changes, hiccups, muscular twitching, convulsion, uremic frost, GI tract ulceration and bleeding (end stage)
  4. Diagnostic evaluation: symptom history, history of kidney disease, lab tests of kidney function, IV pyelography, biopsy
  5. Medical treatment: control of activity, weight, and infections; dialysis; administration of antihypertensive agents; restricted dietary intake of protein, potassium, and sodium; treatment of electrolyte imbalance; vitamin supplementation; kidney transplantation
  6. Complications: uremia, severe infection, coma
  7. Essential nursing care for patients with chronic renal failure
     a) Nursing assessment
        (1) Obtain patient's medical, symptom, drug, allergy, and diet history.
        (2) Assess physical appearance; take vital signs and weight; check skin color and edema; appraise cognition; describe urine.
     b) Nursing diagnoses
        (1) Altered nutrition, less than body requirements, related to anorexia or nausea and vomiting
        (2) Activity intolerance related to anemia
        (3) Potential for infection related to altered immunity
        (4) Fluid volume excess and electrolyte imbalance related to decreased urine output
        (5) Impaired skin integrity related to uremic frost
        (6) Knowledge deficit related to follow-up care
     c) Nursing intervention
        (1) Weigh patient daily; continually assess patient's nutritional status; provide high-quality protein foods; encourage high-calorie snacks between meals; provide pleasant environment at mealtime to counteract anorexia.
        (2) Identify potential sources of excessive fluid, potassium, sodium, and phosphate, including medications, IV fluids, and oral fluids.
        (3) Encourage patient to alternate between periods of activity and rest and to look for opportunities to conserve energy while carrying out activities of daily living.

(4) Rinse skin with warm water and pat dry to remove uremic frost; moisten skin with cream or lotion; change position every 2 hours; inspect for skin breakdown.

(5) Provide information on home care (see Client Teaching Checklist, "Home Care for Patients with Renal Failure").

d) Nursing evaluation

(1) Patient eats prescribed diet and restricts fluids.

(2) Patient tolerates increased activity.

(3) Patient exhibits no sign of infection.

(4) Patient's skin remains intact.

(5) Patient states understanding of self-care.

E. Obstructions (kidneys, ureters, bladder, urethra)

1. Definition: blockage at any point in the urinary tract

2. Pathophysiology and etiology

a) Pathophysiology: development of a stone, tumor, cyst, kink, stenosis, or spasm; urinary blockage by obstruction, leading to distention of kidney pelvis

b) Etiology: cancer, diverticulum in bladder wall, enlarged prostate, traumatic instrumentation, infection, congenital malformation, precipitation of urine salts due to unknown cause

3. Symptoms: abdominal mass, renal tenderness and pain, urine retention (all disorders); slow urine stream, hesitancy, burning, frequency, nocturia (stricture); hematuria, UTI symptoms, pain radiating to genital area, pyuria, ureteral colic, difficulty starting urinary stream, feeling of fullness (stones); palpable prostate on rectal exam

4. Diagnostic evaluation: symptom history; abdominal radiography; retrograde pyelography; ultrasonography; cystoscopy; urinalysis; blood chemistry tests, including analysis of serum calcium and uric acid; biopsy

5. Medical treatment: establishment of adequate drainage (all disorders); dilatation of ureter or urethroplasty (stricture); observation for passage of stone, large fluid intake, surgical removal (stones); prostatectomy

6. Complications: urinary tract infections, peritonitis

7. Essential nursing care for patients with obstructions

a) Nursing assessment: Obtain medical, drug, symptom, and allergy history; send urine sample for analysis.

b) Nursing diagnoses

(1) Pain related to urinary tract obstruction

(2) High risk for infection related to obstruction of urine flow

(3) Hyperthermia related to UTI

(4) Knowledge deficit related to proposed treatment and at-home care

　　　　c) Nursing intervention
　　　　　　(1) Monitor intake and output; catheterize patient as needed.
　　　　　　(2) Administer narcotic analgesic; encourage patient to walk.
　　　　　　(3) Administer prophylactic antibiotics and antipyretic as ordered.
　　　　　　(4) Provide information to prevent future stones (see Client
　　　　　　　　Teaching Checklist, "Home Care for Urinary Calculi").
　　　　d) Nursing evaluation
　　　　　　(1) Patient states that pain is eliminated.
　　　　　　(2) Patient shows no signs of infection.
　　　　　　(3) Patient states understanding of procedures for home care.

F.　Bladder cancer
　　1.　Definition: malignant tumor of the bladder
　　2.　Pathophysiology and etiology
　　　　a) Pathophysiology: formation of superficial tumors or of tumors with
　　　　　　high probability of metastasis
　　　　b) Etiology: associated with cigarette smoking and exposure to toxic
　　　　　　chemicals (aniline dye, paint, rubber)
　　3.　Symptoms: painless hematuria, UTI, pelvic pain, urinary retention,
　　　　urinary frequency, anemia
　　4.　Diagnostic evaluation: cystoscopic exam, biopsy of lesion, retrograde
　　　　pyelography, CT, radiography of pelvis, ultrasonography, kidney
　　　　function lab tests
　　5.　Medical treatment
　　　　a) Superficial tumors: resection or coagulation with transurethral
　　　　　　resectoscope; topical antineoplastic drug injected into bladder by
　　　　　　means of catheter; cystoscopic exam every 3 months for first year,
　　　　　　every 6 months thereafter
　　　　b) Metastatic tumor: cystectomy with urinary diversion procedure

---

✔ CLIENT TEACHING CHECKLIST ✔

Home Care for Urinary Calculi

Explain the following guidelines to patients with urinary calculi.

✔ Follow prescribed diet and medications as directed.
✔ Drink plenty of fluids (at least 10 large glasses daily).
✔ Get plenty of exercise.
✔ Save any stones passed for inspection by physician.
✔ Contact physician if you experience:
　— Hematuria
　— Burning urine
　— Chills or fever
　— Pain
　— Infection anywhere in body
　— Persistent symptoms

6. Complications: metastatic disease, urinary tract infection, peritonitis
7. Essential nursing care for patients with bladder cancer
   a) Nursing assessment: Obtain patient history, and perform physical examination.
   b) Nursing diagnoses
      (1) Pain related to surgery
      (2) Potential for infection related to type of urinary diversion and surgery
      (3) Body image disturbance related to altered body function
      (4) Impaired tissue integrity related to stoma
      (5) Self-care deficit related to surgery and stage of disease
   c) Nursing intervention
      (1) Administer narcotic analgesics as ordered.
      (2) Monitor temperature every 4 hours; monitor vital signs; report any symptoms of peritonitis in patient with ileal conduit or Kock pouch.
      (3) Encourage patient to discuss fears about altered body function.
      (4) Inspect skin around stoma for signs of breakdown or infection each time temporary drainage bag is changed; report excess surface bleeding, color change, or separation of stoma.
      (5) Change dressings promptly; provide good skin care around anal and gluteal areas after ureterosigmoidostomy.
      (6) Assess ability of patient to perform self-care activities; provide any necessary assistance.
   d) Nursing evaluation
      (1) Patient avoids infection.
      (2) Patient begins to accept altered appearance and body function.
      (3) Patient's skin remains intact.
      (4) Patient's self-care needs are met.

G. Prostate disorders (benign prostatic hypertrophy [BPH], prostatitis)
   1. Definition: enlargement or infection of the prostate
   2. Pathophysiology and etiology
      a) Prostatitis
         (1) Pathophysiology: inflammation of prostate gland
         (2) Etiology: infection, prostate enlargement, stricture of the urethra, history of fetal exposure to diethylstilbestrol (DES)
      b) Benign prostatic hypertrophy (hyperplasia)
         (1) Pathophysiology: periurethral hyperplasia that encroaches on and decreases diameter of prostatic urethra
         (2) Etiology: advancing age; possible hormonal imbalance
   3. Symptoms
      a) Prostatitis: perineal or low back pain; fever; chills; urinary urgency, frequency, pain, and burning; nocturia

b) BPH: prostatism (hesitancy, narrowed stream, straining to void, frequency, urgency, nocturia), hematuria, cystitis
4. Diagnostic evaluation
   a) Prostatitis: notation of symptoms; history; digital rectal exam; tests of prostatic fluid (culture, microscopic exam); urinalysis
   b) BPH: digital rectal exam; urinalysis; urodynamic studies; cystoscopy; retrograde pyelography; blood chemistry, including analysis of serum creatinine; measurement of fluid intake and output; determination of prostate-specific antigen (PSA)
5. Medical treatment
   a) Prostatitis: antibiotics, rest, mild analgesic, sitz baths, avoidance of sexual intercourse until disorder is controlled, stool softener, and avoidance of foods and beverages that have diuretic action or increase prostatic secretions, including coffee, tea, alcohol, cola, and chocolate
   b) BPH: catheterization, suprapubic cystostomy, hormonal therapy with antiandrogen and progestational agents, surgical removal of part of gland, transcystoscopic urethroplasty, prostatectomy
6. Complications: sepsis (prostatitis); urinary tract infections, urinary retention, hydroureter, hydronephrosis (benign prostatic hyperplasia)
7. Essential nursing care for patients with prostate disorders
   a) Nursing assessment: Take symptom history, and inquire about urinary pattern; check for signs of distended bladder; examine prostate.
   b) Nursing diagnoses
      (1) Pain related to inflammation (prostatitis)
      (2) Potential for injury related to urinary obstruction (BPH)
      (3) Potential for infection related to urinary obstruction (BPH)
   c) Nursing intervention
      (1) Prostatitis
         (a) Administer broad-spectrum antimicrobial as ordered for 10–14 days, and encourage patient to rest.
         (b) Administer analgesics, antispasmodics, bladder sedatives, sitz baths, and stool softeners as ordered.
      (2) BPH
         (a) Administer hormonal therapy as ordered.
         (b) For nursing management of patient after prostatectomy, see section IV,E of Chapter 15.
   d) Nursing evaluation
      (1) Patient states that pain is controlled with analgesics.
      (2) Patient voids normally after treatment of BPH.
      (3) Patient avoids infection associated with BPH.

1. Gemma, who is 8 years old, has periorbital edema, oliguria, lethargy, and anorexia and is being admitted for treatment of glomerulonephritis. This is Gemma's first hospital experience. Which question would the nurse ask the parents when obtaining a history of the present illness?

   a. "Has Gemma had an ear infection recently?"
   b. "Has Gemma been exposed to chickenpox recently?"
   c. "Has Gemma had a urinary tract infection before?"
   d. "Has Gemma taken any Tylenol within the past 48 hours?"

2. Gemma refuses to eat hospital food, and her mother wants to bring in meals. Which foods would the nurse recommend as appropriate choices?

   a. Cheese pizza and apple juice
   b. A hamburger, french fries, and orange drink
   c. A peanut butter and jelly sandwich and a strawberry malt
   d. Fruit salad, cottage cheese, and fruit punch

3. Which play activity would be appropriate for Gemma during the acute phase of glomerulonephritis?

   a. Baking cookies and cupcakes
   b. Completing jigsaw puzzles
   c. Riding a stationary bicycle
   d. Playing dress-up and house

4. Martin Weller is scheduled to undergo a transurethral resection of the prostate (TURP) tomorrow morning for treatment of benign prostatic hypertrophy. What instruction does the nurse give him about the initial postoperative period?

   a. "Void every 2 hours whether or not you feel the urge to do so."
   b. "Get up and walk to decrease discomfort from bladder spasms."
   c. "Cough and deep breathe every 2 hours to prevent clot formation."
   d. "Expect cherry-red urine that will gradually turn pink."

5. Gail Palen, 35 years old, is admitted for an acute episode of renal colic and diagnostic evaluation of nephrolithiasis. Nursing management of renal colic would include:

   a. Encouraging a fluid intake of 3000 ml/day.
   b. Administering morphine sulfate on a regular schedule.
   c. Straining all urine and assessing for stone passage.
   d. Supplementing the diet with vitamin C and cranberry juice.

6. When monitoring Ms. Palen for complications of renal colic, the nurse would observe for:

   a. Anemia.
   b. Polyuria.
   c. Hypertension.
   d. Oliguria.

7. Ms. Palen will undergo extracorporeal shock wave lithotripsy (ESWL) treatment for the stone tomorrow morning and asks the nurse what the procedure involves. The nurse explains that:

   a. A special scope is passed through the urethra, into the bladder, and up the ureters, where the stone can be captured and removed.
   b. Ultrasound waves are generated in water and are directed at the kidney at a frequency high enough to shatter the stone.
   c. A laser probe is inserted into the renal pelvis via a nephrostomy tube. The stone is visualized and dissolved with a single laser beam.
   d. A probe is inserted into the renal pelvis via cystoscopy, and sound waves are directed at the stone to shatter it.

8. Angela Matos, 36 years old, is being seen in the walk-in clinic for recurrent cystitis. What information does the nurse share with the patient when teaching her about measures to prevent future episodes of cystitis?

a. Drink 1500 ml of fluid each day, including a serving of cranberry juice at bedtime.

b. Take a daily bath, and avoid the use of bath oils and soaps.

c. Take all the medication prescribed, even though the symptoms have subsided.

d. Go to the bathroom and void soon after sexual intercourse.

9. Ida Volmer, who is 72 years old, is experiencing urge incontinence. Teaching her methods for controlling incontinence would include which of the following?

a. Establishing an interval voiding schedule

b. Demonstrating Credé's maneuver

c. Assisting with intermittent self-catheterization

d. Discussing the side effects of bethanechol chloride (Urecholine)

10. Norman Brant, 66 years old, is receiving gentamicin sulfate intravenously for a post-surgical wound infection. Which outcome is included on his care plan for the nursing diagnosis, "high risk for injury related to intravenous antibiotic therapy"?

a. Wound remains clean and moist with healthy granulation.

b. Client reports freedom from pain.

c. Lung sounds remain clear.

d. BUN remains between 10 and 20 mg/dl.

11. Joe Huit, who is 64 years old, has chronic renal failure. The nurse observes the following measurements: BUN 64, hemoglobin 8.8, creatinine 2.4, and a urine output of 250 ml over the past 24 hours compared with a 1000-ml intake. An appropriate nursing diagnosis for this set of data is:

a. High risk for injury related to possible seizure activity.

b. Fluid volume excess related to inability of the kidney to maintain body fluid balance.

c. Anemia related to impaired renal function.

d. Urinary retention related to intake greater than output.

12. Which nursing action would be implemented for Mr. Huit?

a. Insert urinary catheter to promote bladder drainage.

b. Elevate feet when out of bed to promote venous return.

c. Assess lung sounds each shift to monitor fluid status.

d. Supplement diet with protein powder shakes to provide essential amino acids to promote healing.

ANSWERS

1. **Correct answer is a.** When obtaining a history of the present illness, the nurse questions the patient about precipitating factors. Acute glomerulonephritis (AGN) typically occurs 10–14 days after a strep infection. Strep throat or strep-related otitis media is the most common precipitating event.

b. Chickenpox is a herpes zoster virus that is not typically associated with AGN.
c and d. Previous experience of a urinary tract infection and recent use of Tylenol are not pertinent to the history of the present illness.

2. **Correct answer is c.** Dietary modifications in acute glomerulonephritis (AGN) depend on the stage and severity of the disease. Sodium is restricted when hypertension and edema are present, and potassium is restricted during the oliguric period. Protein intake is increased slightly to cover losses. A peanut butter and jelly sandwich and a malt are low in sodium and potassium and are good sources of protein.

a and **b.** Because cheese pizza, apple juice, hamburger, french fries, and orange drink are high in sodium, they are not recommended.

d. A meal consisting of fruit salad, cottage cheese, and fruit punch would not be high in protein.

3. **Correct answer is b.** Bed rest is encouraged during the initial phase of acute glomerulonephritis (AGN), and strenuous activity is restricted until there is no longer any proteinuria or macroscopic hematuria. Age-appropriate activities would include board games, word and jigsaw puzzles, craft projects, and reading.

   a, c, and **d.** Baking, riding a stationary bicycle, and playing dress-up and house are all activities that involve an expenditure of energy that is higher than the bed-rest level.

4. **Correct answer is d.** It is important to inform the patient that his urine will be red during the postsurgical period so that he is not alarmed by its bloody appearance.

   a. A urinary catheter will be in place after surgery to maintain urethral patency and to allow for removal of clots. A continuous normal saline irrigation may be running. Instructions regarding voiding are not given until after the catheter is removed.
   b. Walking does not typically relieve bladder spasms. A B&O (belladonna and opiate) suppository is usually administered for this purpose.
   c. Coughing and deep breathing are important postsurgical activities, but they would not prevent clot formation in a patient who had undergone prostate surgery.

5. **Correct answer is b.** Renal colic is the severe pain associated with ureteral spasms when the ureter is irritated by a stone. Management of the pain experience is best accomplished by administering a narcotic analgesic, such as morphine sulfate, on a regular interval schedule. Antispasmodic medications, including propantheline bromide

(Pro-Banthine) and oxybutynin chloride (Ditropan), are also used.

   a, c, and **d.** Encouraging a high fluid intake, straining the urine, and supplementing the diet with vitamin C and cranberry juice are included in the management of nephrolithiasis but are not direct interventions for the pain.

6. **Correct answer is d.** A stone may occlude the ureter, thereby impeding urine flow from the kidney. This can result in hydronephrosis, a complication that can lead to kidney necrosis.

   a and **c.** Anemia and hypertension are complications of renal failure.
   b. Polyuria is not associated with renal colic. The urine may look rusty as a result of blood in the urine.

7. **Correct answer is b.** Extracorporeal shock wave lithotripsy (ESWL) uses ultrasound to shatter the stone. The patient is placed in a tub of water, and a sensor directed at the kidney generates sound waves that cause the stone to vibrate and break apart.

   a. Passing a scope through the urethra, into the bladder, and up the ureters prior to stone capture and removal is a cystoscopy procedure.
   c. Laser therapy is being developed to treat kidney stones; however, ESWL does not involve laser technology.
   d. Insertion of a probe into the renal pelvis via cystoscopy, followed by shattering of the stone, is a percutaneous ultrasonic lithotripsy procedure.

8. **Correct answer is d.** Bacteria may enter the urethra during sexual intercourse. Voiding soon after intercourse helps flush potential infecting organisms from the urinary tract.

   a. Daily fluid intake of 1500 ml is too low for persons with chronic recurring cystitis. Recommended intake is 2500–3000 ml.
   b. Showers are encouraged instead of tub baths, since sitting in a bath can cause reflux of bacteria into the bladder.

c. Finishing all medication is an appropriate response to a current infection, not a means of preventing future infections.

9. **Correct answer is a.** Urge incontinence occurs as a result of a hypertonic bladder. Patients with this condition cannot hold their urine once they feel the urge to void, and there is a large loss of urine. Methods to control this type of incontinence include bladder retraining on an interval schedule and teaching the patient pelvic floor muscle strengthening (Kegel) exercises.

b, c, and **d.** Credé's maneuver, self-catheterization, and bethanechol chloride (Urecholine) administration are all interventions for urinary retention, not urinary incontinence.

10. **Correct answer is d.** Gentamicin is an aminoglycoside. Because this class of drugs is highly nephrotoxic, the nurse would monitor kidney function closely while the patient is receiving gentamicin. Maintaining BUN, which is a direct measure of kidney function, within normal range is a desired outcome.

a. Wound status is not related to the potential complications of intravenous antibiotic therapy.
b. Freedom from pain is too broad an outcome for potential complications of intravenous antibiotic therapy. Freedom from pain along the cannula site is pertinent to measuring the absence of phlebitis.
c. Clear lung sounds are more appropriately correlated with fluid therapy than with intravenous antibiotic therapy. The amount of fluid administered with intermittent intravenous antibiotic therapy is small and is unlikely to cause fluid volume overload.

11. **Correct answer is b.** The data indicate impaired renal function, which is expected in chronic renal failure (CRF). Because the kidney does not filter or excrete water or waste products, these substances accumulate in the blood, and there is a high risk of fluid volume excess.

a. Seizure potential is related to the buildup of toxic wastes, not renal failure.
c. Anemia is not a NANDA diagnosis.
d. In CRF there is no altered bladder function that would cause urine to be retained. Urine is not being produced in patients with this disorder.

12. **Correct answer is c.** Lung sounds must be assessed to monitor for pulmonary edema, which is a complication of chronic renal failure (CRF).

a. Because this patient can be expected to be oliguric, inserting a catheter would increase the risk of infection and would have no value in the treatment of CRF.
b. Elevating the feet would increase fluid flow to the heart, making the heart work harder. This would be detrimental, since congestive heart failure is associated with CRF.
d. Because protein intake is restricted in CRF, protein supplementation would be inappropriate.

17

Integumentary Function

OVERVIEW

I. Structure and function of integumentary system
   A. Structure of integumentary system
   B. Function of integumentary system

II. General diagnostic tests
   A. Skin cultures
   B. Biopsy
   C. Patch testing

III. General nursing assessments
   A. Patient history
   B. Observation and physical examination
   C. Diagnostic tests

IV. Nursing considerations with selected therapies and techniques
   A. Skin cancer surgery
   B. Facial reconstructive surgery
   C. Rhytidectomy
   D. Laser treatment of cutaneous lesions
   E. Dermabrasion

V. Selected disorders
   A. Pressure ulcers
   B. Psoriasis
   C. Acne
   D. Herpes zoster
   E. Impetigo
   F. Parasitic skin disease
   G. Benign tumors
   H. Skin cancer

NURSING HIGHLIGHTS

1. The nurse who detects and intervenes in early changes in skin integrity has a significant impact on the overall health of elderly and immunosuppressed patients.
2. The nurse should always provide acceptance of and support to patients struggling with disfiguring skin disorders, who may experience profound psychologic distress.

GLOSSARY

comedo—a plug of keratin and sebum within the dilated orifice of a hair follicle (plural, comedones)

cryosurgery—tissue destruction by application of extreme cold

electrodesiccation—tissue destruction by dehydration, accomplished with high-frequency electric current

papule—a skin lesion that is small, solid, and elevated

pustule—a skin lesion that is small, solid, elevated, and filled with pus

urticaria—a vascular reaction of the upper dermis marked by wheals and caused by foods, drugs, infection, or stress; also called hives

wheal—the typical lesion of urticaria; a localized area of edema on the skin that may be accompanied by severe itching

ENHANCED OUTLINE

I. Structure and function of integumentary system

See text pages

A. Structure of integumentary system
   1. Epidermis: the outer layer of cells, which is constantly shed and replaced by new cells moving upward from the dermis
   2. Dermis: the middle layer of the skin, consisting of connective tissue composed of elastic fibers and collagen; also accommodates capillaries, lymph vessels, and sensory nerves
   3. Subcutaneous fat (adipose tissue): the innermost layer of skin, which overlies muscle and bone and is the major site for fat formation and storage

B. Function of integumentary system
   1. Protection: prevention of water loss; barrier keeping foreign substances from entering body
   2. Heat regulation: control of internal temperature by radiation, convection, and conduction

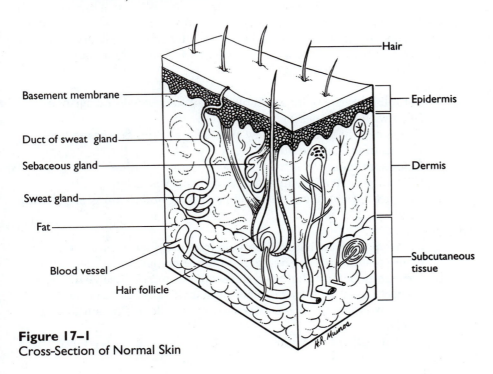

Figure 17–1
Cross-Section of Normal Skin

II. General diagnostic tests

See text pages

A. Skin cultures: study lesions of suspected bacterial, viral, or fungal origin

B. Biopsy: establishes an accurate diagnosis of a skin disorder or assesses effectiveness of treatment

C. Patch testing: identifies allergens by placement of test chemicals in direct contact with patient's skin

III. General nursing assessments

See text pages

A. Patient history: Take medical, allergy, family, drug, and symptom history.

B. Observation and physical examination
   1. Inspect skin, including scalp, hair, and nails.
   2. Examine oral mucous membranes.
   3. Describe and measure skin lesions accurately.
   4. Assist during diagnostic procedures.

C. Diagnostic tests: nursing responsibilities
   1. Skin cultures
      a) Superficial fungal infections: Scrape scales from lesion into clean container for transport to laboratory.
      b) Deeper fungal infections: Assist physician with punch biopsy.
      c) Bacterial infections: Express material from lesion, collect it with a cotton-tipped applicator, and place it in a bacterial culture medium.
      d) Viral cultures: Express and collect vesicle fluid; immediately place culture tube in cup of ice.
   2. Biopsy
      a) Establish sterile field; assemble biopsy equipment and syringe filled with local anesthetic.
      b) Shave patient's hair at biopsy site, cleanse skin, and assist physician with procedure.
      c) Place specimens for culture in sterile saline solution.
      d) Control patient's bleeding, and cover biopsy site.
      e) Instruct patient about means of protecting and cleaning site during healing.
   3. Patch testing
      a) Advise patient to discontinue systemic corticosteroids 48 hours before test but to continue to use topical preparations.
      b) Explain to patient that procedure will require 3 office visits.
      c) Inspect upper back for presence of rash; if skin surface is not suitable, shave hair from alternative sites; clean skin surface with alcohol.
      d) Apply marked test chambers to skin.

e) Instruct patient to keep skin dry and to save, but not to reapply, nonadherent patches.

f) 2 days after patch application, remove chambers, and mark each area of contact with permanent ink; note initial allergic reactions.

g) Assist with final reading of test results in 2–5 days.

IV. Nursing considerations with selected therapies and techniques

See text pages

A. Skin cancer surgery
   1. Caution patient to observe for excess bleeding and constricting dressings.
   2. Advise patient when to report for follow-up (see Client Teaching Checklist, "Home Care Following Skin Cancer Surgery").

B. Facial reconstructive surgery
   1. Prepare patient emotionally for extent of improvement, and explain postsurgical care.
   2. Maintain patent airway after surgery.
   3. Suction secretions as necessary, and cleanse mouth.
   4. Keep head and upper torso slightly elevated.
   5. Maintain cold compresses to reduce swelling.

C. Rhytidectomy (face-lift)
   1. Encourage patient to rest quietly for first 2 postsurgical days.
   2. Elevate head of bed, and discourage neck flexion.
   3. Administer analgesics for discomfort.
   4. Provide liquid or soft diet.
   5. Cleanse skin gently with topical ointment after dressings are removed; comb drainage-matted hair with warm water and wide-toothed comb.
   6. Advise patient not to lift or bend for 7–10 days and to report sudden pain at once.

D. Laser treatment of cutaneous lesions
   1. Argon laser
      a) Apply cold compresses over affected area for 6 hours to minimize edema, exudate, and capillary impermeability.

✔ CLIENT TEACHING CHECKLIST ✔

Home Care Following Skin Cancer Surgery

Explain the following guidelines to patients who have undergone skin cancer surgery.

✔ Avoid unnecessary sun exposure, especially between 10 A.M. and 3 P.M., and wear protective clothing if exposure is unavoidable.

✔ Apply sunscreen and lip balm to block harmful rays; reapply after swimming.

✔ Do not become sunburned.

✔ Do not use sun lamps or commercial tanning booths.

✔ Have moles removed if they are rubbed by clothing.

✔ Watch moles for any change in size, ulceration, bleeding, or exudation.

✔ Have follow-up skin exams for the rest of your life.

          b) Encourage patient not to pick at crusts and to apply antibacterial ointment sparingly until crust separates.

          c) Instruct patient not to use makeup until skin heals.

    2. Carbon-dioxide laser

          a) Cover wound with antibacterial ointment and dressing; teach patient how to care for dressing.

          b) Administer analgesics if necessary; caution patient that pain may occur 3 days after treatment.

          c) Remove dressing after re-epithelialization is complete; apply steroid ointment to reduce scarring.

    3. Pulse-dye laser

          a) Apply ice and antibacterial ointment to treated area, followed by nonstick dressing.

          b) Advise patient to wash crusting with soap and water, reapplying antibacterial cream twice a day.

          c) Advise patient not to use makeup and to avoid exposure to sun until healing is complete.

  E. Dermabrasion (skin peeling)

    1. Apply dressing and ointment after treatment.

    2. Elevate head of bed for first 48 hours to lessen edema.

    3. Remove dressing after 24 hours.

    4. Advise patient to apply prescribed ointment several times daily to prevent hard crusting.

    5. Caution patient to avoid extreme cold and heat, excess straining or lifting, and sunlight for 3–6 months.

See text pages

V. Selected disorders

A. Pressure ulcers (bedsores)

    1. Definition: localized areas of infarcted soft tissue over bony prominences

    2. Pathophysiology and etiology

          a) Pathophysiology: gradual breakdown of skin and underlying tissues caused by sustained pressure on skin that exceeds normal capillary pressure

          b) Etiology: immobility, loss of protective reflexes, edema, friction, malnutrition, anemia, incontinence, altered skin moisture, diabetes, advanced age

    3. Symptoms: redness and break in skin at pressure points, e.g., sacrum, heels, shoulders, and elbows

    4. Diagnostic evaluation: visual inspection

    5. Medical treatment: relief of pressure, application of topical medication, administration of antibiotics, wound debridement, skin grafting, application of Dome-paste bandage

6. Complications: tissue necrosis, gangrene, severe infection
7. Essential nursing care for patients with pressure ulcers
   a) Nursing assessment
      (1) Assess overall skin condition at least twice daily.
      (2) Inspect each pressure site for redness, blanching response, increased warmth, and skin breakdown.
      (3) Evaluate patient's circulatory status.
   b) Nursing diagnoses
      (1) Impaired skin integrity related to immobility
      (2) Pain related to ulcer formation
   c) Nursing intervention
      (1) Prevent pressure areas by frequently changing patient's position to redistribute pressure; encourage patient capable of movement to turn frequently.
      (2) Provide support with pillows or rolled towels; as appropriate, use alternating pressure pad, polyurethane foam, or flotation mattresses or air-fluidized or rocking beds.
      (3) Use well-padded footboard; place extra protection on heels; use polyester sheepskins.
      (4) Elevate patient's upper body to lessen edema.
      (5) Encourage patient in wheelchair to do wheelchair push-ups every 30 minutes.
      (6) Change incontinent patients promptly; wash soiled skin, and lubricate it with mild lotion.
      (7) Provide high-protein diet with protein supplements, and administer iron, vitamin C, and vitamin D.
      (8) Relieve pain with analgesic, if necessary.
   d) Nursing evaluation
      (1) Patient avoids pressure on bony areas.
      (2) Patient demonstrates improved tissue perfusion.
      (3) Patient's pressure ulcer heals.
      (4) Patient states that pain is relieved.

B. Psoriasis
   1. Definition: skin disease characterized by thickened patches of inflamed red skin and silvery scales
   2. Pathophysiology and etiology
      a) Pathophysiology: abnormal proliferation of epidermal cells in outer skin layer
      b) Etiology: unknown, but associated with heredity, environmental factors, drugs, skin trauma, infection, and hormonal changes
   3. Symptoms: patches of reddened skin with silver scales on extensor surfaces of elbows and knees, lower back, and scalp; itching that is usually slight but sometimes severe
   4. Diagnostic evaluation: visual examination of lesions
   5. Medical treatment: control of scaling and itching with coal tar extract, corticosteroids, anthralin, methotrexate, etretinate, triamcinolone acetonide injections, photochemotherapy
   6. Complications: psoriatic arthritis, scarring, infection

7. Essential nursing care for patients with psoriasis
   a) Nursing assessment: Obtain medical, drug, diet, allergy, family, and stressor history; inspect involved areas.
   b) Nursing diagnoses
      (1) Pruritus related to dryness and skin scaling
      (2) Body image disturbance related to disfigurement
   c) Nursing intervention
      (1) Help patient identify and avoid factors that worsen itching.
      (2) Recommend use of light cotton bedding and clothes that allow skin moisture to evaporate.
      (3) Encourage use of hypoallergenic or glycerin soap and tepid bath water; instruct patient to pat skin dry rather than rubbing it.
      (4) Provide information on at-home care (see Client Teaching Checklist, "Home Care for the Patient with Psoriasis").
      (5) Provide emotional support and acceptance; encourage patient to ask questions and express concerns.
   d) Nursing evaluation
      (1) Patient states that pruritus is relieved.
      (2) Patient begins to accept changes in appearance.

C. Acne
   1. Definition: chronic skin disorder caused by inflammation of the hair follicles and sebaceous glands
   2. Pathophysiology and etiology
      a) Pathophysiology: heightened response in sebaceous glands produced by androgenic stimulation
      b) Etiology: interplay of hormonal, bacterial, and genetic factors

---

✔ CLIENT TEACHING CHECKLIST ✔

Home Care for the Patient with Psoriasis

Because the treatment of psoriasis is often prolonged, and exacerbations of the disease often occur, noncompliance with the treatment regimen is often a problem. Provide patients with psoriasis with the following instructions:

✔ Take oral medication and apply topical preparations exactly as prescribed.
✔ Do not use any prescription or over-the-counter drugs without prior approval from physician.
✔ Cleanse skin with mild soap, and avoid the use of perfumes, perfumed soap or lotion, and deodorant soap.
✔ Wash hands thoroughly before and after applying topical medications.
✔ Do not touch affected areas unless applying medication.

3. Manifestations: excessive oiliness of face, chest, and back; presence of comedones, papules, pustules, and cysts
4. Diagnostic evaluation: visual examination, skin culture
5. Medical treatment: skin cleansing with antibacterial abrasive soap; administration of oral retinoids if there is no chance that patient will become pregnant; estrogen therapy for female patients; use of topical and/or oral antibiotics; comedo extraction and pustule drainage
6. Complications: infection, severe scarring, emotional disorders
7. Essential nursing care for patients with acne
   a) Nursing assessment: Obtain medical, drug, diet, allergy, family, stressor, and skin care history; inspect involved areas; document presence of lesions.
   b) Nursing diagnoses
      (1) Impaired skin integrity related to epidermal and dermal tissue disruption
      (2) Body image disturbance related to concern about appearance
   c) Nursing intervention
      (1) Advise patient to wash face with mild soap and water twice a day and to use drying agents and sponge pads, if desired.
      (2) Caution patient to avoid sources of friction and trauma to affected areas.
      (3) Warn patient to avoid manual expression of comedones or pustules to avoid infection.
      (4) Advise patient to use cosmetics, shaving creams, and other toiletries sparingly, if at all.
      (5) Show empathy and acceptance in dealing with patient with acne.
      (6) Explain what is known about the causes of acne and instruct patient to follow treatment regimen every day, even if improvement is not noted at once.
   d) Nursing evaluation
      (1) Patient follows treatment plan.
      (2) Patient discusses concerns about appearance.

D. Herpes zoster (shingles)
   1. Definition: acute viral infection causing painful itchy vesicles along nerve pathways
   2. Pathophysiology and etiology
      a) Pathophysiology: reactivation of the varicella-herpes zoster virus that lies dormant in sensory ganglia after infection with chickenpox
      b) Etiology: immunosuppression
   3. Symptoms
      a) Blotchy skin accompanied by itching, numbness, or pain
      b) Unilateral vesicles that appear along sensory nerve path of head, neck, or trunk within 48 hours
      c) Rupture of vesicles within several days, accompanied by crusting that may cause scarring or skin discoloration
      d) Severe pain along nerve pathways that may persist for weeks, months, or years

    4. Diagnostic evaluation: symptom history, visual examination of lesions, Tzanck test, viral culture

    5. Medical treatment: oral and topical acyclovir; corticosteroid therapy and analgesics to relieve pain; medications to fight itching after crusts are gone; immediate treatment by ophthalmologist for lesions of ophthalmic division of trigeminal nerve

    6. Complications: postherpetic neuralgia, ophthalmic infection and scarring, Bell's palsy, skin necrosis

    7. Essential nursing care for patients with herpes zoster

      a) Nursing assessment: Obtain patient history, and examine face and anterior and posterior trunk.

      b) Nursing diagnoses

        (1) Impaired skin integrity related to viral infection

        (2) Pain related to herpes zoster

        (3) Social isolation related to potential for spread of infection

      c) Nursing intervention

        (1) Instruct patient to practice meticulous skin care.

        (2) Caution patient not to wear tight garments that can further irritate skin and cause additional pain.

        (3) Apply astringent compresses to viral lesions for 20 minutes 3 times a day to promote healing and relieve pain.

        (4) Administer prescribed analgesics if needed to control pain.

        (5) Warn patient to take precautions against spreading infection to others, including avoidance of sexual intercourse until lesions heal.

      d) Nursing evaluation

        (1) Patient's skin integrity is restored.

        (2) Patient states that pain is relieved.

        (3) Patient restricts social interaction to activities that cannot spread disease and understands reason for these precautions.

E. Impetigo

    1. Definition: streptococcal or staphylococcal infection of the skin

    2. Pathophysiology and etiology

      a) Pathophysiology: formation of lesions that begin as small red macules and progress to thin-walled vesicles that rupture and become covered with yellow crust

      b) Etiology: streptococcal or staphylococcal infection, sometimes secondary to herpes simplex, pediculosis capitis, scabies, poison ivy, or eczema; often associated with poor hygiene

    3. Symptoms: erythema, vesicles that form a sticky yellow crust after rupturing

    4. Diagnostic evaluation: visual inspection of lesions

    5. Medical treatment: systemic or topical antibiotics

6. Complications: disseminated infection, acute glomerulonephritis
7. Essential nursing care for patients with impetigo
   a) Nursing assessment: Obtain symptom history, and examine skin lesions.
   b) Nursing diagnoses
      (1) Impaired skin integrity related to bacterial infection
      (2) Social isolation related to potential for spread of infection
   c) Nursing intervention
      (1) Teach patient to use topical antiseptic preparation to reduce bacteria content near site of infection.
      (2) Instruct patient and family to bathe at least once daily with bactericidal soap and to use individual towels and washcloths.
      (3) Keep infected child away from other children until infection resolves.
      (4) Caution patient to avoid scratching area.
   d) Nursing evaluation
      (1) Patient's skin lesions heal.
      (2) Patient states understanding of and maintains hygienic practices that prevent spread of infection to others.

F. Parasitic skin disease
   1. Definition: skin disorder caused by infestation by lice (pediculosis) or itch mite (scabies)
   2. Pathophysiology and etiology
      a) Pathophysiology
         (1) Pediculosis: Severe itching is caused by injection of digestive juices and excrement by louse into human skin; parasite may be head louse, body louse, or pubic louse.
         (2) Scabies: severe itching caused by delayed immunologic reaction to mite or fecal pellets embedded in skin
      b) Etiology
         (1) Pediculosis: sharing contaminated head coverings, hairbrushes, or clothing; close personal contact; sexual intercourse
         (2) Scabies: exposure to objects, animals, or persons contaminated with itch mite
         (3) Both: patients with compromised immunity especially susceptible
   3. Symptoms
      a) Pediculosis: itching, skin irritation
      b) Scabies: intense itching (usually worse at night) with excoriation and burrows usually found between fingers and on forearms, axillae, waistline, nipples, men's genitals, umbilicus, and lower back
   4. Diagnostic evaluation: symptom history, visual inspection
   5. Medical treatment
      a) Pediculosis: washing of hair with shampoo containing lindane or pyrethrin compounds; bathing with soap and water, followed by application of lindane or malathion in isopropyl alcohol
      b) Scabies: topical application of gamma benzene hexachloride and crotamiton

6. Complications
   a) Pediculosis: severe pruritus, pyoderma, dermatitis, epidemic disease
   b) Scabies: secondary lesions, bacterial superinfection, seizures related to improper application of scabicide
7. Essential nursing care for patients with parasitic skin disease
   a) Nursing assessment: Obtain patient history, including demographic and socioeconomic data; inquire about symptoms.
   b) Nursing diagnoses
      (1) Impaired skin integrity related to bacterial infection
      (2) Social isolation related to potential for spread of infection
   c) Nursing intervention
      (1) Instruct patient about proper procedures for cleaning skin and applying medication.
      (2) Teach patient how to disinfect clothing and other possessions with lindane or malathion.
      (3) Alert patient to risk of infecting others.
      (4) Encourage sexually active patient and partner to be examined for presence of coexisting sexually transmitted disease.
   d) Nursing evaluation
      (1) Patient's skin integrity is restored.
      (2) Patient states an understanding of the contagious nature of the disease and takes appropriate precautions.
      (3) Patient is screened for coexisting sexually transmitted disease.

G. Benign tumors (moles, warts)
   1. Definition
      a) Mole (nevus): benign neoplasm of the pigment-forming cells
      b) Wart (verruca): small tumor caused by infection of the keratinocytes by papillomavirus
   2. Pathophysiology and etiology
      a) Pathophysiology
         (1) Mole: may be confined to the epidermis (junctional nevus) or may involve both epidermis and dermis (compound nevus)
         (2) Wart
            (a) Common wart: flesh-colored papule with rough surface
            (b) Flat wart: slightly elevated reddish-brown papule that may multiply on face or hands
            (c) Plantar wart: painful wart on sole of foot
            (d) Venereal wart: sexually transmitted neoplasm that can involve external genitalia, rectum, urethra, vagina, and cervix
      b) Etiology
         (1) Mole: may be congenital or acquired, usually between the ages of 1 and 35
         (2) Wart: infection by papillomavirus

3. Symptoms: none, unless location causes repeated irritation or trauma
4. Diagnostic evaluation: visual inspection; biopsy if there is any suspicion of malignancy
5. Medical treatment
   a) Mole: excision
   b) Wart: excision, electrodesiccation, cryosurgery, topical caustic agents
6. Complications: irritation due to friction or excoriation; malignant melanoma arising from mole
7. Essential nursing care for patients with benign tumors
   a) Nursing assessment: Obtain medical, drug, allergy, and symptom history; examine lesion and its position.
   b) Nursing diagnoses
      (1) Pain related to continuous trauma to benign tumor
      (2) Body image disturbance related to multiplication of flat warts
   c) Nursing intervention
      (1) Inform patient about procedure to be undertaken and about any necessary follow-up care (see Client Teaching Checklist, "Care Following Removal of Mole or Wart").
      (2) Explain any scarring that may follow removal of a wart or mole.
      (3) Discuss the likelihood that benign tumors will return after removal.
   d) Nursing evaluation
      (1) Patient states that pain is eliminated after surgical removal of benign tumor.
      (2) Patient states an understanding of the cause and treatment of benign tumors.

H. Skin cancer
   1. Definition: 1 of several types of cutaneous malignancies that are usually primary and may spread to other parts of the body

---

✔ CLIENT TEACHING CHECKLIST ✔

Care Following Removal of Mole or Wart

To avoid scarring, infection, or other complications, advise patients who have had a mole or wart removed to do the following:

✔ Do not pull or soak scab; allow it to dry up and fall off.
✔ Follow medication regimen exactly as prescribed, and do not apply any other drug or lotion to area.
✔ Follow physician's recommendations about removing and changing bandage.
✔ Contact physician if you experience:
   — Continued bleeding
   — Fever and chills

2. Pathophysiology and etiology
   a) Pathophysiology
      (1) Malignant melanoma: highly malignant, rapidly spreading lesion; associated with good prognosis with prompt diagnosis; associated with poor prognosis after metastasis
      (2) Squamous cell carcinoma: dangerous lesion, often occurring on tongue or lower lip, that tends to metastasize to internal organs
      (3) Basal cell carcinoma: the most common type of skin cancer, arising from epidermal basal cells; good prognosis with prompt treatment
   b) Etiology: prolonged repeated exposure to ultraviolet rays; radiation exposure; long-term ulceration; extensive scar tissue
3. Symptoms
   a) Malignant melanoma: change in color, size, or general appearance of mole or pigmented area
   b) Squamous cell carcinoma: rough scaly tumor
   c) Basal cell carcinoma: waxy tumor with raised pearly border
4. Diagnostic evaluation: visual inspection, confirmed by biopsy
5. Medical treatment: electrodesiccation; surgical excision; cryosurgery; radiation therapy; radical excision of tumor and adjacent tissues, followed by chemotherapy, for malignant melanoma
6. Complication: metastatic growth
7. Essential nursing care for patients with skin cancer
   a) Nursing assessment: Take patient history, including information on exposure to sunlight, radiation, and other risk factors; ask when lesion was first noted; assist with skin biopsy.
   b) Nursing diagnoses
      (1) Impaired skin integrity related to premalignant or malignant skin lesions
      (2) Anxiety related to fear of death or disfigurement
   c) Nursing intervention
      (1) Explain to patient the nature and extent of prescribed treatment.
      (2) Discuss cosmetic changes that may be associated with treatment and the ways in which they can be minimized.
      (3) Encourage patient to discuss fears and to ask questions.
      (4) Teach patient to avoid sun exposure.
   d) Nursing evaluation
      (1) Patient maintains skin integrity by means of prompt medical treatment.
      (2) Patient states a realistic view of disorder and treatment and experiences minimal anxiety.

1. Ms. Rodriguez brings her 4-month-old daughter, Stella, to the clinic. She states that the child's mouth seems to hurt and that there is a "funny-smelling" white coating on her tongue. Nursing assessment of this situation would include:

    a. Asking the mother if there are any household pets.
    b. Obtaining a sample of the plaque for a Tzanck smear.
    c. Visualizing the plaque with a Wood's lamp.
    d. Reviewing current drug use by Ms. Rodriguez and her daughter.

2. Stella Rodriguez, whose primary method of feeding is breastfeeding, is diagnosed as having oral candidiasis. Teaching the mother to care for her infant would include instructions about:

    a. Discontinuing breastfeeding until the infection is gone.
    b. Swabbing the tongue and cheeks with an applicator soaked with nystatin (Nilstat) 4 times a day.
    c. Rinsing the infant's mouth thoroughly with water before each feeding.
    d. Washing toys that the child puts in her mouth with a dilute bleach solution.

3. Lynn Marsh, who is 45 years old, is wheelchair bound as a result of multiple sclerosis. She has a stage II decubitus ulcer on her sacrum. Which finding places her at high risk for impaired wound healing?

    a. Oxygen saturation is 90%.
    b. Hemoglobin level is 13.6 mg/dl.
    c. Current weight is 112 lb.
    d. Serum albumin is 3.0 g/dl.

4. Treatment of Ms. Marsh's wound would include:

    a. Application of a hydrocolloid dressing.
    b. Initiating bed rest until the wound is healed.

    c. Irrigating the wound with 1:1 peroxide/saline solution b.i.d.
    d. Measuring the wound's size and depth daily.

5. Joan Colton, who is 16 years old, has acne vulgaris of the face and back. The doctor has ordered tretinoin (Retin-A) cream, 0.05%, to be applied to affected areas once a day. What information does the nurse teach the patient about the use of this drug?

    a. Apply a thick layer of the drug to cover affected areas thoroughly.
    b. Apply a sunblock of SPF 15 to affected areas during exposure to sunlight.
    c. Discontinue the drug immediately if the skin begins to peel.
    d. Use medicated cosmetic products if make-up is worn.

6. Ann Denning, who is 36 years old, has a herpes zoster infection along the trigeminal nerve route. Clinical monitoring for complications of this condition would include observation for:

    a. Referred pain to the jaw.
    b. Clustered vesicles.
    c. Serous drainage from crusted lesions.
    d. Slurred speech.

7. Ms. Carson calls the telephone triage nurse at the clinic because she thinks that her daughter, Trish, has brought home lice from school. Which response by the nurse is most helpful in assessing the situation?

    a. "Why do you think your daughter has brought home lice from school?"
    b. "Are there scratch marks along your daughter's forearms or red lines between the fingers?"
    c. "Take a look at the nape of your daughter's neck. Do you see tiny red dots?"
    d. "Get a comb and run it through your daughter's hair. Are there tiny white eggs on the comb teeth?"

8. On the basis of the conversation, the nurse determines that it is appropriate to treat Trish for lice. What instruction does the nurse give Ms. Carson?

   a. "Shampoo all family members' hair with lindane (Kwell) 3 times."
   b. "Trish and your other children can return to school within 48 hours."
   c. "Reinfestation is unlikely to occur within the month."
   d. "Boil combs, brushes, and hair accessories for 10 minutes."

ANSWERS

1. **Correct answer is d.** Oral candidiasis (thrush) is common in young infants. It may be a secondary infection caused by the use of antibiotics that are being given directly to the infant, typically for an ear infection, or to the mother. The nurse investigates antibiotic use.

   a. The presence of household pets is not related to thrush, but many animals could play a role in skin rashes.
   b. Tzanck smear is used to diagnose herpetic lesions. A potassium hydroxide (KOH) test is used to diagnose fungal infections.
   c. A Wood's lamp is used to observe skin surfaces.

2. **Correct answer is b.** The mother would be taught to rinse her daughter's mouth with water after feeding and then to apply Nystatin solution around the oral mucosa.

   a. Breastfeeding can continue. The mother is usually given an antifungal cream (such as clotrimazole [Mycelex]) to apply to the breast after feeding and is instructed to wash the cream off before feeding the infant again.
   c. The infant's mouth should be rinsed after the feeding, not before.
   d. Cleaning toys is not a direct intervention for alleviating thrush.

3. **Correct answer is d.** Impaired wound healing can occur when the patient is hypoxic or has decreased tissue perfusion, is anemic, or has protein-calorie malnutrition. A serum albumin level ≥3.5 is required for adequate wound healing.

   a, b, and **c.** These answers are incorrect because the patient's body weight, oxygen saturation level, and hemoglobin level are all within normal range.

4. **Correct answer is a.** The recommended treatment for stage II decubitus ulcers is to alleviate pressure through repositioning and to protect the area from direct pressure and shearing forces by applying a hydrocolloid dressing.

   b. Bed rest predisposes the patient to skin breakdown.
   c. Peroxide is not recommended for use on wounds because it sloughs granulation tissue as well as nonviable tissue.
   d. Measuring wound size is an assessment, not a treatment.

5. **Correct answer is b.** Tretinoin (Retin-A) causes the skin to be photosensitive. A sunblock of SPF 15 or higher is recommended to prevent severe sunburn on areas to which the drug has been applied.

   a. Retin-A must be applied sparingly, as a thin layer.
   c. Skin peeling is an expected effect of Retin-A.
   d. Nonmedicated cosmetics must be used to prevent potential drug interactions with Retin-A.

6. **Correct answer is d.** Bell's palsy, which is characterized by one-sided facial droop, slurred speech, and numbness of the affected side of the face, is a possible complication of herpes zoster infection.

   a, b, and **c.** Referred pain to the jaw, clustered vesicles, and serous drainage from crusted lesions are typically associated with herpes zoster infections and do not represent complications.

7. **Correct answer is c.** Red dots at the nape of the neck or around the ears are characteristic bite marks from lice and are the best means of identifying the condition.

  a. Asking the mother why she thinks her daughter is infested is a nontherapeutic response that does not focus on data collection.
  b. Asking about scratch marks on the forearms and red lines between the fingers would be useful in assessing for scabies.
  d. Running a comb through the child's hair would not be helpful. Lice eggs (nits) stick to the shaft of the hair and do not come off when a regular comb is used. After treatment, nits are removed with a fine-tooth comb.

8. **Correct answer is d.** Brushes, combs, and hair pieces must be boiled to kill the lice and nits and to prevent reinfestation.

  a. Lindane (Kwell) is applied only once. More frequent use can lead to toxic reactions.
  b. The children can return to school once they have been treated with Kwell or permethrin (Nix).
  c. Lice reinfestation can occur at any time.

Medical-Surgical Nursing Comprehensive Review Questions

1. The nurse notes that a patient with burns over 35% of his body begins to perspire and become irritable before dressing changes. The most appropriate nursing diagnosis would be:

   a. Ineffective individual coping related to chronic pain from burn injury.

   b. Impaired adjustment related to long-term hospitalization.

   c. Knowledge deficit related to understanding the need for dressing change.

   d. Anxiety related to anticipation of pain during dressing changes.

2. On the evening before surgery, a patient's temperature suddenly spikes to 101°F. Which of the following nursing actions would be most appropriate?

   a. Retake the temperature in 1 hour.

   b. Give the prescribed acetaminophen (Tylenol).

   c. Report the temperature to the surgeon.

   d. Report the temperature to the night nurse.

3. Which prescribed analgesic would be most appropriate for a patient who is reporting mild incisional pain 3 days postoperatively?

   a. Aspirin (Ecotrin) by mouth

   b. Meperidine (Demerol) intramuscularly

   c. Acetaminophen 300 mg and Codeine 30 mg (Tylenol #3) by mouth

   d. Hydroxyzine hydrochloride (Vistaril) intramuscularly

4. A 10-year-old boy is admitted with a serum sodium of 155 mEq/L. The nurse anticipates that this child may be at risk for:

   a. High fever.

   b. Brain damage.

   c. Muscle cramps.

   d. Tetany.

5. The nurse needs to place an IV cannula. After explaining the procedure to the patient, the nurse begins to look for the best IV site. She assesses the:

   a. Antecubital fossa.

   b. Ankle veins.

   c. Distal arm and hand veins.

   d. Internal jugular vein.

6. James Lim is starting immunotherapy (hyposensitization) injections. He asks the office nurse if his neighbor, who gives herself insulin, can give him his injections. The correct response is:

   a. "The injections must be given here, because you could develop a serious reaction and need emergency treatment."

   b. "After the first 2 injections, you can have your neighbor give you the injections."

   c. "Your neighbor's injections are different, but I can teach her how to give you your injections."

   d. "You will need to have the injections for 6 months, and they should be given in our office."

7. The mother of a 25-year-old patient with HIV infection demands that the nurse tell her if her son has AIDS. The nurse:

   a. Tells the mother that her son does not have AIDS.

   b. States that her son does not have AIDS but has HIV.

   c. Asks the mother why she thinks her son has AIDS.

   d. Refuses because this is confidential information.

8. For which of the following conditions should the nurse implement Universal Precautions?

a. Tuberculosis
b. Influenza
c. Human immunodeficiency virus
d. Infectious mononucleosis

9. When assessing a patient in an intensive care setting, the nurse understands that which of the following has a minimal effect on the host's susceptibility to infection?

a. Nutritional status
b. Presence of multiple invasive devices
c. Mental status
d. Proximity of other patients

10. A radioactive implant was placed in the cervix of Rose Liu, a patient with cervical cancer. She has a supportive husband and 3 young children. The client expresses her feelings of loneliness and isolation to the nurse. The nurse should:

a. Send the patient home in the care of her husband.
b. Ambulate Ms. Liu in the hall after clearing it of others.
c. Allow Ms. Liu's children to visit her for 30 minutes.
d. Discuss Ms. Liu's feelings in the limited time available.

11. While caring for a patient who is at risk for developing superior vena cava syndrome, the nurse should assess for:

a. Shortness of breath and edema.
b. Pulsus paradoxus and edema.
c. Kussmaul's sign and tachycardia.
d. Bruising and abnormal reflexes.

12. Ms. Ann Chu has had a thoracentesis performed to drain a right lower lobe pleural effusion. After the procedure she complains of being short of breath. The nurse's assessment reveals decreased breath sounds in the patient's right lower lobe. These findings most likely indicate:

a. Normal post-thoracentesis symptomatology.

b. Pulmonary edema.
c. Worsening pleural effusion.
d. Pneumothorax.

13. In a conscious patient who has developed an open pneumothorax following a stab wound to the chest, the initial action in emergency intervention would include:

a. Teaching the patient about pant-blow breathing techniques.
b. Placing a towel over the wound so that it is sealed tightly.
c. Telling the patient to exhale and to strain against a closed glottis.
d. Placing the patient in a flat position on the affected side.

14. Three days after being placed in skeletal traction for a fractured pelvis, a 75-year-old patient develops tachypnea, cyanosis, and chest pain that worsens with inspiration. Which of the following conditions is the patient most likely to have developed?

a. Cardiogenic shock
b. Pericarditis
c. Myocardial infarction
d. Pulmonary embolus

15. The nurse working in a coronary care unit observes sustained ventricular tachycardia on the cardiac monitor of Ms. Elizabeth Foster. After the nurse enters her room, Ms. Foster is unresponsive when she is shaken and her name is called; the nurse ascertains apnea after assessing Ms. Foster's breathing. The nurse's initial action should be to:

a. Defibrillate the patient.
b. Initiate cardiac compressions.
c. Begin mouth-to-mouth breathing.
d. Press the emergency call button.

16. When doing discharge teaching for a patient with a newly inserted permanent pacemaker, what information would the nurse be most likely to include in the teaching plan?

a. Pulse rate should remain at about 72/minute.
b. Batteries are rechargeable while in place.

c. Outside electrical interferences are a concern.

d. Pacemaker identification notations are standard.

17. Jerry Botto, a patient with chronic anemia, has a hemoglobin level of 8.8 g/dl. Two units of packed red blood cells are ordered. During administration of the second unit, Mr. Botto develops dyspnea and becomes anxious. The nurse's first actions are to:

    a. Take his temperature and notify the physician.

    b. Stop the infusion and sit the patient upright.

    c. Slow the infusion of blood and start nasal oxygen at 2 L/minute.

    d. Discontinue the blood and infuse normal saline intravenously at a rate of 100 ml/hour.

18. Which of the following actions should the nurse take for Anna Rodriguez, a patient with a high risk for infection development related to decreased immune response?

    a. Place her in a semi-private room.

    b. Bathe her every other day.

    c. Measure her oral temperature once a day.

    d. Remove raw fruits from her diet.

19. A patient with a history of a brain tumor has a seizure as the nurse admits her. During the seizure, which of the following nursing actions represents a patient safety hazard?

    a. Easing the patient to the floor

    b. Remaining with the patient and closing the door

    c. Inserting a padded tongue blade between the teeth

    d. Placing the patient on her side and flexing the head forward

20. 68-year-old Bruce Griffith had a cerebrovascular accident (CVA) 1 week ago. Mr. Griffith has right-sided paralysis and expressive aphasia. In planning his nursing care, which of the following actions would the nurse include?

    a. Positioning Mr. Griffith in bed to prevent contractures and skin breakdown

    b. Ambulating the patient with a walker and supportive shoes

    c. Slowly repeating words and pointing to pictures to communicate with the patient

    d. Performing passive range-of-motion exercises on all extremities every 24 hours

21. Betty Knowles, 78 years old, fell from a standing position on a kitchen chair while cleaning out her cupboards. She sustained an intertrochanteric fracture of the right hip that was repaired under epidural anesthesia with a Massie nail. Nursing actions during the immediate postoperative period would include:

    a. Measuring vital signs every shift.

    b. Positioning the right leg in slight adduction.

    c. Inserting a straight catheter every 8 hours if the patient is unable to void.

    d. Increasing continuous passive motion (CPM) flexion by 5° every 3 hours.

22. Ms. Knowles is receiving clindamycin hydrochloride (Cleocin HCl) by intravenous piggyback every 6 hours. In monitoring for adverse effects of this drug therapy, the nurse would observe for:

    a. Diarrhea.

    b. Oliguria.

    c. Tinnitus.

    d. Tachypnea.

23. For ear irrigation in a conscious adult, correct procedure would have the patient sit or lie with the head tilted toward the side of the affected ear. To insure that the fluid reaches the eardrum, the external auditory canal is straightened by pulling the auricle:

    a. Down and backward.

    b. Straight backward.

    c. Upward and backward.

    d. Down and forward.

24. Which of the following nursing diagnoses would be a priority in planning the home care of a patient who experiences attacks of vertigo?

a. Self-esteem disturbance related to concern about family's reaction to vertigo
b. Sensory-perceptual alteration, kinesthetic, related to attacks of vertigo
c. Ineffective thermoregulation related to neurologic impairment
d. Impaired gas exchange related to inability to breathe during attacks of vertigo

25. A patient with a nasogastric tube that is attached to low continuous suction reports feeling nauseous and is belching. The initial nursing action in this situation is to:

a. Increase wall suction pressure to 80 mm Hg.
b. Irrigate the tube with 30 ml of normal saline.
c. Turn the patient to a side-lying position.
d. Check suction tubing position for dependency.

26. Melinda Peters, a patient with diabetes, is receiving tube feedings at 90 ml/hour to supplement oral feedings. At 7:30 A.M., Ms. Peters received 22 units of NPH and 8 units of regular insulin and ate all her breakfast. At 8:30 A.M., she received a 500-ml continuous tube feeding. Shortly thereafter, she began to vomit. An appropriate nursing action in this situation is to:

a. Give the patient a clear liquid diet for lunch.
b. Turn the tube feeding off 2 hours before lunch.
c. Consult the doctor about continued need for tube feeding.
d. Measure the blood sugar 4 times in the next 2 hours.

27. During an admission assessment, the nurse obtains the following data: diarrhea 2 hours after eating, rectal pain with bright red blood in stools, hemoglobin of 10.4, hematocrit of 35%, and cramping abdominal pain for the past 2 months. On the basis of these data, an appropriate nursing diagnosis would be:

a. Anemia related to gastrointestinal bleeding.
b. Pain related to irritable bowel symptoms.
c. Altered nutrition, less than body requirements, related to diarrhea and malabsorption.
d. High risk for fluid volume deficit related to diarrhea.

28. Teaching a client with diabetes mellitus how to prevent the Somogyi effect would include which of the following information?

a. Administer the evening dose of insulin before bedtime.
b. Eat an evening snack that includes a protein and a carbohydrate.
c. Avoid drinking large amounts of diet soda each day.
d. Do a blood sugar test at 3 A.M., and administer regular insulin as needed.

29. A patient with liver disease has the following laboratory values: hemoglobin 9.6, albumin 3.0, and ammonia 66. For which complication should the nurse monitor the patient?

a. Jaundice
b. Steatorrhea
c. Severe itching
d. Confusion

30. Nursing care for a person with advanced cirrhosis accompanied by ascites would include:

a. Initiating seizure precautions.
b. Encouraging fluids up to an intake of 3000 ml/day.
c. Administering warfarin sodium (Coumadin), 2.5 mg daily.
d. Assessing ventriculoperitoneal shunt function.

31. Which laboratory finding would indicate that levothyroxine sodium (Synthroid), a thyroid replacement hormone, is having a therapeutic effect?

    a. Increased hematocrit (Hct)

    b. Decreased thyroid-stimulating hormone (TSH) level

    c. Increased hemoglobin electrophoresis (Hgb AC)

    d. Decreased thyroxine (T_4) level

32. Carolyn Butler, who has severe hyperthyroidism, reports that she is depressed and embarrassed about the changes in physical appearance that are associated with her disorder. The nurse explains that most of these changes will disappear with effective treatment, but a few can be expected to remain. One of these permanent changes is:

    a. Fine tremors of the hands.

    b. Exophthalmos.

    c. Swelling of the neck.

    d. Flushed face.

33. When teaching a patient how to perform palpatory breast self-examination, the nurse would include which of the following points?

    a. "A semi-reclining position with legs horizontal is recommended."

    b. "Dry skin facilitates manual examination of the breast for lumps."

    c. "You should place a pillow under the breast that is opposite the one that you are examining."

    d. "Lumps are most evident when the breast is flattened and evenly distributed on the chest."

34. When teaching a patient about testicular self-examination, the nurse should inform him that:

    a. Each testis may not be smooth and of uniform consistency.

    b. The testicles are normally the same size.

    c. Enlargement of the testis without pain is significant.

    d. Examination should not take place after warm baths or showers.

35. Rita Leksa has a nephrostomy tube in the left kidney. The nurse has observed no new drainage in the tube for the past 30 minutes. After assessing for kinks in the tube and positioning the patient correctly, the nurse notes that the tube is still not draining. What action would the nurse implement next?

    a. Strip the drainage tubing gently.

    b. Irrigate the tube with 30 ml of normal saline.

    c. Notify the surgeon who inserted the tube.

    d. Observe for drainage for an additional 30 minutes.

36. Jamal Wilson, who is 54 years old, has prostatic cancer and will undergo retropubic prostatectomy tomorrow. Preoperative teaching for this patient includes:

    a. Teaching him to perform perineal exercises.

    b. Demonstrating suprapubic catheter care.

    c. Explaining the need for bed rest until his urine is clear.

    d. Identifying possible surgical complications that will be monitored.

37. Mr. Wilson asks the nurse if he will be impotent after the surgery. Which response is most appropriate?

    a. "Impotence is not a problem, but you may have a brief period of urinary incontinence."

    b. "Impotence is not a complication of the type of prostatectomy you will have."

    c. "Impotence occurs following prostatectomy, but penile implants will be inserted to provide sexual function."

    d. "Impotence may occur with retropubic prostatectomy, but dysfunction will not be evident for several weeks."

38. Tom Owen, 34 years old, had a precancerous lesion removed from his forehead. Postoperative teaching for this patient would include instructions to:

   a. Inspect the skin monthly.

   b. Wear a hat on sunny days.

   c. Avoid washing the area until it has healed.

   d. Apply SPF 10 sunscreen to the face when outside.

39. Wen Chin, 25 years old, is hospitalized for pneumonia. The nurse observes her vigorously scratching her arms and hands and notes red lines between her fingers. Which action should the nurse take?

   a. Provide the patient with an oil-based soap for bathing.

   b. Initiate isolation precautions.

   c. Apply a Burow's pack to the patient's arms for 20 minutes each shift.

   d. Apply hydrocortisone cream (2.5%) to affected areas b.i.d.

ANSWERS

1. Correct answer is d. The patient is exhibiting signs of anxiety caused by anticipating the painful procedure of a burn dressing change.

   a. Ineffective individual coping related to chronic pain does not address the transient symptoms specifically related to the dressing changes.

   b. Impaired adjustment does not address the patient's anticipation of the dressing change.

   c. The patient may or may not understand the need for dressing changes, but the symptoms relate to anxiety in anticipation of pain.

2. Correct answer is c. The temperature elevation is significant and indicates an alteration in the patient's condition. The surgeon needs to know about this change immediately to plan for tomorrow's surgery and to order diagnostic and treatment regimens.

   a and **d.** Retaking the temperature and reporting the elevation to the night nurse should eventually be done, but the first step is to obtain the surgeon's diagnostic and treatment orders.

   b. The surgeon should be called before acetaminophen (Tylenol) is administered. The drug could mask important symptoms, and the surgeon may prefer to order a different antipyretic.

3. Correct answer is c. Tylenol with codeine should effectively relieve mild incisional pain 72 hours after surgery.

   a. Aspirin is not recommended postoperatively, since it can increase the prothrombin time and cause bleeding.

   b. In the first 24–48 hours after surgery, intramuscular narcotics are often required to relieve severe to moderate postoperative pain.

   d. Hydroxyzine hydrochloride is not an analgesic, although it may be given with a narcotic analgesic to potentiate the narcotic's effect.

4. Correct answer is b. In severe hypernatremia, permanent brain damage can occur, especially in children. The damage may be caused by contraction of the brain, resulting in subarachnoid hemorrhages.

   a. Mild temperature elevations may occur, but high temperatures are seldom seen.

   c. Muscle cramps are common in hyponatremia, due to sodium loss and water gain.

   d. Tetany is a symptom of hypocalcemia.

5. Correct answer is c. The most distal site on the arm or hand is used first, so that later IVs can be placed upward on the arm.

   a. The antecubital fossa should not be used, since it would interfere with mobility and the drawing of lab specimens. It may be used if no other site is available.

   b. Veins of the feet and legs should not be used because of a high risk of thromboembolism.

   d. The internal jugular vein is a central vein and may be cannulated by physicians.

6. **Correct answer is a.** Mr. Lim should be observed for 30 minutes after each injection. If an anaphylactic reaction occurs, epinephrine and other life-saving measures are necessary. The neighbor would not be able to provide this emergency treatment.

b and **c.** Immunotherapy injections are usually given on a weekly basis, using gradually increasing concentrations of the allergen. Accordingly, Mr. Lim must be observed after each injection. It would be dangerous to have a lay person administer the injections.

d. Immunotherapy is usually continued over a period of years, depending on the response obtained. Six months would be too short a time in which to decrease the amount of circulating IgE adequately and increase the amount of IgG antibody.

7. **Correct answer is c.** Asking the mother why she thinks her son has AIDS gives her the opportunity to express her fears and allows the nurse to gather information and promote therapeutic communication. The diagnosis of AIDS or HIV could not be disclosed, since the mother's knowledge of this confidential information could cause hardships for the patient.

a and **b.** Medical diagnoses and other confidential patient information cannot be disclosed or discussed.

d. Although the nurse cannot disclose confidential information, this direct refusal would not lead to therapeutic communication and the defusing of a tense situation. The mother has also become the nurse's patient at this time.

8. **Correct answer is c.** According to CDC guidelines, the use of Universal Precautions is necessary to prevent the spread of human immunodeficiency virus, hepatitis B virus, and other blood-borne pathogens.

a, b, and **d.** In these situations, nurse would implement standard infection control procedures such as hand washing and the use of gloves when handling obviously infected materials.

9. **Correct answer is c.** The mental status of the patient would have the least effect on his/her susceptibility to infection.

a, b, and **d.** Nutritional status, presence of several invasive catheters, and the proximity of other patients would all affect the host's susceptibility to infection.

10. **Correct answer is d.** The nurse must limit exposure to the radioactive implant. With careful planning, time may remain to accomplish any necessary treatments and still have meaningful communication with the patient. The nurse cannot spend extra time with Ms. Liu, since radiation overexposure has no immediate symptoms and serious injury can occur.

a and **c.** Patients with radioactive implants cannot be cared for at home. Family members' and other visitors' time with the patient must be limited. Pregnant women and children should not visit or care for these patients.

b. Clients with radioactive implants are often restricted to bed rest to avoid dislodging the implant. It is neither practical nor safe to try to clear the halls to give the patient the opportunity to ambulate without contaminating others. Furthermore, this measure would have little value in helping Ms. Liu cope with her loneliness.

11. **Correct answer is a.** Shortness of breath and edema are the early signs of superior vena cava syndrome, since venous drainage of the head, neck, arms, and thorax is impaired.

b. Pulsus paradoxus is a symptom of cardiac tamponade.

c. Kussmaul's sign is distention of neck veins during inspiration and expiration and indicates pericardial disease.

d. Bruising and abnormal reflexes would not be signs of superior vena cava syndrome.

12. **Correct answer is d.** A potential complication of thoracentesis is pneumothorax. Signs and symptoms include sudden shortness of breath and decreased or absent breath sounds on the affected side. Unequal chest expansion will also be seen, with decreased expansion on the affected side. The patient will also exhibit tracheal shift to the unaffected side.

a, b, and **c.** The findings do not indicate normal postoperative symptomatology, pulmonary edema, or pleural effusion.

13. **Correct answer is b.** In an emergency, anything large enough to fill the wound may be used. It should be placed firmly and held tightly. The patient should also be instructed to inhale and to strain against a closed glottis to assist in lung reexpansion and ejection of air from the thorax. An upright or high Fowler's position will facilitate breathing.

a, c, and **d.** These interventions are not appropriate to the situation.

14. **Correct answer is d.** These symptoms are indicative of a pulmonary embolus. Along with the clinical picture of a patient immobilized in traction, the nurse should realize that elderly patients are at high risk for development of a pulmonary embolus.

a, b, and **c.** The combination of the symptoms in this case rules out the possibility of cardiogenic shock, pericarditis, or myocardial infarction.

15. **Correct answer is c.** Since the patient is pulseless and unresponsive, the CPR protocol requires that she receive insufflations before chest compressions are started so that oxygenated blood will be circulated (**b**).

a. Defibrillation may occur after CPR has begun.
d. The second person to arrive may call for additional assistance.

16. **Correct answer is c.** The patient should be instructed about the risks associated with electrical interference.

a. Depending on how the individual patient's pacemaker is set, a pulse rate of 72 may not apply.
b. The pacemaker must be surgically removed to have the batteries changed.
d. There are different models and brands of pacemakers; there is no "standard" type.

17. **Correct answer is b.** The patient is exhibiting symptoms of circulatory overload. If the transfusion continues, pulmonary edema will develop. To discontinue the source of fluid overload, the transfusion must be stopped first. The patient should sit upright to improve breathing, with the feet hanging down to allow for venous pooling in the legs. This position decreases the amount of circulating blood.

a. The patient's temperature would not be taken first. Body temperature would be more important if a febrile or septic reaction were suspected.
c. The blood transfusion should be stopped. Oxygen may then be ordered and administered.
d. The blood infusion should be stopped, but normal saline should be infused very slowly (25 ml/hour) to maintain an open line for administration of ordered medications.

18. **Correct answer is d.** Removing raw fruits from the diet reduces the client's exposure to potentially harmful environmental microorganisms. All fruits and vegetables should be cooked.

a and **b.** Neither placing Ms. Rodriguez in a semi-private room nor bathing her on alternate days would reduce her environmental exposure to microorganisms. She should be placed in a private room and have a daily bath to reduce the number of microorganisms on her skin.
c. The oral temperature should be taken every 4 hours to assess the patient for signs of infection.

19. Correct answer is c. If a patient has an aura, a padded tongue blade may be inserted in an attempt to prevent biting of the tongue or cheek. Once the seizure has started and the teeth are clenched, nothing should be inserted, since injury to the lips, teeth, or tongue may occur.

a. Easing the patient to the floor is appropriate, since it prevents injury due to falling.
b. Staying with the patient and closing the door is appropriate; the patient has a right to privacy.
d. Placing the patient on her side and flexing the head forward is appropriate, since it allows the tongue to fall forward and drains saliva and mucus, which help to keep the airway open.

20. Correct answer is a. Correct positioning is important to prevent contractures, pressure areas, and decubiti.

b. The patient will not be able to ambulate with a walker, since he has right-sided paralysis. A regimen of physical therapy or rehabilitation needs to be planned. The patient with hemiplegia tends to lose his sense of balance and therefore needs to develop sitting balance before standing.
c. In expressive aphasia, the patient can understand words but is unable to form and return understandable words. Therefore, the patient may use a picture board to communicate. In receptive and global aphasia, the patient will be unable to understand words, and the nurse may use the picture board to communicate with the patient.
d. All extremities should be put through a full range of motion 4–5 times a day. The affected extremities are exercised passively.

21. Correct answer is c. Because epidural anesthesia can block the spinal reflex controlling micturition for several hours after surgery, the nurse must assess for urinary retention. The patient is typically given a straight catheter every 8 hours (or sooner if signs and symptoms of urinary retention

are evident) until spontaneous voiding returns.

a. Upon return to the nursing unit after surgery, the patient's vital signs are assessed every 15 minutes 4 times, every 30 minutes 4 times, then hourly until stable. (Some facilities recommend every-2-hour checks 4 times.) Vital signs are then assessed every 4 hours through the second postoperative day.
b. There are no positioning requirements with a Massie nail as there are with a total hip replacement. The latter requires slight abduction of the operative hip.
d. Continuous passive motion (CPM) flexion is used after total knee replacement surgery.

22. Correct answer is a. Clindamycin hydrochloride is used for infections caused by staphylococcus, streptococcus, or pneumococcus. Although the name of this drug ends in the suffix "mycin," which is characteristic of the aminoglycosides, it does not belong to the aminoglycoside group. A serious adverse reaction to clindamycin therapy is pseudomembranous enterocolitis with *Clostridium difficile* superinfection. The manifestation of this condition is diarrhea.

b and c. Renal toxicity and ototoxicity are the primary adverse reactions that occur with aminoglycoside therapy. Oliguria and tinnitus are the manifestations observed in nephrotoxicity and ototoxicity, respectively.
d. Tachypnea is not associated with clindamycin or aminoglycoside use.

23. Correct answer is c. If the irrigation is to be effective, the fluids must reach the eardrum. Pulling the auricle upward and backward straightens the external auditory canal to achieve this result.

a. Pulling the auricle down and backward is the correct procedure for ear irrigation in children.
b and d. Pulling the auricle straight back or down and forward would not straighten the external auditory canal of an adult.

24. Correct answer is b. A client who has frequent attacks of vertigo has sensory and perceptual alterations that would present a variety of potential problems, one of which would be risk for injury. A nursing diagnosis of sensory-perceptual alteration, kinesthetic, would encompass this problem; nursing interventions could address other vertigo-related problems.

a, c, and **d.** All are incorrect, based on the explanation given in correct answer **b.**

25. Correct answer is d. Because nausea and belching should not occur with nasogastric (NG) suctioning, there is probably a problem within the system. The system should be assessed in the following order: Observe for dependent position of the tubing, which causes resistance to flow; check suction unit function by disconnecting drainage tubing from the NG tube and listening for a swish and gurgle sound; check for placement of the NG tube by injecting 10–15 ml of air and listening for a swish and gurgle with a stethoscope placed over the epigastric region; aspirate for gastric content, and feel for resistance to pull; and irrigate with 30 ml of normal saline only after tube placement has been verified.

a. The overall functioning of the system must be evaluated before any change in wall suction pressure can be made.
b. It would be inappropriate to irrigate the tube until tube placement has been verified.
c. Since the underlying problem in this case is a suction system malfunction, changing the patient's position would not relieve nausea and belching.

26. Correct answer is c. Considering that Ms. Peters is also receiving oral feedings, the rate of the tube feeding is too high. Her emesis was probably caused by reflux as the result of a too-full stomach. Checking for tube feeding residual prior to serving breakfast would have helped the nurse determine whether it was safe to give the meal. Since the patient has eaten all the food on her breakfast tray, the doctor should be consulted

about possible adjustments to the tube feeding rate and about the continued need for the tube feedings.

a. Clear liquid diets are indicated in situations in which emesis is related to viral infections. There is no reason to suspect that infection is present in this case.
b. Although it may appropriate to turn off the tube feeding 2 hours before lunch, this action would have to be ordered by the patient's doctor.
d. Since the tube feeding will continue at 90 ml/hour, the patient will have sufficient food to cover the morning insulin dose, and no special blood sugar monitoring needs to be done.

27. Correct answer is d. These manifestations indicate fluid loss. When fluid is lost in large amounts through diarrhea, the potential exists for fluid volume deficit. Increased hematocrit and elevated sodium and BUN levels would confirm the actual fluid volume deficit.

a. Although the low hemoglobin level indicates that anemia does exist, anemia is not a NANDA diagnosis.
b. Acute pain does exist, but the related statement is not given in correct NANDA format. The patient's pain is related to cramping, not the disease condition.
c. The data presented in this situation are not sufficient to support a diagnosis of altered nutrition. A weight comparison would be needed to confirm altered nutrition, although the data presented indicate a potential for altered nutrition.

28. Correct answer is b. The Somogyi effect results in nighttime hypoglycemia that typically occurs at about 3 A.M. It is followed by a progressive rebound of blood sugar level toward morning. This condition is precipitated by an imbalance among food intake, medication use, and altered patterns of exercise. Prevention of the Somogyi effect focuses on maintaining a consistent blood sugar level by means of ingestion of 5–6 regularly scheduled, calorically balanced meals per 24-hour period; maximization of medication effectiveness; and performance of daily exercise. The last meal each day should include a protein and a complex carbohydrate.

a. Insulin administered before bedtime can result in nighttime hypoglycemia.
c. Drinking diet beverages would not cause the Somogyi effect.
d. Performing a blood-sugar assessment at 3 A.M. would confirm the presence or absence of the Somogyi effect but would not prevent it from occurring.

29. **Correct answer is d.** The patient's high blood ammonia level will eventually result in encephalopathy associated with liver disease, of which confusion is the primary manifestation. A low albumin level causes edema and ascites formation. A low hemoglobin level will manifest as pallor, increased pulse and respiration rate, fatigue, and dizziness.

a, b, and **c.** These laboratory values do not in themselves suggest the presence of jaundice, steatorrhea, or severe itching, although the patient may be experiencing each of these signs and symptoms.

30. **Correct answer is a.** Besides ascites, complications of advanced cirrhosis include portal hypertension, bleeding esophageal varices, bleeding tendencies, jaundice, portal-systemic encephalopathy (PSE), and hepatorenal syndrome. PSE is caused by an accumulation of ammonia in brain cells, a condition that interferes with normal brain function and physiologic activity. Seizures may occur as a result of impaired electrical conduction in the brain.

b. Because fluid volume excess is present in advanced cirrhosis, fluids are limited to 1000–1500 ml/day.
c. Liver disease is associated with impaired production of coagulation factors, resulting in bleeding tendencies. Accordingly, vitamin K, not warfarin (Coumadin), is given.
d. A peritoneovenous, or LeVeen, shunt is placed to control ascites in advanced cirrhosis. A ventriculoperitoneal shunt is used to drain fluid from the brain in hydrocephalus.

31. **Correct answer is b.** Levothyroxine sodium (Synthroid) is a thyroid replacement hormone. In hypothyroidism, thyroid-stimulating hormone (TSH) levels are very high, while thyroxine levels (T_4) are low. When thyroid function is replaced, TSH level decreases and T_4 level increases.

a and **c.** Increased HCT and increased Hgb AC levels would not be related to Synthroid replacement therapy.
d. An increase in T_4 would indicate that Synthroid is having a therapeutic effect.

32. **Correct answer is b.** Exophthalmos, or bulging eyes, is normally a permanent change that is associated with hyperthyroidism. The nurse should give Ms. Butler the opportunity to discuss this change and, if appropriate, should refer her to a counselor.

a, c, and **d.** Hand tremors, neck swelling, and flushing of the face can be expected to resolve after successful treatment of hyperthyroidism.

33. **Correct answer is d.** Lumps are most easily detected by palpatory examination when the breast is flattened and evenly distributed on the chest wall.

a and **c.** The best position for palpatory breast self-examination is a supine position, with the side to be examined elevated on a blanket or pillow.
b. Wet skin facilitates manual breast examination for lumps.

34. **Correct answer is c.** Enlargement of the testis without pain is a significant diagnostic finding.

a. The normal testicle is smooth and uniform in consistency.
b. It is not abnormal for one testis to be larger than the other.
d. Testicular self-examination is best performed after a warm bath or shower, when the scrotum is relaxed.

35. **Correct answer is c.** A nephrostomy tube is placed in the renal pelvis of a kidney. Urine should flow continuously from the tube into the drainage system. If no drainage is observed after assuring the patency of the tube, the nurse may irrigate the tube with 3–5 ml of sterile normal saline only when there are physician's orders to do so. If no drainage is observed within seconds after irrigation, the surgeon who placed the tube must be notified.

a. The nephrostomy tube should never be stripped, since damage to the kidney may result from the negative pressure created by stripping.
b. The tube should be irrigated with no more than 20 ml of normal saline.
d. An additional 30-minute delay could prove dangerous to the patient.

36. **Correct answer is a.** Perineal exercises are important in facilitating urinary sphincter control after removal of the urethral catheter.

b. A suprapubic catheter is not used after a retropubic prostatectomy because the bladder is not surgically incised in this approach.
c. Bed rest is usually implemented for the operative day, after which the patient may be up as tolerated unless there is gross hematuria. If a continuous normal saline irrigation is running, the nurse adjusts the flow rate so that the drainage remains a light pink color.
d. It is the surgeon's responsibility to discuss the surgical procedure and possible surgical complications with the patient.

37. **Correct answer is b.** Impotence is not a problem with suprapubic or retropubic prostatectomy, although it does occur with the perineal approach owing to pudendal nerve damage. The pudendal nerve stimulates erection and orgasm.

a. Transient urinary incontinence would not be expected to follow retropubic prostatectomy.
c and **d.** Impotence does not follow retropubic prostatectomy.

38. **Correct answer is a.** Persons who have had precancerous or cancerous lesions removed need to be taught to observe their skin for new lesions on a monthly basis. A hand-held mirror is useful for observing areas that cannot be directly observed.

b. The cause of skin changes is ultraviolet (UV) light, which is equally intense on cloudy and sunny days. Accordingly, the patient should wear a hat whenever he is outside.
c. The surgical area needs to be kept clean and dry. Gentle patting of the area with a washcloth and warm water helps remove normal skin oils and dirt. A bandage can be worn over the wound for protection.
d. A sunblock of SPF 15 or greater should be used.

39. **Correct answer is b.** Vigorous scratching of the arms and hands and red lines between the fingers indicate an infestation with scabies. The patient needs to be isolated and treated with lindane (Kwell).

a. An oil-based soap would normally be used to remove crusts or scales.
c and **d.** A Burow's pack and hydrocortisone cream would normally be used to treat inflammatory skin conditions.